Narcissism in Personality, Pathology and Psychotherapy

This timely volume questions our understanding of the highly current concept and phenomenon of narcissism, working from a broad psychotherapeutic perspective.

Making a strong case for revising the formal diagnostic criteria of narcissistic personality disorder, this work argues for an approach that includes not just grandiose but also vulnerable manifestations of narcissistic pathology. It documents how inconsistent applications of the concept of narcissism have caused confusion in the field, creating a need for new definitions and deeper understanding. In doing so, this book offers specific suggestions for how best to treat people with narcissistic personality pathology in modern relational psychotherapy, whilst also discussing the notion of healthy forms of narcissism.

Presented with insights from deep clinical experience and a broad theoretical base, this title offers a key resource for treatment professionals working with narcissistic patients, those currently living with narcissism and anyone with an interest in this deeply fascinating topic.

Carsten René Jørgensen is PhD and professor of clinical psychology at Aarhus University, Department of Psychology, trained in group analytic psychotherapy and (since 2001) attached to the Clinic for Personality Disorders, Aarhus University Hospital, Skejby. He has worked with intensive psychodynamic psychotherapy for more than thirty years – both as a therapist and a scientist – and is one of Scandinavia's leading researchers in the field of identity, identity disturbances, and borderline and narcissistic personality disorders.

Narcissism in Personality, Pathology and Psychotherapy

Carsten René Jørgensen

Routledge
Taylor & Francis Group
LONDON AND NEW YORK

Designed cover image: Getty Images/Eoneren

First English edition published 2026
by Routledge
4 Park Square, Milton Park, Abingdon, Oxon OX14 4RN

and by Routledge
605 Third Avenue, New York, NY 10158

Routledge is an imprint of the Taylor & Francis Group, an informa business

First Danish edition published by Hans Reitzels Forlag 2025

British Library Cataloguing-in-Publication Data
A catalogue record for this book is available from the British Library

Library of Congress Cataloging-in-Publication Data
A catalog record has been requested for this book

ISBN: 978-1-041-25070-8 (hbk)
ISBN: 978-1-041-24109-6 (pbk)
ISBN: 978-1-003-74496-2 (ebk)

DOI: 10.4324/9781003744962

Typeset in Optima
by Taylor & Francis Books

To Vibeke, Mathilde, Johanne and Anna

Contents

Tables

Acknowledgements

I wish to thank the many – who naturally must remain anonymous – who have shown me the profound trust of sharing their innermost thoughts, feelings and experiences, whether as part of our joint psychotherapeutic effort or in the interviews I conducted in connection with various research projects. Your contribution has been invaluable for the creation of this book. Without it, the book would never have been possible. Thank you!

Thanks to the private foundation JP-fonden and Aarhus University's research fund, which made it possible for me to write parts of the book in Prenzlauer Berg, Berlin, and at the Sandbjerg Estate in the southwest of Denmark.

1 Introduction

This is a fake heading: delete at typesetting stage

Modern Western culture and modern human beings are often described as narcissistic (Lasch, 1979). Narcissism has been called the borderline disorder of our time, because narcissistic disorders are as similarly stigmatized and as poorly understood as borderline personality disorder was a few decades ago (Choi-Kain, 2020). In particular, what some perceive as young people's self-centred and self-absorbed behaviour on social media (SoMe) may be regarded as narcissistic. Many prominent politicians and business leaders have also been characterized as narcissists, with US President Donald Trump as a strong candidate for the most full-blown narcissist of them all. The term 'narcissism' is often used to single out individuals that we do not like, for various reasons, classifying them as psychologically disturbed and driven by excessive self-love, self-satisfaction and a tendency for socially unacceptable behaviour. Used in this sense, 'narcissism' is a highly normative, moralizing and vague term that serves to pathologize, stigmatize and marginalize individuals whose behaviour defies the norms in certain contexts and who appear unlikeable due to self-absorption and an urge to control and take advantage of others. This usage associates narcissism with sinful self-absorption and seemingly excessive self-satisfaction. And indeed, some of the people who are labelled as narcissists do act in ways that most people would find socially unacceptable.

As the following chapters will discuss in more depth, narcissism is related to an individual's self-image and self-esteem, which may become distorted in a positive or negative direction by narcissistic disturbances. This is especially true of people who have a narcissistic personality disorder, as their self-image and self-esteem may differ dramatically from how others perceive them. Further, it can be argued that a certain level of narcissism – attention to how we appear to and are perceived by others – is part of normal psychological development and functioning.

The Irish writer Oscar Wilde's Gothic novel *The Picture of Dorian Gray* (1891/2022) describes some of the key elements of the common understanding of narcissism. Dorian Gray, who is also described as 'Narcissus' in the book

DOI: 10.4324/9781003744962-1

(p. 15), is a beautiful young man who is immensely preoccupied with his youth, his looks and how he is perceived by others. He sits for a self-portrait, and when it is first revealed to him, it is like a revelation. He likes to sit in front of the painting, overwhelmed by his own beauty (p. 114); on one occasion, he even kisses the lips of his own portrait (Rank, 1911, p. 411). However, he is also worried about losing his beauty as time goes by and age takes its toll, while the painting will remain unchanged. He is concerned that others will only like him 'Till I have my first wrinkle, I suppose' (Wilde, 1891/2022, p. 28). 'If it were only the other way! If it were I who was to be always young, and the picture that was to grow old! For that – for that – I would give everything! Yes, there is nothing in the whole world I would not give! I would give my soul for that!' (p. 28). Dorian sells his soul, and in return his body remains forever young, while his portrait ages – only the painting shows his soul, the effects of age and his shame over his many amoral acts. He pays a high price, however. He is no longer a complete human being and is incapable of intimate contact with others, since all he can bring to the interaction is his seemingly perfect, youthful facade. The rest is hidden, split off, hidden in a locked room where he keeps his self-portrait, which no one else is allowed to see.

Dorian briefly falls in love with an actress, but it soon turns out that he is only in love with her perfect ability to portray characters on stage, not in her as a person – a complete human being. When she drops her act and is simply 'herself', she is no longer perfect in his eyes, and he can no longer love her: 'Without your art, you are nothing [...] What are you now? A third-rate actress with a pretty face' (Wilde, 1891/2022, p. 96). He treats her with disparagement and contempt and rejects her so completely that she is driven to suicide by their break-up. When this happens, Dorian's only concern is how selfish he considers her act – he feels no compassion with her and does not appear to have any insight into how his actions affected her (p. 108). However, there is one tiny crack in Dorian's pervasive narcissistic egotism: he is aware that he is incapable of feeling the tragedy of the events (p. 107). He is incapable of loving others because he is so self-absorbed. He appears to love himself so intensely that he has lost both the ability and the desire to love others (Rank, 1911, p. 421). In the course of the narrative, he acknowledges this: '"I wish I could love," cried Dorian Gray [...] But I seem to have lost the passion and forgotten the desire. I am too much concentrated on myself. My own personality has become a burden to me' (Wilde, 1891/2022, p. 210).

Not just excessive self-satisfaction: Vulnerable and grandiose narcissism

Many of the people who are labelled and stigmatized as despicably self-satisfied by being described as narcissists are in fact anything but satisfied with themselves. Their self-worth or self-esteem is not nearly as strong or positive as their facade would suggest or as reflected in our own immediate reactions to their often loud and grandiose facades. Contrary to the more popular usage and understanding of the concept, narcissism is far from primarily about excessive self-satisfaction or self-infatuation. It is in part related to self-esteem and the capacity for love and involves the ability to engage in emotional contact with self and others, to look beyond oneself, to see and sense others, and to sense what is happening in other persons – and in one's own psyche. Narcissism cannot be reduced to self-satisfaction and grandiose gestures but also involves vulnerability: a fragile self-image and fragile self-esteem that require persistent and explicit confirmation from others, even in persons who may outwardly appear remarkably self-confident and convinced of their own excellence.

Narcissistic disturbances can be manifested in a wide variety of ways. On the one hand, it may involve grandiose and megalomaniacal fantasies of own grandeur, importance and entitlement to special treatment – combined with attention-seeking behaviour and limited empathy and interest in others – which may be seen as an attempt to boost a fragile self-image. On the other, it may produce a high level of vulnerability and a strong urge to withdraw from close interpersonal contact. This may be combined with an urge to protect the vulnerable self by embracing exaggerated and unrealistic perceptions of own mental prowess and significance or, alternatively, seeking refuge in an inner universe shaped by fantasies of self-reliance and independence. This distinction between grandiose and vulnerable manifestations of pathological narcissism is a key point in the present book: narcissism can in no way be reduced to overtly grandiose perceptions of own importance and high and seemingly iron-clad self-esteem.

We need to move beyond the widespread simplistic and exclusively negative notion of narcissism that typically dominates the understanding of the concept, both among the general public and in parts of the literature. As with the similar use of the term psychopathy, clearly disturbed narcissistic and psychopathic partners, bosses and leaders do exist, but we need to be much more precise and careful with our use of these important psychological and psychiatric terms instead of applying them loosely to shame and marginalize individuals whom we dislike, for various reasons, by labelling them as psychologically disturbed and radically different from ourselves.

The term 'narcissist' is almost always used about someone else, not self-referentially. In most cases, it is used as a derogatory label, as part of a problematic attempt to ostracize or 'other' someone that the person using the term does not like, is repulsed by or, perhaps, feels inferior to. The 'narcissist' is implicitly or explicitly identified as a radically different 'other', someone who deviates from the norm in a negative and morally dubious or reprehensible way – perhaps because they are or appear too self-satisfied, self-assertive and intimidating in their insistence on being unique and entitled to privileged treatment. This judgement overlooks how people with narcissism, especially severe narcissism, struggle with relational difficulties, painful loneliness, impaired functioning in several areas, perhaps depression-like symptoms, emotional distress and sometimes suicidal ideation behind what is perhaps a 'loud' and grandiose facade. As the self-psychologist Ernest Wolf (1996, p. 23) puts it, in our modern Judaeo-Christian culture, when we encounter someone who appears self-righteous, arrogant, conceited and obstinate, it can be a challenge to meet them without prejudice and thus see past their grandiose and seemingly infinite 'self-infatuation' to their underlying inability to love themselves and others. It is easy to perceive narcissism, especially in its grandiose manifestations, as a reflection of repulsive selfishness and self-sufficiency and thus fail to see the tormented human being behind the narcissistic defences or facade.

People with severe narcissism typically have a high degree of ambivalence, and they need for us to see who they are and how they are really doing behind their grandiose or timid facade. They need for us to maintain emotional and psychological contact with them, even when their fragile and shameful sides are disclosed and they feel the urge to withdraw from contact or to attack anyone they perceive as a threat to their established – often inflated and unrealistic – self-image and identity. To the extent that we are able to see the fragile and vulnerable self behind what may be a loud and grandiose – or perhaps evasive – facade, the easier it will be for us to empathize with the person behind this immediate presentation, who is typically tormented by destructive shame, including fragile self-esteem and a painful sense of emptiness or lack of meaning.

The term 'narcissism' is more commonly used to stigmatize and ostracize people than as a basis for understanding what certainly may be a psychological disorder: a very severe personality disorder that it can be difficult to treat, even for highly specialized and experienced therapists. This book is motivated by a deep-felt hope of contributing to a more substantial, nuanced and empathic understanding of individuals with pathological narcissism, who, behind their arrogant facade or less obvious avoidance of deeper, authentic contact with others, struggle with profound psychological distress, despair, loneliness and a yearning to be able to truly love and be loved. In a session, a patient with narcissistic personality disturbances said – clearly emotionally moved and moving – that what she wanted most of all was to love and be loved but that she had never (yet) had that experience. She was convinced that she was so damaged and so toxic to others that her situation could never change: she felt she was doomed to remain in her present state of deep emotional loneliness, incapable of entering into equal relationships, and that no one and nothing could possibly change this. Fortunately, change is indeed possible, although it may require long-term intensive psychotherapy (cf. Rosenfeld, 1987, p. 149).

Dependence and self-reliance

Narcissism can be said to simultaneously conceal and reveal our fundamentally human dependence on each other, including admiration and empathically acknowledging mirroring of our self and being from significant others. On the one hand, the grandiose self-perception that is characteristic particularly of immature and disturbed narcissism signals a self-sufficient, cold and arrogant quality that may, at first glance, be taken for a basic independence of others – a sense that the grandiose self does not need anyone else. On the other hand, these grandiose perceptions often spring from poorly met needs for empathic mirroring and approval of the self, particularly in early relations. They reflect the attempts of a deeply fragile self to deal with their – possibly unacknowledged – vulnerability and to stabilize their fragile self-esteem by constructing grandiose perceptions of their own significance and invulnerability. This psychological dynamic is at play both in individuals with very explicit grandiose perceptions and in individuals in whom these self-perceptions appear more discreet and, at first glance, seem to be limited to the person's inner life and fantasies about their own significance and related entitlement to privileged treatment; often interpreted as vulnerable manifestations of narcissism (see Chapter 2.3).

As the concept of narcissism is generally defined in the present book, it may, in principle, be applied to universal psychological processes, dynamics and challenges that are experienced by everyone, to varying degrees. To some extent, narcissistic needs and personality traits are a common and normal part of being human that does not, in itself, represent a psychological disorder requiring treatment. This includes narcissistic needs such as the need to feel seen and valued and the need for healthy self-esteem. Thus, narcissism is also related to how we see ourselves and, not least, our feelings and opinions about ourselves, which can be quite painful and associated with self-hatred and destructive shame in individuals with pathological narcissism. Thus certain aspects of human self-esteem and the capacity to regulate these feelings in a balanced way are closely related to narcissism.

When it comes to more pronounced narcissistic traits, as narcissism reaches a more problematic level, including actual narcissistic personality disorders, it is important to note that in this case, too, we are dealing with different individuals, whose perceived human difficulties and challenges cannot be reduced to the narrow and clear-cut category of any psychiatric diagnosis. There is much to suggest that we ought to adopt a dimensional view of narcissism and, indeed, of many other psychological disorders, understanding them as phenomena or clusters of psychological processes that exist in a variety of degrees along a spectrum of psychological functioning. More specifically, this implies that people may have varying degrees of narcissism, and that there is rarely a clear-cut line that defines when this tips over into a problematic condition that constitutes an actual psychological disorder. Thus, when a particular way of being and acting becomes maladaptive or perhaps pathological may depend on multiple factors in the socio-cultural context of the person's life (see Chapter 3.1).

Narcissism is a complex concept, and it can be challenging to formulate a precise, condensed and fairly unambiguous definition that might achieve broad consensus. In part, these challenges stem from the highly varied use of the term across different disciplines and the fact that its meaning has changed and been watered down somewhat over time. The *Oxford English Dictionary* defines narcissism as excessive self-love or vanity, self-admiration and self-centredness. The dictionary also associates narcissism with a state where a person achieves emotional or even erotic satisfaction by admiring and being intensely absorbed in themself. Finally, in some contexts, narcissism is viewed as an early stage in normal psychological development that a person may regress to later in life, as part of a psychological disorder. From a psychological perspective, this description of narcissism is not far off the mark. However, it is far from exhaustive, in part because it reflects a fairly narrow and purely descriptive definition that focuses mainly on the problematic and grandiose aspects of narcissism. Its focus is on pathological elements of narcissism, which is also the dominant focus of this book.

Healthy and normal narcissism

It is debatable whether it is most helpful to speak of healthy or normal narcissism, or whether the concept of narcissism should be reserved for more problematic and actually pathological conditions and behaviours. However, the notion of healthy or normal narcissism is typically used to refer to a predominantly positive self-image and high but also generally realistic self-esteem, which are key aspects of the emotional foundation of our ability to function as autonomous persons with individual agency. Healthy narcissism enables us uphold our own personal boundaries, needs and opportunities for self-expression without seriously violating other people's boundaries. Normal narcissism is also associated with the ability to set realistic goals and ideals for our lives and, not least, maintaining realistic and balanced confidence that we can achieve them with reasonable effort (agency), perhaps with appropriate aid and support from others, including well-functioning social communities and institutions. Healthy narcissism helps us contain and regulate self-conscious feelings, such as shame, pride, inferiority and perceived humiliation. More generally, it may also be seen as a psychological resource and a source of resilience. Finding that we are entitled to our own private space, thoughts, boundaries, feelings and intentions may also be seen as a concrete manifestation of healthy and normal narcissism, provided it does not lead to behaviour that violates or restricts someone else's freedom and personal integrity. Healthy narcissism may be viewed as enabling the development of a resilient sense of individuality, as the self lives out and defends their individuality without violating other people's boundaries (cf. the mature and well-integrated superego; Charim, 2022, p. 27).

Thus, healthy narcissism is associated with a realistic and predominantly positive self-image that includes both strengths and weaknesses. The person accepts their own strengths and weaknesses, integrating them into a coherent and nuanced self-image that includes a realistic awareness of their own human vulnerability and the development of balanced confidence in – and dependence on – others. This is quite different from grandiose perceptions of independence, invulnerability and self-reliance or excessive dependence on others and continuous confirmation. Healthy narcissism is associated with predominantly positive opinions and feelings about one's own self and body that promote healthy self-respect, self-acceptance and self-compassion (Kernberg, 1998, p. 83 ff.; Ronningstam, 2021, p. 4). This stable and positive self-esteem is rooted in the internalization of positive experiences with others who have approved of and confirmed the self as valuable and lovable (Diamond, et al., 2022, p. 6); it helps the self deal with the fact that it contains both positive and negative elements, to varying degrees.

Healthy narcissism will also be manifested in balanced and reality-based pride in one's own actual competencies and achievements. This is different from the exaggerated and egocentric pride or arrogance that is common in grandiose manifestations of pathological narcissism – and which is one of Christianity's seven deadly sins – possibly accompanied by self-deprecation and self-hatred driven by unrealistic and shameful negative self-perceptions that are more common in vulnerable manifestations of pathological narcissism. Healthy and balanced narcissism is also important for our courage to explore unknown parts of the world, handle challenges, deal with criticism and perceived defeat and overcome traumatic experiences (Ronningstam, 2005, p. 31) without lapsing into grandiosity, paranoid delusion or attacks on others (Maroda, 2022, p. 76).

Our ability to handle rejection from others and to accept approval and praise for our own real achievements and qualities without being overwhelmed by shame or fantasies of omnipotence also springs from healthy narcissism (Ronningstam, 2005, p. 72). It can also be argued that healthy narcissism helps us to contain, regulate and cope with perceived frustration, humiliation and other painful emotions, just as it can help us tolerate, understand and regulate anger and hate in connection with perceived (narcissistic) injury, defeat and shameful events (Ronningstam, 2021, p. 4). Healthy narcissism helps us protect ourselves from emotional injury and nurture our true self: our innermost core of more private and vulnerable thoughts and feelings. Healthy narcissism is the basis of extroversion, confidence in self and others, and courage to be and reveal oneself and engage in close emotional and psychological contact with others. This close emotional connection inevitably involves lowering one's guard, opening up to the other and thus leaving oneself open to injury, humiliation, loss and other forms of emotional pain.

As a phenomenon and as a driver of psychological organization, narcissism is associated with our attempts and ability to strike the right balance between different needs and considerations in our individual lives as well as in our interactions with others. This includes, for example, how we strike the right balance between our self-perception and how we are perceived by others, including how we react if we find that there is too big a gap between the two. How much emphasis do we wish to place on others' perceptions and opinions of our ways of being and acting? And to what extent are we able to observe and appraise ourselves from outside, from someone else's perspective, and what significance do we place on this: do we perhaps want to revise our self-image and behaviour in light of feedback from others and their expressed perception of us?

Needs for freedom and relatedness

Thus, narcissism is also related to our efforts to balance our need for self-assertion (autonomy) with our need to be integrated into well-functioning social communities (dependence), including how much emphasis we place on our own needs versus those of others. The latter relates to our expectations of individual freedom and self-expression versus our concern for social community, norms and values that go beyond our own narrowly individual needs in the moment. The American psychoanalyst Sidney Blatt (2008, p. 15 ff.) has described how every human being has two fundamental tasks in their psychological development and how we each need to strike the right balance between these two, dialectically connected developmental tasks and the underlying basic psychological needs they represent: developing meaningful reciprocal interpersonal relationships that are as mutually satisfying as possible – a task that is associated with our basic human need for interpersonal relatedness – and establishing a differentiated, integrated, realistic and essentially positive sense of self and individual identity – a task that is associated with personal identity and the basic human need for individual integrity, self-definition and individuality.

As we develop a capacity for interpersonal relatedness, we gain experience with being dependent on and merging with significant others and with affiliation, intimacy, love, cooperation, submission and intersubjectivity, and physical and sexual contact (Blatt, 2008, p. 15 ff.). To the extent that these experiences have been largely positive, they enable us to establish and be present in situations characterized by even very deep interpersonal relatedness without perceiving any narcissistic threat or injury. Similarly, the development of a healthy capacity for self-delimitation is associated with mainly positive experiences with individuation and separation; experiences with control, dominance, power, autonomy, the expression of individuality, agency, initiative and industry. In narcissistic disorders, these two developmental tasks have failed, to some degree, and – at times severe – imbalances have emerged between the person's pursuit of their needs for self-delimitation, autonomy and independence, on the one hand, and their needs for interpersonal relatedness, dependence and close emotional contact with others.

Narcissism is also related to our attempts to strike an appropriate balance between, on the one hand, what we believe we are entitled to and deserve by virtue of who we are, our accomplishments and our (real and imagined) social status and, on the other hand, what we have actually accomplished and how others view it. This balance also relates to our tendency to evaluate and compare ourselves, who we are and our accomplishments, being and identity with others – including how we react to and deal with inevitable occasional setback, being outperformed by and seeing others receive more attention, admiration and approval than we do. When this happens, are we happy, maybe even proud, for them or on behalf of the human community – or do we, rather, experience injury, envy and rage over seeing others being and receiving approval for something we feel that we are or deserve credit for? This may also be described as narcissistic injury or perhaps envy, a common feeling among many people with narcissistic disorders. Do we react to that with narcissistic rage, for example when we feel humiliated, overlooked, ridiculed or shameful over being viewed as inadequate or inferior? These are all experiences that may feel like a severe threat to an already fragile and unstable self-esteem, and the narcissistic rage may be regarded as an attempt to defend or restore a positive self-image and self-esteem.

Narcissism and identity

Our identity is associated with who we are in our own eyes as well as in the eyes of others (Jørgensen, 2008, 2020), while narcissism, as mentioned earlier, relates to what we are worth in our own and others' eyes: our self-esteem and self-regard and our sense of being seen and approved by others. Because narcissism and identity are so closely related, identity disturbances and narcissistic disturbances will be interrelated to some degree, particularly in their more severe forms. We all contain some degree of vulnerability and uncertainty about our own sense of who we are, how we are perceived by others and what we are worth: our identity and self-esteem. Fundamentally, narcissism is about individuals' – and, to some extent, social groups' – self-image, identity, self-esteem and social status as well as their perception of others, including what we do to enhance and defend our self-esteem, identity and social status when we feel that these core aspects of our psychology are fragile or threatened. Narcissism relates to our capacity to regulate our self-esteem and handle social emotions, such as shame, guilt and pride. Healthy narcissism may be understood as an internal reservoir of positive self-esteem that we can draw on in difficult situations, when our self-image and identity are being challenged. To some degree, we all contain fantasies and illusory narratives about ourselves, our identity, who we are and our significance. One of the problems for individuals with pathological narcissism is that, for various reasons, they take these fantasies and ideas about themselves deadly seriously and insist that they reflect reality – at the expense of their capacity for valid and nuanced understandings of reality and for engaging with others (Mitchell, 1988, p. 195 ff.).

As fundamentally social creatures, we all need to have our identity, person and ways of being noticed and approved by others. Genuine approval can only come from autonomous subjects who are separate from us and whom we recognize as fundamentally equal to us (Honneth, 1992; Hegel, 1807/2019). Another implication – and a highly significant one in this context – is that any (apparent) approval that is expressed under coercion or which comes from someone we generally view as inferior, unreliable or subject to our control is virtually worthless for meeting our need to have our self and our identity confirmed.

Thus, one of the tragic dimensions of the grandiose aspects of narcissism in particular is that the more the person succeeds in subjugating and controlling the people around them in order to compel them to show attention, admiration, respect and approval, the more these others are reduced to objects bereft of subjectivity, and the person's relationship with them is characterized by alienation and inauthentic contact. To the extent that this narcissistic perversion of interpersonal relations is 'successful', it also ruins any chance for the person to experience true approval of their real self, as this would require an equal relationship with a clearly separate and autonomous other. As a result, the narcissistically disordered self becomes even more isolated and lonely in their solipsistic inner universe and grandiose perceptions of the world.

Grandiose narcissism drives others away and makes them pull back. Thus, the self achieves the opposite of what it so desperately needs and has an even harder time achieving the genuine interpersonal contact, positive attention and approval that are so vital for stabilizing the self's identity and fragile self-esteem; a form of contact that could also help detoxify destructive shame and enhance the self's capacity for dealing with criticism, shame and other painful emotions. As human beings, the only way we can find ourselves and develop our uniquely human capacity for self-reflection is by letting go of our urge to control the other. By setting the other free and accepting the human subject's fundamental autonomy (separateness in relatedness), we become able to see and find ourselves in the other's mirroring and reactions to our self. This lets us meet our own ways of being and acting as subjects in interaction with the other and the world in general.

In persons with grandiose narcissism, the important dialectic balance between pursuing the need for autonomy versus the need for interpersonal relatedness has collapsed. The self is dominated by an exaggerated – and destructive – urge for self-definition, control and power at the expense of the self's capacity and need for relatedness, dependence and intimate contact with others who are separate from and beyond their control (Blatt, 2008, p. 178 ff.). The self has an excessive preoccupation with its own power and status and a persistent need to mark its own value, driven by underlying feelings of – and anxiousness related to – inferiority, worthlessness and shameful inadequacy. Naturally, the person may also seek solitude in an attempt to achieve and ensure maximal freedom and independence. The key is whether this solitude is associated with psychological pain and accompanied by an inadequate capacity for engaging in close contact with others and is thus pathological and may require treatment.

Many different meanings of narcissism

As outlined so far, the concept of narcissism has been defined very broadly and applied in fundamentally different ways. To this day, we still have not arrived at any real consensus about the precise meaning of the term. It could be argued that narcissism may refer more generally to at least the seven following psychological phenomena, which to some degree overlap and are interrelated:

- Narcissism as an early stage or a separate line of normal psychological development (before the clear separation of self and other), where developmental processes may become arrested, in which case we may speak of a form of developmental delay, if not a fixation, in the development of normal psychological maturity. The person may also later return (regress) to this earlier, more primitive stage of development and ways of psychological functioning. This understanding, which must now be regarded as inadequate, is rooted in Freud's early interpretation of narcissism (see Chapter 2.1) and Kohut's self-psychological theory of narcissism (see Chapter 3.3).
- Narcissism used as a term for certain forms of non-pathological behaviour, typically behaviours that contain clear elements of and are driven, to some extent, by an exaggerated view of the person's own significance (grandiosity), (primarily emotional) lack of empathy and interest in others, and self-centred, egocentric behaviour and sense of entitlement to privileged treatment. In some – but far from all – cases, this behaviour serves to stabilize or enhance vulnerable self-esteem (see Chapter 2.3 about high-functioning narcissism); in more popular interpretations of the concept of narcissism, it is associated with inflated self-esteem and self-infatuation.
- The term narcissism used in attempts to define and describe certain forms of intrapsychic and intersubjective psychological functioning and personality organization, where the core dynamic impetus is the person's fundamentally vulnerable self and self-esteem. The person has a profound need for others and their admiration, confirmation and approval but denies or seeks to repress this need out of fear of growing dependent on others or of being revealed as fragile, inadequate and weak in their own and others' eyes. In this view, narcissism refers to a fundamental preoccupation with and insecurity about the significance of the person's own self, tensioned and eternally varying between the self as highly significant versus insignificant, between omnipotence and impotence. This concept of narcissism describes a person characterized by profound insecurity, an unstable self-image (identity) and fragile self-esteem, accompanied by a similarly profound need for continuous and explicit recognition, positive feedback, confirmation or even admiration from others. In this view, narcissism is associated with a fundamental

psychological conflict or tension between grandiose perceptions of the self and either unconscious or more consciously acknowledged vulnerability, fragility and perceived (shameful) inferiority of the self. Thus, narcissistic grandiosity is seen as a form of facade, a psychological defence intended to cover up the vulnerability and precariousness of the underlying true self. This view is mainly seen within certain areas of psychoanalysis and clinical psychology (see Chapter 3).

- The term 'narcissism' used to describe certain personality traits or dimensional personality properties in otherwise well-functioning young people and adults and in people with some degree of maladaptive, perhaps even socially problematic, functioning, without necessarily having an actual psychological disorder. In this sense, we may also speak of accentuated or excessive narcissism or a narcissistic personality style manifested, for example, as pronounced self-enhancement, self-positioning, self-absorption as well as a lack of interest in and belittling and arrogant behaviour towards others. These features may be more pronounced and occur with greater frequency in certain age groups and (sub)cultures than others (Ronningstam, 2021, p. 4) and have also varied over time in our cultural history. This understanding of narcissism is mainly seen in social and personality psychology (see Chapter 2.2).
- Narcissism as a fairly distinct and often quite severe personality disturbance (see Chapter 3.1) that can be challenging to treat in psychotherapy. Pathological narcissism and narcissistic personality disorder (NPD) are typically associated with both psychological vulnerability and a grandiose self-image, while the relative severity and visibility of this vulnerability and grandiosity may vary considerably over time and across individuals. Furthermore, in this understanding, these two elements are regarded as dynamically linked, in the sense that grandiose notions, self-promotion and high apparent self-esteem may be activated and intensified in an attempt to escape, deal with, conceal or compensate for fragile self-esteem and shameful negative perceptions of the self as being inadequate, inferior or threatened (see Chapter 3.2). On the other hand, extreme self-criticism and self-hatred may also fuel perfectionism, an urge for control and an intense struggle for attention and admiration from others. In situations where this clearly fails, the person's narcissistic vulnerability may become apparent in the form of a collapse of self-esteem, explicit self-hatred, intense dependence on explicit approval from others, depressive symptoms, suicidal ideation and suicide attempts.
- The concept of 'narcissism' applied – often in fairly vague terms – to describe a culture, historical period or social character or a generation of (usually) young people or, at least, people who are younger than the attributor. Typically, this use of the term has an undercurrent of (culturally conservative) moralizing dismissal and limited empathic understanding of the culture or group that is labelled as narcissistic. Young people may also categorize each other and their own generation as narcissistic and, thus,

as 'immature' or 'problematic'. The present book cannot claim entirely to avoid some aspects of these, potentially problematic, views. However, it does attempt mainly to use 'narcissism' as a way to describe and understand, rather than to pathologize, pass moral judgement on or marginalize groups or cultural trends.

A common feature of the many different applications of the concept of narcissism is that it deals, to varying degrees, with the human ability to generate, maintain and defend a predominantly positive and reasonably realistic – but in narcissistic disorders obviously unrealistic – self-image. Narcissism is associated with the fundamental human need for attention, approval and admiration from others and with the development of the ability to strike a suitable balance between self-conscious affects, such as shame and pride in our own personal characteristics and accomplishments. All of this is related to how we perceive ourselves, how we are seen and perceived by others, the compatibility of these two perceptions and the emotional impact of any disparities between them.

Narcissism could also be viewed as related to our emotional and cognitive interest in ourselves. In some cases, this interest is so underdeveloped that we become self-effacing and eager to please, at the expense of our own needs; in others, it is so powerful that we become excessively self-centred and selfish and lose the ability to take an interest in others that goes beyond their role in meeting our own needs for attention and confirmation.

In extension of this understanding, narcissism also relates to human empathy and the ability of normally functioning individuals to strike a suitable balance between their own and others' needs, between pursuing their own short-term needs and their concern for social communities and our shared home: Planet Earth. This stands in contrast to the remarkable hubris of some individuals and cultures and their pursuit of their own, narrowly defined immediate needs with no apparent awareness of the long-term implications of their behaviour for the global climate, social balances and long-term survival. Such behaviour can arguably be described as narcissistically disordered if we, momentarily, allow for a slightly broad definition of what falls under the definition of narcissistic disorders.

Chapter overview

The following chapter begins with a review of the roots of the concept of narcissism in Ovid's classical story of the young Narcissus and Sigmund Freud's introduction of narcissism as both an aspect of human psychological development and a severe psychological disorder. Next, it argues that we need to distinguish between different understandings of the concept, with particular emphasis on the very different definitions and understandings of narcissism in social and personality psychology, on the one hand, and psychoanalysis and clinical psychology, on the other. These differences may lead to confusion between fundamentally different phenomena, all – perhaps somewhat misleadingly – referred to as narcissism. We also need to distinguish between grandiose and vulnerable manifestations of narcissism and attempt to understand the dynamic relationship between them. The chapter concludes with an outline of the main elements of what might be called the core of narcissism and a brief discussion of the close relationship between narcissism and shame.

Chapter 3 discusses how we might best capture and describe the main elements of pathological narcissism, including narcissistic personality disorder (NPD). Since pathological narcissism often coincides with a wide range of related psychological disorders, the text discusses ways of distinguishing NPD from other personality disorders and related symptom disorders in practice. Further, the chapter addresses some possible causes of pathological narcissism based on a wide range of empirical studies of various elements and implications of pathological narcissism, including relational difficulties, attachment disorder, risk of suicide, narcissism in leaders, and connections between narcissism and aggression/violence.

Next, the chapter describes the key elements of the two most important contributions to our understanding of normal and pathological narcissism: Heinz Kohut's model of narcissism, based on self psychology, and Otto Kernberg's model, based on his object relations theory. Kohut and Kernberg laid the foundations of the psychoanalytic understanding of narcissism and are still considered the two principal figures in this field. They both have their roots in psychoanalysis, but in relation to key themes, they represent two fundamentally different approaches to how we should understand pathological narcissism and approach psychotherapeutic treatment of patients with this disorder. As these differences remain a source of persistent professional disagreement in the field, they are important to consider. The chapter is rounded off with a brief discussion of how John Steiner's theory of some people's urge to construct 'psychic retreats' and avoid close emotional contact with themselves and others can help shed light on common strategies for psychological survival in individuals with severe narcissistic pathology

Chapter 4 describes how psychotherapists can meet and help individuals with pathological narcissism. The main focus is on the typical manifestations of pathological narcissism in the psychotherapeutic space and in interactions with the therapist, including the patient's transference and the therapist's countertransference. This discussion is not intended as yet another manual or a collection of specific techniques in the treatment of narcissism. Rather, it aims to outline a relational or intersubjective approach to the understanding and treatment of pathological narcissism. It contains numerous recommendations for practising a dynamic relational approach in understanding and engaging with commonly occurring situations in encounters with patients with pathological narcissism. Further, it argues for the need to remain mindful of how one's own narcissism and narcissistic needs might come into play in the psychotherapeutic process. Thus, therapists should adopt a psychotherapeutic stance not just towards the patient's ways of being and acting in the therapeutic space but also to their own ways of being and acting in their interactions with the patient.

References

Blatt, S. J. (2008). *Polarities of experience: Relatedness and self-definition in personality development, psychopathology, and the therapeutic process*. American Psychological Association.

Charim, I. (2022). *Die Qualen des Narzissmus: Über freiwillige Unterwerfung* [The torments of narcissism: On voluntary submission]. Zsolnay.

Choi-Kain, L. (2020). Narcissistic personality disorder: A coming of age. *Journal of Personality Disorders*, 34, 210–213.

Diamond, D., Yeomans, F. E., Stern, B. L., & Kernberg, O. F. (2022). *Treating pathological narcissism with transference-focused psychotherapy*. Guilford.

Hegel, G. W. F. (2019). *The phenomenology of spirit* (P. Fuss & J. Dobbins, Trans.). University of Notre Dame Press. (Original work published 1807)

Honneth, A. (1992). *Kampf um Anerkennung: Zur moralischen Grammatik sozialer Konflikte* [Struggle for recognition: On the moral grammar of social conflicts]. Suhrkamp.

Jørgensen, C. R. (2002). *Psykologien i senmoderniteten* [Psychology in late modernity]. Hans Reitzel Forlag.

Jørgensen, C. R. (2008). *Identitet: Psykologiske og kulturanalytiske perspektiver* [Identity: Perspectives from psychology and cultural analysis]. Hans Reitzels Forlag.

Jørgensen, C. R. (2020). *Identitetskriser: Veje og vildveje for det fragmenterede moderne menneskes identitet* [Identity crises: Paths and detours for the identity of fragment modern people]. Hans Reitzels Forlag.

Kernberg, O. F. (1998). *Ideology, conflict and leadership in groups and organizations*. Yale University Press.

Lasch, C. (1979). *The culture of narcissism: American life in an age of diminishing expectations*. Norton.

Maroda, K. J. (2022). *The analyst's vulnerability: Impact on theory and practice*. Routledge.

Mitchell, S. A. (1988). *Relational concepts in psychoanalysis. An integration*. Harvard University Press.

Rank, O. (1911). Ein beitrag zum Narzissmus[A contribution to Narcissism]. *Jahrbuch für psychoanalytische Forschungen*, 401–426.

Ronningstam, E. (2005). *Identifying and understanding the narcissistic personality*. Oxford University Press.

Ronningstam, E. (2021). *NPD Basic: A brief overview of identifying, diagnosing and treating narcissistic personality disorder* (4th Ed.). McLean Hospital, Harvard Medical School.

Rosenfeld, H. (1987). *Sackgassen und Deutungen: Therapeutische und antitherapeutische Faktoren bei der psychoanalytischen Behandlung von psychotischen, Borderline und neurotischen Patienten* [Dead ends and interpretations:

Therapeutic and antitherapeutic factors in the psychoanalytic treatment of psychotic, borderline, and neurotic patients]. Verlag Internationale Psychoanalyse.

Wilde, O. (2022). *The Picture of Dorian Gray*. Ryerson University. https://pressbooks.library.torontomu.ca/thepictureofdoriangray/ (Original work published in 1891)

Wolf, E. S. (1996). *Theorie und Praxis der psychoanalytischen Selbstpsychologie* [Theory and practice of psychoanalytic self psychology]. Suhrkamp Verlag.

2 From normal to pathological narcissism

Towards a dimensional understanding

2.1 The history of the concept of narcissism

Graeco-Roman mythology: Ovid's story of Narcissus

The concept of narcissism has roots in Greek mythology. There are several different interpretations of the myth about the young hunter Narcissus (Latin) or Nárkissos (Greek). Chief among them is Sigmund Freud's (1914/1957b) introduction of the concept of narcissism as a lens for understanding core processes in human psychology, psychological development and certain psychological disorders, particularly narcissistic personality disorder. Perhaps the most prominent version of the myth about Narcissus is the one authored by the Roman poet Ovid circa 10 BCE (Ovid, ca. 10 BCE/2004). Narcissus is the son of the river nymph Liriope and the river god Cephissus (Kephfissos). He is conceived when his father rapes his mother, which we may imagine – at the risk of being a little too concrete and modern in our interpretation of the stories from Greek mythology – will have influenced Narcissus' relationship with his parents in a profoundly negative way. For example, a mother might develop an extraordinarily complicated relationship with a son who is the result of a sexual assault; consequently, Narcissus may not have received the empathic and validating mirroring from his mother (and his father) that is necessary to enjoy a normal psychological development and avoid developing a narcissistic disorder.

Shortly after Narcissus' birth, his mother, Liriope, consults the blind seer Tiresias, who predicts that the boy will live to ripe old age 'so long as he never knows himself' (Ovid, ca. 10 BCE/2004, p. 109). This stands in stark contrast to the maxim engraved at the entrance to the Temple of the Oracle of Delphi, 'Know thyself', which encourages human beings to know themselves, in part to keep us from violating established boundaries and to remind us that we are merely human, not divine. Arguably, because we are inevitably confronted with and thus get to know ourselves when we are in close contact with others, Narcissus has to forgo and avoid close contact with others and thus, in practice, forgo living a full life in order to live 'to a ripe old age' (Shoshani et al., 2006, p. 515). Ovid further writes, 'empty

DOI: 10.4324/9781003744962-2

words, as they long appeared, but the prophet was proved right. In the event, Narcissus died of a curious passion' (Ovid, ca. 10 BCE/2004, p. 109). What Ovid tells us from the outset of his story is that Narcissus will go mad and die once he sees and gets to know himself. From a modern intersubjective understanding of narcissism, the seer's prediction means that Narcissus cannot enter into real relationships with others, as intimate emotional and psychological contact with others inevitably involves encountering and recognizing oneself (Ermann, 2020, p. 16).

The young Narcissus is known for his extraordinary beauty, and 'Legions of lusty men and bevies of girls desired him' (Ovid, ca. 10 BCE/2004, p. 109), 'but the heart was so hard and proud in that soft and slender body, that none of the lusty men or languishing girls could approach him' (p. 109.). Narcissus is incapable of loving and cannot return another's passion. The young nymph Echo, who is incapable of initiating a conversation but can only repeat someone else's last statement, falls in love with Narcissus: 'The closer she followed, the flames of her passion grew nearer and nearer, as sulphur smeared on the tip of a pine-torch quickly catches fire when another flame is brought into close proximity' (p. 110). Arguably, Echo will never be able to engage in a mature and equal intersubjective relationship, because she has completely given up herself – she is not a subject but a subjectless mirror; an echo, bereft of vitality, repeating what the other – Narcissus – says. One day, Narcissus, exhausted from hunting, has been separated from his companions and cries out, 'Is anyone there?' to try to reconnect with his hunting party. Echo, who has followed him into the woods, replies, '… one there?'

After calling out to each other for some time, with Narcissus becoming increasingly confused by the strange replies from Echo, who can only repeat what he just said, Narcissus makes one more attempt to make his interlocutor show themself. He calls out, 'This way! We must come together.' Echo, delighted, replies, 'We must come together!' – her reply carrying a different and potentially more erotic meaning than Narcissus' statement. Then she bursts out from hiding 'arms outstretched to fling them around the shoulders she yearned for' (p. 111). Narcissus appears to shrink away in horror and flees as he calls out, 'Hands off! May I die before you enjoy my body' (p. 111).

Thus, Narcissus is quite insensitive, unempathic, aggressive and almost sadistic in his rejection of Echo, who, we must imagine, is overwhelmed by shame as Narcissus meets her passion with intense contempt. This constitutes a narcissistic injury of Echo, triggered by Narcissus' obvious disgust and intense rejection of her love: 'Scorned and rejected, with burning cheeks, she fled to the forest to hide her shame and live thenceforward in lonely caves' (p. 111). Here she dries up and withers, until 'nothing remained but voice and bones […] Buried away in the forest, seen no more on the mountains, heard all over the world, she survives in the sound of the echo' (p. 112). After suffering a severe narcissistic injury, as her love was met by cold contempt, she withdraws from the world. In almost masochistic fashion, she isolates herself, fades away and is petrified: 'for her bones (so they say) were transformed to stone' (p. 111 ff.). Echo is far from the only admirer whom Narcissus rejects in this intense and insensitive manner. In fact, he turns away 'Legions of lusty men and bevies of girls' (p. 109). In other versions and interpretations of the myth, it is the young man Armeinias who is so contemptuously rejected by Narcissus.

Finally, 'one of his scorned admirers lifted his hands to the heavens: "I pray Narcissus may fall in love and never obtain his desire!" His prayer was just and Némesis heard it' (Ovid, ca. 10 BCE/2004, p. 112). The Greek goddess Nemesis represents a form of higher justice and inflicts retribution and revenge when human beings have committed hubris: acting with arrogance before the gods and violating the divine laws. With his offensive rejection of others, Narcissus has earned the punishment of the gods: he is doomed to fall in love with himself and thus barred from ever obtaining the object of his desire. He must experience the same hopeless love as the many he has spurned. Narcissus has met his admirers' declarations of love with cold disdain. He shows contempt for love (Green, 2004, p. 83), and his despicable response to Echo's love is punished with painful and hopeless self-infatuation (Rank, 1911, p. 407).

One day, Narcissus, once again exhausted from a long day of hunting, lies down by a spring in the forest, 'The place looked pleasant, and here was a spring! Thirsty for water, he started to drink, but soon grew thirsty for something else' (Ovid, ca. 10 BCE/2004, p. 112). Mirrored in the spring, he sees a beautiful youth; unbeknownst to him, what he sees is his own reflection, and he is immediately enthralled. 'His being was suddenly overwhelmed by a vision of beauty. He fell in love with an empty hope, a shadow mistaken for substance' (p. 112). Overcome by this vision, he freezes: 'All that his lovers adored he worshipped in self-adoration. Blindly rapt with desire for himself, he was votary and idol, suitor and sweetheart, taper and fire – at one and the same time' (p. 113). What Ovid describes is that Narcissus, without being fully aware of it, is both the subject and the object of his own love. His own self is both source and target of this passionate adoration. Narcissus seeks to be close to the object of his desire but is doomed to fail, because it is his own fleeting self-image reflected in the surface of the water. As soon as he touches the reflection in the water, the surface is disturbed, and the image disappears. 'Those beautiful lips would implore a kiss, but as he bent forward the pool would always betray him. He plunges his arms in the water to clasp that ivory neck and finds himself clutching at no one' (p. 113). Narcissus is unable to distinguish between himself and others (his perceptions of self and others). He cannot separate himself from others nor realize that what he sees (and loves) in 'the other' in the water's surface is not another but himself: his own projective ideas about another.

Narcissus loses himself in his infatuation with the reflected image. He loses his ability to take care of the necessities of life: 'Nothing could drag him away from the place, not hunger for food nor need for sleep. As he lay stretched out in the grassy shade, he never could gaze his fill on that fraudulent image of beauty; and gazing proved his demise' (p. 113). Narcissus grows increasingly desperate over his inability to understand and consummate his desire: '"Wise old trees," he exclaimed, "has anyone loved more cruelly? [...] I've looked and have longed [he sees his own reflection but has not yet realized what he sees]. But looking and longing is far from enough. I still have to find!"' (p. 114), as he cannot achieve physical contact with the object of his love and consummate their connection. He calls out to the boy in the water, 'Come out to me here, whoever you are! Why keep eluding me, peerless boy? When I seek you, where do you steal away?' (p. 114). This passage, like others in the myth, clearly show that the infatuation may be seen as homosexual in nature, as Narcissus chooses himself and his own sex as the object of his love. In addition, it also demonstrates that Narcissus is clearly incapable of understanding his own desire and, not least, of consummating it, which he cannot do in a relationship to himself but only in a relationship with another human being. Despairing, he says, 'When my arms reach out to embrace you, you reach out too. I smile at you, and you smile at me back' (p. 114). Thus, in a sense, he finds that his love or infatuation is requited but only at a distance, never physically and never in the sort of real intersubjective contact that is a condition of true interpersonal love.

Suddenly, much too late, Narcissus realizes that the object of his overwhelming infatuation is his own reflection; that it is himself:

> I know you [the boy in the water] now and I know myself. Yes, I am the cause of the fire inside me, the fuel that burns and the flame that lights it. [...] All I desire I have. My wealth has left me a pauper. [...] I wish my love were not here! – a curious prayer for a lover.
>
> (p. 115)

Narcissus acknowledges that self-love is a poor form of love, and he wishes that the object of his love were not himself but a tangible other; not his own fleeting reflection. He also seems to realize, unconsciously, that genuine love is only possible if the object of desire is clearly separate from oneself. This painful insight makes Narcissus wish he were dead: 'Death will be easy to bear, since dying will cure my heartache' (p. 115). This passage may also be seen to express that when Narcissus realizes that he can neither have, possess or become his ideal (self-)image nor separate from it, he wishes to end his life (Diamond et al., 2022, p. xii).

In Ovid's interpretation, Narcissus goes mad once he realizes that he is infatuated with himself and that this infatuation can never be consummated: 'With that he turned distractedly back to his own reflection; his tears were troubling the limpid waters and blurring the picture that showed in the ruffled pool. When he saw it fast disappearing, "Don't hurry away, please stay! You cannot desert me so cruelly. I love you!"' (Ovid, ca. 10 BCE/2004, p. 115.). In despair that he can never be with his love, Narcissus rips his clothing and strikes himself. He fades away, like Echo – and 'gone was the physical vigour and all he had looked at and longed for, broken the godlike frame which once poor Echo had worshipped' (p. 116).

> His final words, as he gazed once more in the pool, rang back from the rocks: 'Oh marvellous boy [...]' [...] He rested his weary head in the fresh green grass, till Death's hand gently closed his eyes still rapt with their master's beauty. Even then, as he crossed the Styx to ghostly Hades, he gazed at himself in the river.
>
> (p. 116)

Not even as he slips into death is he able to give up his infatuation with his own reflection, which he now sees in the river Styx, the boundary of the land of the dead and never-ending darkness. Narcissus dies, and where he lay, there is only 'a flower with a trumpet of gold and pale white petals' (pp. 116–117): a narcissus.

Sigmund Freud's introduction of narcissism

The concept of narcissism was first applied in psychology and psychiatry by the British sexologist Havelock Ellis in 1897. He wrote about auto-eroticism, including masturbation and sexual daydreams, both of which involve sexual arousal that does not involve real others, only the person themself. The first to engage in a more fully elaborated application of the concept in psychology was Freud, in his 1914 paper 'On narcissism: An introduction' (1914/1957b). And psychoanalysis remained the main arena for developing our understanding of narcissism until the 1970s, when certain social and personality psychologists began to use and explore what should primarily be seen as narcissistic personality traits (see later). In psychoanalysis, the focus is not just on specific and observable personality traits but also on (the degree of) personality organization and dynamic psychological processes underlying observable traits and behaviour.

In his classic treatise 'On narcissism: An introduction', Freud (1914/1957b) proposes an understanding of narcissism framed by intrapsychic psychology and, to some extent, personality structure and based on his drive theory – which we must now recognize as being largely untenable. The article is far from one of Freud's clearest or best-written, which probably stems in part from the fact that it is part of Freud's dispute at the time with certain younger psychoanalysts, including Carl Gustav Jung, who with increasingly substantial arguments rejected parts of his drive theory. Furthermore, it conflated what might be called sexual and vital drives, thus causing unnecessary confusion about Freud's understanding of narcissism, among other topics (Lacan, 1975/1988, p. 149 ff.). Freud sought to defend his untenable drive theory by supplementing the object-directed sexual drive with a drive directed at the own self, which is further eroticized; this in turn makes it almost impossible to distinguish between his somewhat abstract notions of sexual drives, vital drives and self-preservation drives (Küchenhoff, 2003, p. 151). Furthermore, Freud's treatise on narcissism represents a sort of transition between his early id or drive theory and his more nuanced ego psychology and also contains initial stages of both object relations theory and self psychology, which were later developed by, among others, Melanie Klein, Otto Kernberg and Heinz Kohut (Zabel, 2019, p. 29) (see Chapters 3.3 and 3.4).

Freud (1914/1957b) imagines that human beings contain a certain amount of (broadly defined sexual) drive energy that the ego can invest either in itself or in external objects, primarily in relations with other human beings. Here, we should recall that Freud's article on narcissism predates the development of his structural personality model (Freud, 1923/1990), where the ego is defined as a distinct element of the personality like the id and the superego. What Freud refers to as the ego in his treatise on narcissism more or less corresponds to what we now call the self (Wolf, 1996, p. 21). According to Freud, the more (drive) energy the ego invests in itself, the less it will have left to invest and engage in relations with others, and vice versa. Or, as Freud (1914/1957b, p. 76) puts it, there is 'an antithesis between ego-libido and object-libido. The more of the one is employed, the more the other becomes depleted'.

One concrete implication of this is that if the self invests too much of its mental energy (libido, vital/sexual drive) in others, its self-esteem and capacity for self-preservation will suffer. Conversely, it also means that an overly one-sided focus on the self and withdrawal of interest in others, with the purpose of investing all of one's mental energy in solipsistic attention to oneself, may undermine the capacity for contact with others. In the worst case, this may lead to psychotic states, where all forms of intimate emotional contact with others becomes disrupted. According to Freud (1917/1963, p. 531), this also includes melancholy, where the self's mental energy (libido) has been withdrawn to and invested in the ego via what Freud calls narcissistic identification, and the ego has become its own primary object. Here, Freud sees narcissism, narcissistic withdrawal from the world and death wish as interconnected (Rosenfeld, 1987, p. 145). Today, rather than referring to Freud's concept of a semi-biological death wish, we would speak of the existence of more psychological and severely destructive, including self-destructive, forces in individuals with a severe narcissistic disorder that may hamper or almost completely block the ability to establish any close emotional contact with others. These destructive forces will generally become meaningful and understandable as these individuals' often severely traumatic history is uncovered in psychotherapy – and thus should not be attributed to any speculative death wish.

The core idea in Freud's introduction of the concept of narcissism is that the self, in an attempt to bolster its – possibly fragile – self-esteem, may become overly focused on its own needs and show limited interest in what others might need. Among other implications, this egocentricity will weaken the self's capacity for deep and genuine contact with others. Here, severe narcissistic disorders are thus not regarded as conditions that are mainly about excessive self-love. Rather, they are related to a basic inability to love and be in contact with others and, to some extent, to connect with large areas of one's own emotions.

As early as 1939, Karen Horney, one of the forerunners of relational psychoanalysis and a founder of a separate understanding of 'feminine psychology' (Horney, 1967), sharply rejected Freud's drive-theory-based understanding of narcissism. She writes that

> the postulate that an instinct is the generating cause prevents a perception of the meaning and significance which particular trends have for a personality. According to my view, narcissistic trends are not the derivative of an instinct but represent a neurotic trend, [...] an attempt to cope with the self and others by way of self-inflation.
>
> (Horney, 1939, p. 99)

This represents a much more relational understanding of, especially, the more grandiose manifestations of narcissism as attempts to protect the self in interactions with others. She also does not believe that 'narcissism is an expression not of self-love but of alienation from the self. [...] [A] person clings to illusions about himself because, and as far as, he has lost himself' (p. 99 ff.). In Horney's assessment, a person with pronounced narcissistic traits is 'alienated from self as well as from others' (p. 100). Thus, as much as possible – even past the point of obviously dissocial behaviour and psychopathy – we should meet persons with narcissistic disorder with empathic understanding, kindness and caring rather than moral condemnation and social exclusion.

Today, most people would agree that Freud was fundamentally wrong in understanding love of self and others as a zero-sum game (Fiscalini, 2004, p. 103). Rather, love of self and others would mutually strengthen each other until a certain point, at which the narcissistically disordered person's attention might become too exclusively focused on one of the two, idealizing or devaluing self and/or others as an object of either grovelling admiration or contempt. It is not the case that human beings have a finite supply of love and compassion, such that the greater our self-esteem and the more compassion we feel with ourselves, the less we have to give to others – on the contrary, to a certain point. However, low self-esteem, shame, self-hatred and lack of compassion with one's own self can hamper our ability to connect emotionally with and love others.

Primary and secondary narcissism

Another central aspect of Freud's understanding of narcissism is that he basically views it as part of normal psychological development; a view that was later continued in self psychology (Kohut, 1971), among other schools of thought. Freud identified two types of narcissism: primary narcissism, which, simply put, refers to the child's investment in their own primary objects (above all, the mother) during the earliest phase of life, when the infant has not yet developed clearly distinct awareness of self and others (Jacobson, 1964, p. 15). According to Freud (1914/1957b), this primary narcissism occurs before the child is capable of clearly distinguishing between self and others. This understanding of primary narcissism rests on the assumption of an original symbiosis of mother and infant. Arguably, it relates narcissistic issues to an inadequate distinction between self and others, me and not-me. This constitutes a form of narcissistic organization (Rosenfeld, 1971) or pathological personality organization (Steiner, 1993) that may hamper the establishment of mature relations with real others (clearly distinct from the self) and result in distorted perceptions of reality (Roth, 2008, p. 9).

Freud never offered a precise description or definition of primary narcissism (Balint, 1968, p. 40), but in a more abstract sense, we should imagine Freud's understanding of primary narcissism as a near paradisiac state characterized by an oceanic feeling of bliss, where the self's world consists solely of the symbiotic relationship with the mother, all basic needs are met, the pleasure principle reigns supreme, and the self may experience a sense of omnipotence and perfection. This state persists until the person (the infant) has to confront external realities – the reality principle – and the fact that we cannot develop into mature human subjects without breaking free from this primary infantile narcissistic state and symbiosis. We may also see it as an archaic (nostalgic) narcissistic dream or fantasy that it might be possible to return to this state or restore a universe where the omnipotent self has all their needs met. This virtual Nirvana, where all forms of frustration and desire are eliminated, is akin to death in some regards: a mental death where more complex elements of human psychology (often associated with ambivalence) have been suspended or do not exist. In terms of a more specific phase in human psychological development, it is not viable to speak an original symbiotic relationship between mother and infant (Stern, 1985).

Later, Freud (1921/1940, p. 69) attempts to link primary narcissism with a form of autistic state, in which the self imagines that its needs can be met more or less independently of others. In this state, the self also abandons any need of others; cf. an illusory notion of the self's near total independence of others, except, perhaps, of the primary object – typically the mother or, perhaps, God. Today, we must join Rosenfeld (1981, p. 197) in viewing Freud's concept of primary narcissism as a description of very primitive object relations, where fantasies of omnipotence, in particular, play a prominent role: the other is seen and treated as a part of the self (cf. inadequate self-other differentiation and the purely internal object) and is used to evacuate and contain undesirable aspects of the self, including via projective identification (Jørgensen, 2018/2019, p. 249 ff.). In relation to adults with severe personality pathology, primary narcissism should thus be viewed as a mental state where the capacity for establishing real relationships with external objects is almost completely or partially blocked (Britton, 2003, p. 145).

In the normal course of development, the child, according to Freud, will gradually overcome their primary narcissism and shift their attention from their own self to the external reality and invest their mental energy, or drive, energy in others. However, if this normal progression is derailed for some reason, this may result in what Freud describes as secondary narcissism, as the child or young person withdraws their (drive) energy to their own self, once again focusing the bulk of their attention on themself, at the expense of taking an interest in others (Freud, 1914/1957b, p. 74 ff.). This is a disturbed and regressive form of narcissism that – again, according to Freud – should be attributed mainly to psychotic states and which cannot be treated through psychoanalysis (or psychotherapy), because patients with this 'narcissistic neurosis' (Freud, 1917/1963, p. 424) have withdrawn from relations to others to such a degree that they are unable to develop the transference (emotional investment) in the relationship to the therapist that is a key condition of effective psychoanalytic treatment (Ermann, 2020, p. 34).

According to Freud, the recurrence of key elements of the patient's interpersonal difficulties that is common in the patient's transference and interactions with the therapist (Freud also speaks of 'transference neuroses') does not occur in narcissistic neuroses, corresponding to psychotic states (see Freud, 1917/1963, p. 480 ff.). Today, we would reject this view, which should be seen in relation to the fact that Freud never developed the very significant distinction between narcissism as a form of absence of close relations with others (cf. primary narcissism and pronounced grandiosity) versus narcissism as a way of relating to others, albeit in some cases in a severely disturbed way (cf. object relations) (Symington, 1993, p. xi) that we see in individuals with severe narcissistic personality disorders. Freud's attempts, based on drive theory, to explain the underlying psychological dynamics of narcissism must generally be viewed as clearly untenable. However, some parts of his descriptions of the phenomenology of narcissism remain enlightening, in the sense that severe narcissistic disorders are, in part, related to egocentric preoccupation with oneself and one's own needs at the expense of genuine interest in others, including severe empathy deficiencies, particularly with regard to emotional empathy.

The narcissistic character

In a small treatise introducing a form of human typology with a focus on the organization or fate of the human libido or drive/vital energy, Freud (1931/1957a) briefly introduces a particular narcissistic type: individuals who are independent, who are focused on self-preservation (own needs), who do not seem susceptible to anxiety and whose ego has access to large amounts of aggression, manifested – for better or worse – in readiness for activity (p. 218). According to Freud, individuals with a narcissistic character often appear as 'personalities' who are suited to offering support and to others; they may become leaders and thus promote cultural change, but they may also do great damage to the established system, including the social and moral order (p. 218). Here, Freud's understanding of the concept of narcissism seems somewhat ambiguous or incomplete, in the sense that individuals with a narcissistic character, according to Freud, have the capacity both to become important leaders and to take destructive action that harms other people and social communities.

In extension of this view, the psychoanalyst Wilhelm Reich (1933/1949, p. 201), a contemporary of Freud's, writes about the phallic-narcissistic character, which he describes as arrogant and self-confident with considerable aggression, manifested in part by anticipating attacks on the self by attacking the other and by contempt for others. Reich also describes how the phallic-narcissistic character strives for leading positions and struggles to submit to other people's leadership and agendas: when someone with a phallic-narcissistic character is compelled, for some reason, to submit to someone else's agenda, they will typically try to cope with or compensate for this by exerting dominance and control over others who are perceived to be 'on lower rungs of the ladder' (p. 201), such as their spouse, children or colleagues. This apparent superiority may be viewed as a defence against unacceptable experiences of own vulnerability and inferiority (Altmeyer, 2000, p. 34).

According to Reich (1933/1949, p. 202) the phallic-narcissistic character is much more common among men, whose relationship with women will often disturbed by conscious or unconscious contempt for the female sex. This is also manifested in their sexuality, which, according to Reich, is often driven by an urge to prove their potency and to dominate, degrade or even 'destroy' the woman (p. 203) as a form of revenge over perceived letdowns or defeat. According to Reich (p. 201), these men are often physically attractive, with a particularly masculine appearance and behaviour. Thus, Reich too paints a rather mixed and ambivalent picture of the narcissistic character, which, on the one hand – in its undisturbed (Reich would say 'unneurotic') manifestations – may be associated with positive agency and leadership abilities but, on the other hand, is also often associated with acts and perceptions of self and others that are destructive, particularly to other individuals, groups and social structures.

The narcissistic object choice

In his early writings, in a short note about the development of human sexuality, Freud also introduces the – somewhat peculiar, from a contemporary point of view – claim that narcissism is a key aspect of the development of male homosexuality (perhaps also bisexuality), based on the homosexual preference for a sexual object of the same sex as himself. Freud views this as a sort of intermediate stage in the development from autoeroticism to mature object love (Freud, 1905/1949, pp. 222; see also Freud, 1911/1958, p. 60; 1917/1963, p. 377 ff.); the homosexual object choice is thus viewed as a transitional stage but also as a narcissistic fixation on the path to the more mature object love (Schmidt-Hellerau, 2021, p. 17). Freud also speaks of the so-called narcissistic (immature) object choice – choice of love and sexual object – where an individual seeks what they are (themself), what they once were or what they would like to be (Freud, 1914/1957b, p. 88). Like most of his contemporaries, Freud apparently did not have sufficient imagination to associate mature love and sexuality with anything, really, besides a heterosexual relationship.

More generally, it could be argued that the early psychoanalytic understanding of narcissism conflates at least four levels or potential forms of narcissism: 1) sexuality directed at the self, 2) excessive emotional investment in one's own self (self-love) at the expense of emotional involvement in others (love of and genuine interest in others), 3) egocentric focusing on or excessive attention on oneself (own experiences, needs, particular qualities), including the inability to see the self and the world from someone else's perspective, and 4) positive feelings for oneself or a level of self-esteem that, in the case of a narcissistic disorder, may be at odds with reality in terms of excessively positive (grandiose) or excessively negative self-esteem (self-hatred) (Westen, 1990, p. 186 ff.).

Freud's narrow understanding of narcissism, based on one-person psychology, may be interpreted to mean that individuals with very immature or disturbed narcissism are so absorbed in themselves, their own needs and their own inner life that they are incapable of entering into a relationship with someone else. However, as the psychoanalyst Sydney Pulver (1986 [1970], p. 107) pointed out, even before the development of the modern, more intersubjective and relational understanding of narcissism, we should rather view key aspects of disturbed narcissism as expressions of an immature way of relating, in which the individual's pervasive interest in their own self and their own immediate needs causes their perception of others to become reduced and distorted – coloured by the person's own egocentric needs and projective ideas – and risks compromising the person's psychological and emotional differentiation between self and others and their emotional investment in others.

An important element in understanding narcissism through a Freudian lens hinges on whether the young person or adult regulates their self-esteem in age-appropriate ways or, rather, seeks to stabilize their fragile self-esteem through behaviours that might be regarded as age-appropriate early in life but which must be viewed as immature or even disturbed later in life (cf. Kernberg, 2004a, p. 49). This may be manifested, for example, as the rigid conviction of being unique (grandiosity) and a resulting insistence on being entitled to special treatment; as narcissistic rage or a sense of injustice and victimhood when the self does not receive the expected level of attention and admiration from others; or an egocentric lack of gratitude when others actually do help and support the self. When pathological narcissism makes it difficult to show authentic (unlike insincere, manipulative) gratitude, this probably stems in part from the fact that gratitude may be associated with being in a subordinate position in relation to benefactor (perhaps also with envy; cf. O'Shaughnessy, 2008, p. 88), an unbearable situation, in particular in predominantly grandiose narcissism. Genuine gratitude requires giving up one's sense of omnipotence and acknowledging that others may offer something good, perhaps even something that one needs (Lear, 2024, p. 131). A similar relational issue of feeling placed in a subordinate position may also play a role in the apparent absence of guilt and shame in pathological narcissism.

Narcissism and ego ideal

However, Freud (1914/1957b) also proposes a slightly different understanding of the development of human narcissism; one in which the focus is on the individual's establishment of an ego ideal which it loves the same way it once loved itself (in primary narcissism) and which it continuously strives to realize as a form of yearning for narcissistic satisfaction and perfection. As the Austrian philosopher Isolde Charim (2022, p. 29) puts it, Freud's concept of narcissism primarily concerns the relationship between the internal and the external world. She also sees it as characteristic of late modern human psychology that we voluntarily submit to our own ego ideal – an ego ideal that we largely, if unknowingly, adopt from contemporary culture – at the same time as we do everything in our power to realize (become) this ego ideal, unaware that this is basically impossible, since our real ego will always have deficiencies compared with our internalized ego ideal. The ego ideal is unattainable, impossible to fully realize, and a person with predominantly grandiose narcissism will make an (illusory) attempt to resolve this impasse by merging their ideal self with their real self (see Chapter 3.4).

People living in late modernity establish an internal ego ideal which they continually hold their own real ego up to while attempting to overcome the gap between the two. In Freud's (1914/1957b, p. 94) words: 'What he projects before him as his ideal is the substitute for the lost narcissism of his childhood in which he was his own ideal.' The ego ideal is 'the heir to the original narcissism in which the childish ego enjoyed self-sufficiency' (Freud, 1921/1940, p. 110). At the same time, the ego ideal can offer some internal consolation and compensation for deficiencies in the real ego and thus become part of a psychic retreat (see Chapter 3.6), a sanctuary for the self when it finds itself unable to live up to the demands and expectations of the outside world (cf. narcissistic imbalance and injury), 'that a man, when he cannot be satisfied with his ego itself, may nevertheless be able to find satisfaction in the ego ideal which has been differentiated out of the ego' (Freud, 1921/1940, p. 110). In simplified terms, the inadequate (real) ego comforts itself with its own elevated moral and other ideals which it projects for itself and for others to see and which it perceives as a part of itself, essentially saying, 'I have such lofty goals and moral standards for myself and my life, which I continuously to everything to realize, which in itself makes me special.' Thus, the ego ideal is both part of the ego, as part of the ego's own projected ideas and goals, and not part of the ego, as something that the ego is not (yet) but strives to become (Charim, 2022, p. 38).

Narcissism or the individual's investment of its mental energy in itself thus shifts from the early childhood self to 'this new ideal ego' (Freud, 1914/1957b, p. 94). At the same time, according to Freud (1914/1957b, p. 94), we should see this as an attempt to reclaim 'the narcissistic perfection of his childhood' in 'the new form of an ego ideal'. He writes about the psychological maturation of the ego and the related development in narcissism:

> The development of the ego consists in a departure from primary narcissism and gives rise to a vigorous attempt to recover that state. This departure [from primary narcissism] is brought about by means of the displacement of libido [drive energy; we might also say a displacement of mental attention and focus] on to an ego ideal imposed from without; and satisfaction is brought about from fulfilling this ideal.
>
> (Freud, 1914/1957b, p. 100)

Freud thus introduces a process or an authority in human psychology that persistently observes or monitors the ego and compares it (the real ego) with its ego ideal or an internal (perhaps internalized) standard (Wright et al., 1989, p. 218); an ideal that also contains social aspects: 'it is also the common ideal of a family, a class or a nation' (Freud, 1914/1957b, p. 110).

By establishing the ego ideal, the person also internalizes the (generally patriarchal) social order – a process that is thus a core aspect of the human ability to function in social groups (Verhaeghe, 2017, p. 39). However, unlike the superego, which, simply put, consists of a set of moral prohibitions and directions – an intrapsychic psychological representative of prevailing norms and ideas about what is right/permitted and wrong/prohibited, established through internalization of the prevailing social order – the ego ideal is a more individual entity. It is an individually developed model that, without offering very specific directions, requires the ego to develop its own particular individuality and acts as a driver of a persistent effort to improve and optimize itself, its identity and its chances of earning the admiration and approval of others (Charim, 2022, p. 45 ff.).

In extension of this understanding, Charim (2022, p. 48) views narcissism in late modern societies as the tyranny of the ego ideal, which is constantly pushing us on, preventing us from ever feeling content and at ease with considering ourselves adequate, 'good enough'. The goal we strive for is not external – an external object that we might seek to acquire or possess – but something that we strive to become. When we fail – as we must, since the ideal can always be further perfected – we feel inadequate and shameful, perceiving our failure as a blow to our self-esteem (Jørgensen, 2023/2024). As a result, we may experience a psychologically painful narcissistic crisis. These narcissistic dynamics may shed some light on the powerful emotional forces behind late modern people's constant striving for self-optimization and the realization of (unrealistic) heroic ego ideals. This ambition comes with considerable risk of overburdening and exhausting us and leading to psychological and physical collapse, and it points to shame as a core affect in narcissism (see Chapter 2.4).

2.2 Lack of conceptual clarity: Fundamentally different understandings of narcissism

Simply put, we may distinguish between two important and largely separate traditions or pillars in the study of narcissism: one that is based on general psychology and relies mainly on quantitative research methods and one that is more theoretically founded and is based on work with clinical populations, including psychotherapeutic work with people with various forms of narcissistic disturbances. One key challenge in the study of narcissism is that while psychoanalysis and clinical psychology, on the one hand, and the fields of social and personality psychology, on the other, use the same term, it far from always refers to the same phenomenon. In some regards, narcissism is defined, understood and operationalized very differently within the two branches of psychology. In social and personality psychology, narcissism is mainly considered a part of the normal personality spectrum. Practitioners speak of varying degrees of narcissistic traits and are primarily interested in non-pathological manifestations of grandiose narcissism, which they believe can be assessed through self-report questionnaires.

Clinical psychology, and some forms of psychoanalysis, tend to use 'narcissism' more as a term to capture various degrees and forms of psychological disturbance and are sceptical of the use of relatively simple quantitative questionnaires to capture its central elements. Many psychoanalysts also use the term to refer to certain dynamic intrapsychic processes that may be manifested, for example, in different ways of being and acting. The questionnaires used to describe personality traits and disturbances in quantitative research can only capture these processes to a certain degree, typically a very limited degree. In psychoanalysis, grandiosity is not necessarily viewed solely as a personality trait – a relatively stable personal characteristic that is the focus of personality psychology's interest in individual differences – but also, in some cases, as a defence against narcissistic vulnerability and an attempt at self-regulation: the fragile self using a grandiose inflated self-image and omnipotent behaviour to escape perceived inferiority and low self-esteem (Ronningstam, 2012, p. 946). Similarly, dissocial behaviour and aggressive attacks on others by individuals with severely malign narcissism and general dissociality are viewed as attempts to escape low self-esteem and emotional dysregulation (Pincus, 2023, p. 636). Thus, rather than being viewed primarily as a personality trait, these behaviours are understood as ways of being that are driven by pathological internal psychological processes.

Attempts to quantify narcissism

Due to the fundamentally different understandings of narcissism, most of the quantitative questionnaires for self-reporting narcissism and narcissistic personality traits that have been developed in the fields of social and personality psychology provide only limited and rather imprecise assessments of the sorts of elements that psychoanalysis and parts of clinical psychology regard as key aspects of more severe narcissistic disorders. This includes, for example, the most widely applied instrument, the Narcissistic Personality Inventory (NPI) (Raskin & Hall, 1979; Raskin & Terry, 1988), which has little or no ability to capture more vulnerable and disturbed manifestations of narcissism (see Chapter 2.3).

Until around 2010, the vast majority of the quantitative studies of narcissism conducted in the fields of social and personality psychology relied on NPI (Wright & Edershile, 2018, p. 74), which almost exclusively captures certain non-pathological aspects of grandiose narcissism – that is positively associated with self-esteem and negatively associated with shame (Pincus & Lukowitsky, 2010, p. 425). Several studies suggest that it does not capture the same phenomenon as later instruments developed for measuring less adaptive, including more vulnerable, manifestations of narcissism (Miller & Campbell, 2008, p. 462). In recent years, however, a few instruments have been developed for quantitative assessments of narcissism that, in various ways, attempt to bridge the gap between the understandings of narcissism in social and personality psychology versus clinical psychology. One example is the Pathological Narcissism Inventory (PNI) (Pincus et al., 2009). However, none of these quantitative instruments really manage to overcome the very significant differences in the basic understanding of narcissism that separates these two traditions in narcissism research.

The primary goal of narcissism research in the fields of social and personality psychology is to uncover grandiose and non-pathological narcissistic personality traits. This is typically pursued via large-scale questionnaire studies based on non-clinical populations, very often university students, who are typically easy to recruit for university researchers but are not necessarily very representative of the general population. In recent years, this approach has been supplemented with more experimental methods that seek to actualize the participants' narcissism by subjecting them to relatively trivial injuries to their self-image and self-esteem and either observing or asking them to report their reaction. Simply put, these studies will at best be able to uncover relatively trivial manifestations of non-pathological narcissism, but it will not always be clear to what extent their findings can be generalized to the population at large, including, in particular, to people with severe narcissistic disorder. Although these studies may hold merit, they are not necessarily very helpful in furthering our understanding of pathological narcissism. However, with the recent development of questionnaires that also seek to include more pathological elements in their measures of narcissism, we have, in principle, moved closer to being able to include quantitative methods in the study of pathological narcissism.

Qualitative differences between normal and pathological narcissism

In relation to this issue, we need to address at least two other questions pertaining to our fundamental understanding of the phenomenon of narcissism. One is whether it is possible to apply an exclusively dimensional understanding of narcissism, meaning that the forms of narcissism we see in normally functioning individuals are, in every significant regard, the same as the ones we encounter in individuals with severely pathological narcissism. Or whether we need to consider certain key qualitative differences between normal and pathological narcissism – differences that are reflected in the fundamentally different understandings of narcissism in social and personality psychology versus parts of clinical psychology and psychoanalysis. An initial answer would be that we need to apply a basic qualitative distinction between a normal and a pathological spectrum of narcissism. In extension of this point, we need to consider whether we should base empirical studies of pathological narcissism on people who actually have these disorders rather than conducting large-scale studies where university students and other non-clinical populations fill out questionnaires that include various dimensional measures of pathological narcissism. In extension of the answer to the first question above, the initial answer to this second question must be that empirical studies of pathological narcissism should to a significant degree be based on clinical populations: individuals diagnosed with pathological narcissism (NPD). We should furthermore, at the very least, be very cautious about applying findings from social and personality psychology studies of young university students to expand our understanding of people with severe narcissistic personality disorders.

Currently, there are not many empirical studies that involve patients with NPD. The few existing studies typically include a broader group of people with personality disorders, with a minority – often a very small minority – having an NPD diagnosis (Pincus, 2023, p. 631). This clearly presents a fairly serious problem. In addition, when people with pathological narcissism are actually included in empirical studies, their diagnosis is typically based on the narrow definition of NPD in the *Diagnostic and Statistical Manual of Mental Disorders* (*DSM*) system (Pincus et al., 2009, p. 371). In practice, this means that they often only include people with predominantly grandiose manifestations of NPD, which is the main focus of the *DSM* system's diagnostic criteria for NPD. More vulnerable manifestations of narcissism are not included, as they are not captured by the *DSM* system's NPD diagnosis, or only to a very limited degree (see Chapter 3.1).

Overall, it is notoriously difficult to arrive at a consensus about the definition, operationalization and development of valid methods for empirical studies of a complex and multifaceted psychological phenomenon such as narcissism. Naturally, this does not mean that we should not continue to pursue this goal. However, we need to be aware that in our efforts to build consensus about a common understanding and empirical operationalization of narcissism and develop practically applicable tools for quantitative research, we may simplify our understanding and, thus, the phenomenon of narcissism so much that we would end up creating new and serious problems for ourselves.

Although studies based on students and other non-clinical populations use questionnaires designed to capture pathological narcissism, it is far from given that the participants who get the highest scores for pathological narcissism in these studies are comparable to patients diagnosed with pathological narcissism. Hence, the findings of studies such as these cannot be directly generalized and applied to enhance our understanding of pathological narcissism. Moreover, there is a risk of fairly problematic circular reasoning, as we first seek to narrow pathological narcissism down to quantified answers to simple questions in a questionnaire and then define or equal pathological narcissism to a high score in these simple quantitative inventories (Brown & Tamborski, 2011). The most promising path to a deeper and more nuanced understanding of pathological narcissism is probably to conduct more qualitative studies based on participants diagnosed with narcissistic disorders and on experiences from psychotherapeutic work with pathological narcissism (Jørgensen & Bøye, in prep.).

On the other hand, it could also be argued that the psychoanalytic understanding of the phenomenology and underlying internal psychological processes of narcissism primarily contains theoretical and relatively abstract elements that are not, or only sparingly, operationalized in ways that make them applicable to the type of quantitative empirical studies that dominate empirical personality psychology. From some perspectives, this must be regarded as a problem.

The relationship between grandiose and vulnerable narcissism

One specific example of this occurs in the psychoanalytically informed notion that grandiose aspects of narcissism may cover up and serve as elements in a defence against internal vulnerability and fragile self-esteem (Ackerman et al., 2017, p. 358). Sometimes, this is referred to as the 'mask model', which views grandiose perceptions as a protective mask or facade to cover up underlying or more fundamental narcissistic vulnerability and inferiority.

Several studies have attempted to operationalize this model by distinguishing between explicit and implicit self-esteem. While researchers measure the former through self-reporting, they believe that the latter can be captured through various experimental methods, including association tests (Bosson et al., 2008). From a psychoanalytic perspective, the applied methods appear somewhat primitive and are hardly capable of assessing complex unconscious processes. Thus, there is reason to doubt that indirect (association) measures of (so-called) self-esteem can actually capture unconscious or not immediately consciously available self-experiences and self-assessments (Krizan & Herlache, 2018, p. 22). Generally, it does not seem readily possible to develop reliable quantitative instruments for charting a phenomenon as complex as implicit or unconscious self-esteem (Miller et al., 2017, p. 301).

It should be noted, however, that so far, it has not been possible to present convincing empirical support for the 'mask model', even though a small number of studies do seem to support certain aspects of it (Kuchynka & Bosson, 2018). A few studies found that a high score on measures of grandiose narcissism correlate with perceptions of the self as inadequate and vulnerable to rejection (Biberdzic et al., 2023), which may support an understanding of a grandiose narcissistic self-image as a defence against underlying or covert narcissistic vulnerability. In this understanding, vulnerability and grandiosity are not seen as two distinct categories of narcissism but are instead dynamically related phenomena that may manifest themselves in and dominate an individual at different times and in different contexts. Further, studies have found that narcissistic personality disorders (NPDs) are associated with more extensive implicit or underlying shame compared to borderline personality disorders (BPDs) and non-clinical control groups (Ritter et al., 2014). This too may be associated with fragile and poor self-esteem behind what may be a very grandiose facade.

Furthermore, most of these studies have the same problems as most of the more quantitative narcissism research, and we need more in-depth qualitative studies of the inner life and subjective experiences of people with pathological narcissism (Kuchynka & Bosson, 2018, p. 90; Jørgensen & Bøye, in prep.). However, studies of the mask model based on patients who are in psychotherapy or other forms of psychiatric treatment also involves certain challenges. Patients in psychiatric treatment will often have a higher likelihood of NPD with a relatively higher emphasis on vulnerable manifestations, as they have sought help and are in treatment, while persons with a relatively higher occurrence of grandiose manifestations of NPD will often be underrepresented in psychiatric populations.

Conversely, there would probably be a higher share of predominantly grandiose pathological NPD profiles in forensic psychiatry and in prison populations, as individuals with a higher occurrence of grandiose manifestations of NPD would, on average, be expected to be somewhat less likely to seek help and would thus primarily be found in institutions based on some degree of non-voluntary participation, including court-mandated treatment (Miller et al., 2017, p. 305 ff.). Furthermore, we should expect the manifestations of grandiose narcissism found in studies based on psychiatric patients and prison inmates to be far more extreme and pathological than the manifestations found in studies based on university students and other non-clinical populations.

Degree of pathology makes a difference

A meta-analysis of correlations between vulnerable and grandiose manifestations of narcissism in various populations lend some support to this point (Jauk et al., 2022). Thus, grandiose and vulnerable narcissism have been found to be uncorrelated, seemingly representing two separate phenomena in the case of low and moderate (non-pathological) levels of grandiose narcissism. In the case of high (pathological) levels of grandiose narcissism, on the other hand, a relatively strong correlation was found between grandiose and vulnerable narcissism. This finding suggests that the psychological processes at play in low versus high levels of grandiose narcissism are fundamentally different, including that narcissism may vary between grandiose and vulnerable manifestations in the case of pathological levels of grandiose narcissism (Jauk et al., 2022, p. 717). Thus, findings from studies – typically from the fields of social and personality psychology – based on persons with low or moderate levels of grandiosity will probably not provide valuable insights into persons with pathological levels of grandiose narcissism, including NPD (see also Grijalva et al., 2015b).

The findings of this meta-analysis suggest that, on the one hand, we can distinguish between two separate personality traits in the general population that have come to be identified under the – somewhat problematic and potentially misleading, from a clinical point of view – labels of grandiose and vulnerable narcissism. On the other hand, pathological narcissism, which is found in clinical populations and, in particular, in individuals with severe personality pathology, may be manifested as both grandiose and vulnerable narcissism. In this understanding, vulnerable and grandiose narcissism are closely related and should not be regarded as two separate personality traits. Rather, it seems that pathological narcissism alternately, and to varying degrees, manifests itself as vulnerable and grandiose forms, which thus do not constitute stable, mutually exclusive personality traits. We also find (Jauk et al., 2022, p. 716 ff.) that the level of vulnerable narcissism increases in connection with high levels of grandiose narcissism, while the level of grandiose narcissism is not similarly seen to increase in individuals with high levels of vulnerable narcissism.

To the extent that future studies arrive at the same finding in larger clinical studies based on persons with personality disorders (see Fossati et al., 2015, p. 421), this might imply that pathological vulnerable narcissism is more likely to occur without significant elements of pathological grandiose narcissism – where the grandiose defence may have collapsed – while high levels of grandiose narcissism is far more likely to be accompanied by pathological vulnerable narcissism, presumably because severe pathological grandiose narcissism should be viewed, in a dynamic understanding, as an attempt to protect a vulnerable self that is struggling with severe narcissistic imbalances. However, there is reason to assume that some individuals with high-functioning grandiose narcissism or severe malignant narcissism accompanied by psychopathy do not, or only to a very limited extent, contain (or manifest) elements of vulnerable narcissism.

Because the basic understandings of and attempts to operationalize narcissism differ so much in certain regards, findings from narcissism research from the perspective of social and personality psychology cannot be directly applied to psychoanalysis and clinical psychology, or vice versa. If we want to attempt to implement the findings anyway – as this book does to some extent – we need to bear in mind what differentiates the two understandings of narcissism. The fields of social and personality psychology place a much higher emphasis on predominantly grandiose (but not necessarily pathological) elements of narcissism, including arrogance, (at least superficially) high self-esteem and self-reliance (autonomy), need for attention, social dominance, reduced empathy and a tendency to exploit others.

Clinical psychology, on the other hand, focuses much more on the more vulnerable aspects and manifestations of narcissism, including unstable and fragile self-esteem, emotional instability, dependence on others, insecure attachment and more internalizing symptoms of psychological dysfunction, such as shame and depression (Hatemi & Fazekas, 2018, p. 874; Rohmann et al., 2012) along with an intense focus on severely disturbed manifestations of grandiose narcissism. Thus, in psychoanalysis and clinical psychology, the concept of pathological narcissism is not limited to narcissistic personality disorder (NPD), as defined in the *DSM-5*, which does not account sufficiently for the more vulnerable elements and manifestations of narcissistic disorders (see Chapter 3.1).

Narcissism as a personality trait

Attempts have been made to bridge the gap between the study of personality disorders in social and personality psychology versus clinical psychology by conceptualizing the individual personality disorders based, in particular, on methods from trait psychology. These attempts have involved the classic five-factor model (Big Five) for understanding the basic elements of human personality (Saulsman & Page, 2004, p. 1056). More specifically, there have been attempts to identify differences and similarities between the individual personality disorders by examining how people with specific personality disorders describe themselves in questionnaires designed to measure the five core personality traits of agreeableness, neuroticism, extroversion, openness and conscientiousness (Mortensen et al., 2017). Each of the five personality traits can be broken down to facets or components. For neuroticism, for example, the constituent aspects include anxiety, vulnerability, impulsivity, depression and irritability. The basic goal of this effort has been to measure, describe and understand personality disorders exhaustively as extreme variants of these five normal personality dimensions. Whether this is a tenable idea is clearly debatable. As a minimum, such an approach to narcissistic personality disorder, for example, can certainly not stand alone.

A small number of reviews and meta-analyses of these studies of possible connections between the five common personality traits and personality disorders have been published. They conclude that personality pathology is generally associated with relatively low levels of kindness/agreeableness in interpersonal relations and high levels of neuroticism, which may be regarded as a rough measure of the degree of pathology: psychological instability, vulnerability and anxiety. This is also the case for narcissistic personality disorder, although here, the correlation with low agreeableness is the most pronounced (Saulsman & Page, 2004), while various analyses argue both for and against a possible connection between NPD and neuroticism. The latter point may be explained by the fact that an elevated score for narcissism may be found both in high-functioning individuals (with accentuated grandiose traits) and in individuals with severe psychological disorders, who would be expected to have significantly higher scores on simple self-reported measures of neuroticism. This is supported by studies which found grandiose narcissism to be negatively associated with neuroticism, while vulnerable narcissism, on the other hand, correlated with higher levels of neuroticism (Miller & Maples, 2011, p. 74 ff.).

However, findings of correlations with vulnerable narcissism are based on a very small number of studies and must generally be regarded as having a significantly weaker foundation than correlations with (largely non-pathological) grandiose narcissism. Furthermore, some analyses suggest that narcissistic personality disorder may also be associated with a high degree of extroversion (Saulsman & Page, 2004, p. 1068). This is also meaningful, considering that a broad understanding of NPD also includes relatively high-functioning individuals with predominantly grandiose narcissism – individuals who will often be extrovert and assertive. Some studies also suggest that vulnerable narcissism has a negative correlation with extroversion (Miller & Maples, 2011, p. 74 ff.).

One meta-analysis supports the correlation between NPD and low agreeableness, while it did not find any significant correlation between NPD and any of the other four personality traits from the five-factor model, including extroversion and neuroticism (Samuel & Widiger, 2008, p. 1330). It also found that indications of NPD are clearly correlated with virtually all the facets or dimensions of agreeableness. More specifically, this means that NPD is associated with lower trust, altruism and straightforwardness in interpersonal interactions (p. 1331) and with a single facet of neuroticism: angry hostility. In relation to these attempts to establish an empirical link between common personality traits and personality pathology, it is generally important to note some fairly serious methodological problems, including that the studies typically rely on measures of personality disorders that either focus almost exclusively on grandiose manifestations of NPD or primarily capture non-pathological aspects of narcissism (Saulsman & Page, 2004, p. 1073). Moreover, indications of personality pathology are typically measured via questionnaires, not interviews, which have a much higher degree of validity, and many of the studies included in the presented meta-analyses involved non-clinical populations, often university students, which makes them rather problematic to use as a way to shed light on severe personality pathology, such as NPD.

Generally, the identified correlations between personality traits and possible manifestations of personality pathology are stronger in studies based on non-clinical populations than on clinical ones (Saulsman & Page, 2004, p. 1077). This is remarkable and indicates that, as a minimum, we should be cautious about using these studies as a basis for delimiting and understanding NPD. Overall, the five-factor model and other models and theories that focus on common personality traits thus do not appear to be very well suited to capturing the particular and defining aspects of narcissistic personality disorder, although they may be included in more general descriptions of potential commonalities of more or all types of personality disorders.

The fields of social and personality psychology have also presented numerous analyses of what is often called the core dimensions or facets of narcissism as personality traits. Based on these studies, it has been argued that interpersonal antagonism (Miller et al., 2017) or self-centred antagonism (Crowe et al., 2019) is perhaps the most central element of narcissism as a personality trait or as a common dimension of the personality. This interpersonal antagonism includes several dimensions or facets, including lack of empathy, exploitativeness, arrogance, manipulativeness, reactive anger and distrust (Miller et al., 2017, p. 296 ff.). These features are clearly present in pathological grandiose narcissism, but they are far from given in pathological vulnerable narcissism. Furthermore, studies from social and personality psychology have found that grandiose manifestations of narcissism are associated with low agreeableness and high extroversion (possibly also attention-seeking), while more vulnerable manifestations of narcissism are more closely associated with reactive anger and dependence on others for validation of the self (Crowe et al., 2019, p. 1160 ff.) and with neuroticism (or anxiousness) (Miller et al., 2018).

These studies further point to at least two other factors or traits associated with narcissism: high neuroticism, particularly including shame and need for admiration (and related to more vulnerable manifestations of narcissism) and assertive exhibitionism, which includes a number of facets, such as grandiose fantasies and authoritativeness (Miller et al., 2017, p. 296 ff.). However, high-functioning narcissism, in which grandiose traits are the most prominent, are more likely to be negatively associated with neuroticism, while vulnerable narcissism is more likely to be associated with the absence of extrovert traits and assertive behaviour or agency (Watts et al., 2013, p. 2380). The fields of social and personality psychology have introduced several other possible factors related to narcissism as a common personality dimension, including distrustful self-reliance and attention-seeking (Crowe et al., 2019, p. 1164), both of which are associated with more grandiose aspects of narcissism.

Problems in studies of personality traits

In addition to the previously described challenges stemming from the fact that these analyses of narcissistic personality traits are based on quantitative self-report questionnaires on narcissistic traits completed by predominantly normally functioning participants – including the many issues involved in self-reporting traits that the respondents are not necessarily fully conscious of and which they may perceive as morally reprehensible, which may lead to under-reporting – studies from the fields of social and personality psychology also tend to be based on sophisticated statistical analysis of purely quantitative data. This means that studies are more removed from the phenomenology of narcissism, which reduces their practical applicability, particularly for aiding our understanding of the individual human being struggling with a severe narcissistic disorder.

Furthermore, self-report studies of how the self appears to and is perceived by others rely on the notion that individuals are capable of making nuanced and valid assessments of this – a problematic assumption for people with narcissistic disorders who typically have considerable difficulties in this very area (Crisp & Gabbard, 2020, p. 9). If we wish to gain insight into and understand the phenomenology of narcissism, in particular the internal and interpersonal psychological processes in individuals with more severe narcissistic disorders – the subjective experience of living in an internal and relational universe characterized by narcissistic dynamics, including its manifestation in real-life interactions with others (including therapists) – psychoanalysis can offer far more nuanced and in-depth analyses that also offer insight into helpful psychotherapeutic approaches to individuals with severe narcissistic disorders (see Chapter 4).

2.3 The main features of narcissism

In speaking of narcissism, we need to be aware of at least two levels or dimensions of the concept. On a more theoretical level, we should distinguish between what narcissism 'is', i.e., its defining characteristics, versus its many different manifestations and, not least, disturbances in people's narcissistic balances or narcissistic pathology, including narcissistic personality disorders (NPDs), in people's cognitions, emotions, behaviour and interpersonal interactions (Pincus & Roche, 2011, p. 32). In trying to determine what narcissism 'is', we need to consider how narcissism fundamentally relates to self-image, self-esteem, vulnerability to shame and need of others' attention and approval, which may play out and be manifested in human behaviour in a wide variety of ways, depending on the developmental stage and level of personality organization.

One of the factors that differentiates pathological narcissism from the more 'normal' version of narcissism is that individuals with pathological narcissism are characterized by dysregulated self-esteem and compromised affect regulation. This includes significant problems with containing and regulating painful affects, such as shame and envy. Interpersonal relations and other people are primarily used as a means to enhance the person's own fragile self-esteem at the expense of reciprocity and possibilities of establishing more intimate relationships and close psychological and emotional contact with others (Ronningstam, 2005, p. 69). Generally, it is not possible to define a clear-cut line between healthy/normal and pathological narcissism that makes it possible to determine when 'normal' narcissistic behaviour turns pathological, and vice versa. We have to accept a certain grey area in between clearly pathological and clearly non-pathological narcissism (Crisp & Gabbard, 2020, p. 144).

Narcissistic spectrum

In addition to this mainly theoretical distinction between what narcissism is and how narcissistic processes and imbalances may be manifested in people's ways of being and acting in the world, we should consider and attempt to describe a spectrum of narcissism (Walter & Bilke-Hentsch, 2020, p. 52) ranging from 1) normal and healthy narcissism to 2) a state characterized by varying degrees of accentuated narcissistic traits that will often be observable in exceptionally extrovert and assertive individuals to 3) different degrees and manifestations of narcissistic personality disorders (NPD), where, as mentioned above, it will be helpful to distinguish between two fundamentally different manifestations of NPD: a 3a) predominantly vulnerable and a 3b) predominantly grandiose manifestation of pathological narcissism or NPD. Some have argued that these vulnerable and grandiose manifestations should rather be seen as more temporary narcissistic positions or self-states that the individual alternates between to varying degrees (Huprich & Malone, 2022, p. 230).

Alternatively, they may be viewed as two separate and dynamically related dimensions of narcissism, one involving a vulnerable self and vulnerable self-esteem and one primarily involving grandiose notions, from internal, quiet traits to very overt ones that clash with reality. In this understanding, the former is associated, in part, with hypersensitivity to criticism, avoidant behaviour, more overt distress, mainly covert grandiosity and a timid and inhibited approach to the world, while the latter primarily involves overt attention-seeking and socially charming (in the eyes of some) behaviour, low observable anxiety, a more explicit sense of entitlement and exploitative behaviour (Levy, 2012, p. 887).

Arguably, Kernberg's description of 4) malignant narcissism, bordering on dissocial personality disorder, or perhaps even 5) dissocial personality disorder and psychopathy, can also be related, to some extent, to very severely disturbed narcissism; in this sense, it should be regarded as a very extreme manifestation of narcissistic disorders. However, Kernberg's malignant narcissism will not be further discussed here, as it borders on disorders that are very difficult or impossible to treat psychotherapeutically in practice, due to the pronounced dissocial and psychopathic traits (see, however, Chapter 3.1 on diagnosing narcissistic pathology).

We may distinguish between at least three main manifestations of accentuated narcissism or narcissistic traits – ranging from potentially pathological to severely pathological narcissism (Russ et al., 2008; see also Wink, 1991), see Table 2.1 1) a mainly grandiose and usually pathological manifestation that involves an inflated self-image, self-absorption and controlling/intimidating behaviour in interpersonal interactions; 2) a predominantly more vulnerable, timid and shame-driven manifestation characterized by outwardly low and fragile self-esteem; however, behind this often inhibited, passive, submissive and easily injured facade, the person typically has varying degrees of grandiose notions or fantasies about their own uniqueness, importance and expectations as well as (frequently dashed) hopes that others will see and recognize this; and, finally, 3) a high-functioning form of narcissism that should not generally be regarded as pathological. In addition to these three central manifestations of narcissism, Ronningstam (2005) has described a psychopathic manifestation of narcissism related to Kernberg's malignant narcissism; both are severely pathological forms of narcissism.

Vulnerable and grandiose narcissism

In this context, vulnerable manifestations of narcissism refer to a level of narcissistic vulnerability that should be regarded as being, to varying degrees, pathological and which may require treatment. In principle, however, the concept of narcissistic vulnerability may also be applied much more broadly, to include varying degrees of feelings of inferiority, lack of self-confidence, a generally insecure attachment style and a tendency to become overwhelmed by destructive shame in response to what others would perceive as fairly innocent self-exposure. Predominantly grandiose manifestations of narcissism are typically accompanied by arrogance and more or less overt aggressive behaviour towards others. These elements are typically absent in vulnerable and timid manifestations, which instead typically involve an inclination to avoid (deeper) interpersonal contact for fear of rejection, associated with hypersensitivity to perceived threats to the fragile self (Ronningstam, 2005, p. 72). Individuals with predominantly vulnerable narcissism find contact with others both emotionally and mentally demanding; interpersonal contact is exhausting to them, and thus they often seek to minimize close contact with others (Britton, 1998, p. 47).

This distinction between predominantly grandiose and vulnerable manifestations is sometimes described as a distinction between overt versus more covert or 'masked' pathological narcissism or between thick-skinned and thin-skinned narcissism. It also relates to professional debates about whether the central and defining elements of pathological narcissism should be very specific and observable or if they might also, to varying degrees, involve internal psychological processes and the structural organization of the personality (Caligor et al., 2015, p. 416). However, to someone who has developed an eye for the more vulnerable manifestations of narcissism, there is little to suggest that it would be clinically meaningful to distinguish categorically between overt and more covert variants of pathological narcissism, as both variations on pathological narcissism will always manifest themselves in varying ways in the affected individuals' subjective experiences, emotional reactions and behaviour.

Pathological narcissism will almost always manifest itself as a mix of thin- and thick-skinned elements, of vulnerable and grandiose elements (Diamond et al., 2022, p. 62). Even persons characterized by pronounced grandiosity will often feel inadequate and as imposters, behind their grandiose appearance, and their grandiose self-image is unstable and at risk of collapse in the face of defeat or if others fail to admire or recognize their grandiose self (Caligor et al., 2020, p. 113; Diamond et al., 2022, p. 8). Thus, the term 'covert narcissism' seems, most of all, to be a relic from an outdated, overly narrow understanding that views narcissism as being exclusively dominated by grandiose self-perceptions, while vulnerable narcissism is not attributed the same significance (cf. the formal diagnostic criteria for NPD; see Chapter 3.1).

Historically, there has been little consensus on whether pathological narcissism or, as a minimum, NPD only includes openly grandiose manifestations of narcissism – a view that has been and, unfortunately remains, the basis of the formal diagnostic criteria for NPD in the *DSM-5* – and on whether there might be two clearly defined categories of narcissism, a grandiose and a vulnerable form, that should be understood and treated as distinct and fundamentally different disorders. As mentioned earlier, however, there does seem to be an emerging professional consensus that the symptom picture presented by the vast majority of patients with NPD alternates to varying degrees between grandiose and vulnerable elements or manifestations of pathological narcissism (Biberdzic et al., 2023, p. 2). The perspective of the present book is that we should view grandiose and vulnerable symptoms as manifestations of the same underlying disturbance of the personality organization or structure. In practice, it is proving more challenging to reach a consensus on, and drawing a clear distinction between, 'normal' and pathological narcissism. In fact, it could be argued that we ought to reserve the concept of narcissism for pathological narcissism, which requires treatment.

Dynamic psychological understanding of the relationship between vulnerability and grandiosity

Most clinicians who work with patients with pathological narcissism will presumably have experienced how, behind their inflated facade, patients with symptoms dominated by grandiose narcissism contain a shameful and strictly self-monitoring self (child), just as patients with a predominantly depressive and vulnerable narcissistic symptom picture similarly contain grandiose ideas about who they might be or become (McWilliams, 2011, p. 178). Even in patients with a strong dominance of grandiose narcissism, feelings of inadequacy and a painful feeling of being an imposter (Caligor & Stern, 2020, p. 113) – cf. the grandiose facade as just that, a facade – are not seen as reflections of the person's true self. Transference in patients with predominantly vulnerable narcissism can suddenly tip over into rage, grandiosity and toxic contempt for the therapist, while a seemingly impenetrable facade of arrogance, contempt and indifference to the therapist in the predominantly grandiose patient may suddenly collapse, as the patient is overwhelmed by shame, and their transference becomes dominated by intense sensitivity and vulnerability to the therapist's thoughts and opinion about the self (Gabbard & Crisp, 2018, p. 88). This may happen as a reaction to criticism or if the grandiose self does not receive the attention, validation and admiration from others that it yearns for (Crisp & Gabbard, 2020, p. 144); see Chapter 4.2.

These types of experiences suggest that vulnerable and grandiose manifestations of pathological narcissism are dynamically related. For a theoretical understanding of these dynamic psychological connections, we may turn to, among others, Kohut's concept of a vertical split of the personality (see Chapter 3.3) and Kernberg's description of identity diffusion and primitive defence mechanisms centred on splitting in patients with borderline personality organization – a typical personality organization in patients with pathological narcissism. As it will briefly be discussed later (see Chapter 3.4), identity diffusion is associated with the insufficient integration of conflicting and highly polarized identity elements or perceptions of self and others. One implication of this is that the person may alternate, confusingly, between excessively positive (idealizing, grandiose) and unrealistically negative (devaluing) perceptions of self (and others), just as their self-esteem may become destabilized (Crowe et al., 2019, p. 1152; Caligor & Stern, 2020, p. 112 ff.).

Kernberg (1975, p. 229) also writes about alternating ego-states, as an ego that is dominated by a grandiose self-image may suddenly be overwhelmed by a negative self-image and require help to stabilize their dysregulated self-esteem. The dominance of grandiose (idealized) self-perception – accompanied by dissociation or the splitting-off of negative (devalued) self-components, which are then perhaps projected onto others – will often be associated with a certain stabilization of the identity, compared with patients with borderline personality disorders (see Chapter 3.1). This more stable identity will, unfortunately, often appear as inauthentic and fake to others and, in many cases, also to the patient themself.

The patient may attempt to conceal or suppress narcissistic vulnerability, insecure self-esteem and destructive shame behind a facade of extrovert self-assertion, grandiosity and condescension towards others (Ronningstam, 2021, p. 4 ff.). Like a grandiose self-perception, a grandiose, arrogant, self-reliant and emotionally unapproachable appearance may be an attempt to regulate and stabilize inherently unstable self-esteem (Ronningstam, 2012, p. 945; Pincus, 2023, p. 636). Similarly, avoidance of close contact with others and perceptions of independence and self-sufficiency may be attempts to protect a vulnerable self from what might happen in encounters with others that confront it with other aspects of itself and with reality. Thus, the grandiose facade is often fairly unstable and might crack when challenged in interpersonal encounters, as the narcissistic vulnerable self emerges from behind the grandiose facade. In extension of this point, Britton (1998, p. 51 ff.) has pointed out that patients with predominantly grandiose or thick-skinned narcissism may contain certain schizoid characteristics, in the sense that it will often be difficult to establish close emotional contact with these patients, who may furthermore tend to focus consistently on 'factual', 'objective' and 'rational' aspects of life, as a defence against being emotionally affected, losing control (cf. fear of internal and external chaos) and thus reveal themselves as vulnerable, weak and shamefully inadequate.

Closely related to these dynamic psychological connections between grandiose and vulnerable manifestations of narcissism, the self-psychologist Andrew Morrison (1989, p. 64 ff.) has introduced the concept of a dialectic of narcissism, as the self swings between two poles. At one pole, the self feels special, with a unique identity, and is characterized by exhibitionism and perhaps (particularly in pathological variants) arrogance and grandiosity. In this state, the self strives to detach and differentiate from others and to develop and defend its own autonomous self. The other pole is characterized by a self that feels very small and insignificant and has a strong urge to merge with an idealized other in an attempt to strengthen its threatened and vulnerable self. Morrison's distinction is related to Blatt's (2008) description of the basic human need for self-definition and embeddedness in social communities (see above). According to Morrison, a patient with pathological narcissism may swing between extreme versions of these two poles. At any given time, one pole will typically be in the foreground, appearing to dominate, but this can change in an instant (Morrison & Stolorow, 1997, p. 71), corresponding to fluctuation between grandiose and vulnerable manifestations of pathological narcissism.

Similarly, Michael Balint (1968, p. 68; 1959, p. 37 ff.) speaks of an *ocnophilic* versus a *philobatic* orientation in the approach to external objects. While the former describes the self that only feels safe when in close contact with the object – clinging to it and feeling insecure and lost when it does not have access to it (originally the mother) – the latter experiences external objects as unreliable, insignificant or maybe even dangerous to the self, withdraws from or writes them off and displays a high degree of autonomy and self-reliance (Greβ et al., 2002, p. 95). A self with an *ocnophilic* orientation uses the object to keep the self together and stabilize a fragmented self – the object is not loved – while a self with a *philobatic* orientation is characterized by pseudoautonomy and denies its yearning for and dependence on others. In their more extreme forms, both orientations or positions in relation to external objects represent psychopathology (cf. vulnerable versus grandiose narcissism). Balint (1968, p. 68) views this as a basic fault in the personality organization resulting from inadequate satisfaction of the need for primary affection in early relations.

Arguably, the *ocnophilic* orientation, with its profound need for attachment and merging with others (the object), is driven by fear of loneliness and alienation from others. In itself, it may lead to fear of losing oneself, one's freedom and one's own identity as a result of the pronounced inclination to submission and self-surrender that it involves. On the other hand, the *philobatic* orientation, with its (pseudo-)self-reliance and pronounced urge for freedom, autonomy and detachment from others, may be driven by fear of losing oneself and one's identity in contact with others and may thus in itself result in painful emotional loneliness, contactlessness and alienation from others (Shoshani et al., 2006, p. 508). As mentioned earlier, both poles in this dynamic interplay between different relational constellations represent fundamental psychological and relational needs. The art is to strike the right balance between them – a developmental task that failed in individuals with pathological narcissism. We all have to accept some degree of self-surrender, loss of autonomy and restrictions on our urge to be ourselves – fully authentic with no filter whatsoever – in order to adapt in interpersonal relationships and social communities. Similarly, we also need to maintain boundaries and be able to be alone in order to hold onto ourselves and function as mature, independent subjects. This is a difficult balancing act and one that persons with pathological narcissism have failed to master.

High-functioning narcissism

As mentioned earlier, in addition to the two general manifestations of pathological narcissism – grandiose and vulnerable – we may also identify a high-functioning variant of narcissism. This form is not normally pathological but is characterized by clearly accentuated narcissistic personality traits and behaviours that are common, for example, in leaders, prominent politicians, cultural figures and others with high-visibility roles in the public space or social positions with relatively high social status and authority. They are typically charismatic, extrovert and dominant individuals who display a high degree of authority and competence within their field and who may also, in fact, have achieved extraordinary accomplishments. As long as they continue to perform well and receive admiration and recognition for their achievements, this may help them maintain an internal narcissistic balance. However, this balance may be jeopardized and even collapse when they experience serious setbacks or when they are no longer in a position that garners the same degree of positive attention and recognition. They often appear – and much of the time, they are in fact – socially well-adjusted and good at navigating in social contexts (particularly the more formal ones); they are charming and affable and 'the life of the party'.

In some cases, however, especially when seen from a distance, they may also appear to have based their remarkable self-esteem and their ability to become the centre of attention on a slightly inflated belief in their own abilities and significance. Sometimes, this may be accompanied by a sense that there is little substance behind their shiny and seemingly well-functioning (and high-performing) facade. Or, perhaps, that their apparently high self-esteem is not quite genuine but is mainly a cover for a different, less impressive reality (see Table 2.1). The high apparent self-esteem may become unstable if it is not explicitly and continually recognized and admired (Crisp & Gabbard, 2020, p. 144); the self may have a strong need for continual success, confirmation and admiration.

When people with narcissistic traits who appear to be socially and professionally very well-functioning move towards a state where their fundamentally narcissistic personality organization begins to be problematic, behind their high-performance facade they may struggle with a lurking subjective sense of emptiness and boredom and find it difficult to establish and handle close emotional and psychological interpersonal contact and closeness (Kernberg, 2004a, p. 51). In relation to this point, it is important to remember that purely physical-sexual contact and very action-oriented contact related to practical activities are far from the same as emotional and psychological contact, and in a sense both may work fine in the absence of close emotional contact. However, over time, these types of contact may begin to seem hollow and unsatisfactory and may give rise to feelings of meaninglessness and emptiness if they are not complemented by other relationships characterized by close emotional contact.

Persons with high-functioning narcissism bordering on pathological narcissism may also struggle to understand – and seem remarkably disinterested in – their own and others' inner worlds. Their capacity for mentalizing may be fragile and unevenly developed. If they seek treatment, they may maintain good formal eye contact, appear interested in the therapist, and express recognition and appreciation of the therapist's work. However, these expressions will often lack emotional depth, and they may also generally try to keep the conversation on an intellectualizing and rational level where they are not truly emotionally affected or come into contact with their narcissistic vulnerability. On the surface, they may appear to be interested in the therapist's knowledge and the conveyed insights into the psychology of the self, but they do not actually take the insights in and seem mostly interested in therapy as a venue for obtaining knowledge that they can use in various contexts without undergoing personal change. Often, at least part of the self will try to convince the therapist that they are actually doing great and do not need help – instead, what they really want is for the therapist to confirm and admire their high apparent level of functioning (Gabbard & Crisp, 2018, p. 85 ff.).

As mentioned earlier, the field suffers under a vague and very broad use of the concept of narcissism, and it is debatable whether the high-functioning variant of narcissism – in some cases bordering on highly accentuated and socially problematic manifestations of narcissistic traits or perhaps an overly positive self-image combined with very high self-esteem and expectations of admiration from others – should be relabelled and understood without reference to narcissism. We will never be able to draw a clear-cut line between, on the one hand, accentuated narcissistic traits that stay within the boundaries of what is socially acceptable and which may also serve as a significant driver of human creativity, agency and ability to lead the way and act as an inspiring visionary or leader and, on the other hand, what should be considered pathological and destructive for the affected individual, the people close to them and the social communities they are a part of or may consider themself a leader of.

Furthermore, some researchers have argued that vulnerable manifestations of narcissism should instead be seen as representing malignant or problematic (self-degrading) self-regard associated with depressive and masochistic personality traits (Pedone et al., 2023). The main problem with these attempts to redefine vulnerable manifestations of narcissism as representative of masochistic, internalizing or depressive personality traits is that, like most understandings of narcissism based on personality psychology, they are based on studies of personality traits that are large (in terms of the number of participants) but methodologically relatively primitive (in part because personality traits are solely measured through self-report questionnaires) involving participants randomly selected among the general population or among university students (see, e.g., Huprich et al., 2018), that is, non-clinical populations. At the very least, it is problematic to use findings from these types of studies as a basis for classifying and understanding more pathological narcissism.

Table 2.1 Proposal for defining characteristics in the three most central manifestations of accentuated narcissistic traits and disordered narcissism (see also Miller et al., 2017; Russ et al., 2008; Pincus & Lukowitsky, 2010; Caligor et al., 2015; Ronningstam, 2005, p. 72 ff.; Russ & Shedler, 2013, p. 35 ff.; Rosenfeld, 1987, p. 370 ff.).

	Grandiose narcissism	*Vulnerable narcissism*	*High-functioning narcissism*
Observable appearance	'Thick-skinned'; appears unaffected by criticism – or reacts with great intensity to perceived threats to self-image and self-esteem; lack of capacity for nuanced and balanced self-criticism; often very limited curiosity about and insight into own motivations and inner life	'Thin-skinned'; very vulnerable to and has strong reactions to criticism, feels rejected and overlooked by everyone; avoids becoming the centre of attention in order to protect the self from criticism; vulnerable to fragmentation, dissociation	Often charismatic, 'takes up a lot of room'; exhibitionistic, attention-seeking, autonomous, elitist, arrogant; covert vulnerability to criticism and lack of recognition; fear of being ordinary; typically at best only shows pseudo-curiosity about and pseudo-insight into own inner life
Relational behaviour	Manipulative, extrovert; dominant, controlling, aggressive reactions to perceived criticism and narcissistic injury; externalizing defence	Timid, inhibited, passive, reserved, self-effacing, strong urge to protect own private space; often characterized by intense and obvious shame, despair; internalizing defence; dependent	'Leader', air of authority, dominant, seeks power over/influence on others; assertive, high agency, efficient use of own skills; in some cases sexually and otherwise provocative, invasive, intimidating, injurious towards others
Emotional appearance	Feels/appears superior, arrogant in relation to others; lacks capacity for emotional and psychological closeness; often chronic sense of emptiness and boredom; underlying but denied destructive shame	Very vulnerable to feeling unfairly treated, misunderstood; proneness to narcissistic injury and previous traumatic attacks on self-regard, perhaps accompanied by suppressed rage; often clear signs of being unhappy, depressive, inhibited, despairing; pronounced self-pity	Extrovert, socially competent, innovative, good sense of humour; in some cases emotionally lonesome; no one, or only very few people, can get close to the self, struggles to deal with emotional closeness; in some cases deeper-seated experience of emptiness, meaninglessness and boredom

	Grandiose narcissism	*Vulnerable narcissism*	*High-functioning narcissism*
Self-esteem	Obviously inflated self-esteem; exaggerated view of own abilities, accomplishments, qualities and importance; unrealistic self-image, inflated self-regard; grandiose and omnipotent facade conceals underlying identity diffusion and fragile self-esteem	Often obviously vulnerable/low self-esteem, more covert grandiose fantasies of the self's uniqueness as defence against low self-esteem, anxiety and loneliness; may feel superior in relation to others in some areas; only revealed after closer/longer contact; often clear signs of identity diffusion	High self-esteem, feels superior to others, at times exaggerated faith in own abilities and importance; increased risk of cynicism towards others and unethical behaviour; no indication of severe identity disorder
Regulation of self-esteem	Attempts to escape low self-esteem through self-centred, intimidating, invasive behaviour – physically, emotionally and/or sexually; deficits in the superego increases the risk of shameless behaviour; often absence of guilt over harming others; guilt is externalized, others are blamed for the problems and setbacks of the self; often associated with dissocial behaviour	Often obvious problems with regulating self-esteem and negative affects; intense self-criticism, especially in connection with lack of achievement of sometimes unrealistic goals and self-standards; persistent fear of failure, humiliation, being revealed as inadequate, inferior; very conditional self-esteem, dependent on persistent accomplishments and confirmation	Often perfectionist, perhaps a 'workaholic' in order to prove their worth, given that self-esteem is, to some degree, conditional on persistent accomplishments; others are primarily seen as sympathetic admirers of the performance and superior qualities of the self – injured, wronged, aggressive, devaluing when others do not meet this expectation
Empathy	Lack of empathy; solely instrumental interest in others as a source of admiration and confirmation of the grandiose self	Self-focused need for others to stabilize the fragile self-esteem can lead to a lack of empathy and genuine interest in others – but also to adaptation to others' expectations and needs	Tendency to use and exploit others to attain own goals, a lack of genuine interest in and empathy for others; often covered up by good social skills and charisma
Need for others	Need for others to persistently show respect for and clearly recognize (submit to) the self and its uniqueness; pseudo-self-reliance characterized by (often unacknowledged) envy, denies need for/dependence on others	Basic distrust of others; persistently vigilant and sensitive to signs that others look down upon or do not recognize the self; combined with a large need for care, persistent empathic mirroring and explicit confirmation	Imagines that others look up to/admire the self; appears self-reliant without any significant need for others; tends to surround themself with sycophants /unquestioning supporters; has difficulty accepting advice and help from peers; possibly strong idealization of selected others, personal role models, 'heroes'

	Grandiose narcissism	*Vulnerable narcissism*	*High-functioning narcissism*
Social status of the self	Focused on own social status, power, others' admiration/respect for the self; pronounced feelings of entitlement to special treatment – increased risk of unethical behaviour, urge to bend rules and laws to own advantage, and criminal conduct	Often submits to others, masochistic traits; may feel like an outsider without close relations – may submit to idealized other in an attempt to boost self-esteem; in some cases striving for uniqueness through extraordinary victimhood	Competitive; prepared to take risks – in some cases acts impulsively; sometimes so focused on own image and achieving attention and admiration from others that it hampers actual performance; often has feelings of entitlement to special treatment and feelings that not all norms and rules apply to the self
Related problems	Increased risk of dissocial, psychopathic and paranoid traits and abuse – in more extreme cases, the boundary towards psychopathy becomes porous (cf. also malignant narcissism)	May approach borderline and, to some extent, evasive and dependent personality disorders (perhaps social phobia), albeit with the absence of grandiose notions and typically with clearly better personality organization without identity diffusion – except in the case of BPD	May struggle to maintain high self-esteem if the recognition that the person expects and feels they deserve from others is absent – and in case of lacking success and perceived defeats – in that case risk of depressive breakdown; increased risk of certain types of substance abuse
Need for/ seeking help	Disinclined to seek help until the grandiose self-image collapses, causing depression, suicidal ideation, severe substance abuse; possibly externalizing problem behaviour, including interpersonal aggression	Often lowest functioning level; more inclined to seek help, typically for internalizing symptom disorders (anxiety, depression, self-harm, suicidal behaviour) or interpersonal difficulties (cf. high comorbidity with BPD)	Often associated with good well-being and low risk of psychological disorder – provided the high performance level is maintained and is recognized by others

The borderlands of pathological narcissism

When we observe descriptions of manifestations of narcissism, particularly grandiose manifestations, in social and personality psychology, it is important to bear in mind that even though many of these descriptions may indicate that these are ways of being and acting in the world that are problematic and potentially painful, both to the affected person and to others, and which are associated with increased risk of developing a psychological disorder, they are not necessarily representative of an actual psychological disorder or disturbance. Rather, they are probably representative of a certain accentuation of narcissism-related themes in the perception of self and others and in how the self acts in interpersonal interactions. The same is true of manifestations of high-functioning narcissism.

Psychiatric diagnoses, with the diagnosis of NPD as the most relevant in this context (see Chapter 3.1), seek to capture psychological disorders. Only when several narcissistic traits or manifestations of narcissism are present simultaneously and to a pronounced degree should we consider whether they represent a psychological disorder that requires treatment. In addition, we should consider that the vast majority of the existing descriptions of narcissism and its manifestations are very focused on the decontextualized individual. In some cases, this can be problematic, because human ways of being and acting are always already embedded in and, to some extent, spring from or are enhanced by an interpersonal, social and cultural context that should also be included in our understanding and assessment of narcissistic traits and ways of being.

High-functioning narcissism is not inherently associated with severe psychological difficulties. On the contrary, there is evidence suggesting that (predominantly grandiose) narcissism – presumably up to a certain, not clearly pathological level – is associated with lower risk of developing a psychological disorder and with assertiveness and confidence in one's own ability that may help lay the foundation for improved quality of life and a good basis for realizing one's own ideas about a good life (Dashineau et al., 2019; Blasco-Belled et al., 2023; Miller et al., 2007). In this sense, we may also speak of a more or less mature and reality-matched narcissism, associated with a predominantly positive, stable and realistic self-image, self-esteem and pride in own real achievements and valuable characteristics, which may lay the foundation for creativity, the ability to be comfortable in one's own skin and the ability to handle criticism. We should also consider the consequences that the ways of being and acting that are characteristic of persons with high-functioning narcissism may have for other individuals and for social communities. So far, this perspective has only received limited attention in the diagnostic criteria for NPD, but it should arguably be included in future revisions of our diagnostic systems (Miller et al., 2022, p. 409).

Considering grandiose and vulnerable narcissism, we should note that the distinction between these fundamentally different manifestations is far from clear-cut and that the individual may alternate between them, to varying degrees. Furthermore, some individuals will be bordering on high-functioning narcissism, where it is far from always clear whether, or in which areas and in relation to what, a given person should be regarded as high-functioning or not (pathological). A few studies based on university students and other non-clinical populations suggest that within a narrow timespan (up to a few hours), an individual may fluctuate between predominantly grandiose and predominantly vulnerable manifestations of narcissism. In these studies, we also see that persons with a predominant tendency for grandiosity are more likely to also show manifestations of vulnerable narcissism, while persons who predominantly show signs of vulnerable narcissism typically have a low level of grandiosity; again, within a short timespan (Edershile & Wright, 2021b). In relation to this point too, we should bear in mind that we cannot necessarily generalize these findings from non-clinical populations to persons with NDP.

Grandiose and vulnerable – or thick-skinned and thin-skinned – manifestations of narcissism in particular may also be viewed as psychological positions or functional modes that the individual may alternate between. As such, they should not be seen as elements in a clear-cut schematic breakdown into fundamentally different types of narcissism (Rosenfeld, 1987, p. 370 ff.; Bateman, 1998). Grandiose and vulnerable manifestations of pathological narcissism should thus be regarded as two phenotypical manifestations of the same underlying narcissistic pathology (Cain et al., 2008, p. 650), and we should abandon our tendency to associate narcissism mainly with its grandiose manifestations and to perceive grandiose and vulnerable manifestations of pathological narcissism as two distinct categories and separate disorders. However, some professionals still argue that grandiose and vulnerable narcissism should be viewed as separate categories of NPD (Russ & Shedler, 2013, p. 33 ff.). Focusing more on concrete categorizations based on observable symptoms and behaviours than on the possible underlying psychological processes that drive the different symptoms or manifestations of NPD may make it seem more meaningful to suggest the existence of two more distinct subcategories of NPD.

The degree of disturbance or pathology is further related to how pronounced, rigid and pervasive the narcissistic traits and modes of functioning are in the specific person's life, including the severity of any problems they cause for the individual or for others. Thus, the key here is that we should not be speaking of two or three fundamentally different forms of narcissism but of different degrees and manifestations of narcissism that are dynamically interconnected. They should be understood as analytical categories seeking to capture how narcissism may manifest itself, with an emphasis on elements in one of the three outlined categories. This means that it will rarely be meaningful to assign a person squarely to one of the two categories, either grandiose or vulnerable narcissism. Furthermore, individuals whose narcissistic manifestations fall mainly into one of the three categories of grandiose, vulnerable or high-functioning narcissism may exhibit very different levels of psychosocial functioning, which may furthermore fluctuate considerably over time and across social contexts, such as romantic relationships or close relations versus social contexts characterized by more superficial interpersonal contact.

It is also important to point out that in several areas, severe narcissistic disturbances that are captured by the psychiatric diagnosis of narcissistic personality disorder are decisively and qualitatively different from the much more normal and commonly occurring narcissistic traits that are the focus of social and personality psychology – although we still need to speak of narcissism as a dimensional phenomenon on a continuum. There are significant and crucial differences between having several, perhaps even relatively pronounced narcissistic traits and having a severe narcissistic personality disorder. Still, there will always be people who exist in a border zone, so that it may not be easy to determine whether they have an actual psychiatric disorder requiring treatment. In those cases, one of the key factors that the clinician should focus on is the quality and stability of the individual's basic personality organization. At the same time, pathological narcissistic difficulties that require treatment cannot be reduced to the formal diagnostic criteria for narcissistic personality disorder (see Chapter 3.1). Pathological narcissistic imbalances and traits occur in a much broader group of patients, including, in particular, patients with other personality disorders than NPD and, not least, other cluster B personality disorders, especially evasive, dependent and schizotypal personality disorders.

Commonalities of narcissism: From accentuated to pathological narcissism

As mentioned earlier, narcissism relates to how the person perceives themself and imagines that others see and perceive the self (self-images); how the individual regards themself and senses that others regard them; what feelings the person has for themself – whether they are ashamed or proud over who and what they are (self-esteem); how the person handles differentiation from and connectedness with others, including how they handle dominance, submission and control in interpersonal relationships and is able to establish and be in contact with others and with their own inner life; and, finally, how the self handles consideration of their own and others' boundaries and needs. Table 2.2 lists some of the core themes or dimensions of narcissism along with suggestions for how they might be imbalanced or disturbed in persons characterized by pathological narcissism.

Across the three manifestations of narcissism outlined above, it is possible to identify several potentially problematic commonalities that may be more or less pronounced. While they are typically less prominent in high-functioning narcissism, they may still have considerable – mostly negative – impact on the individual's inner psychological life, subjective experiences and behaviour. Among these commonalities and specific manifestations of narcissistic imbalances and difficulties that should be included in the assessment of potential psychopathology – especially in the diagnostic assessment of narcissistic personality disorder (see Chapter 3.1) – the following are of particular relevance (Caligor, 2013, p. 72; Ackerman et al., 2017):

Table 2.2 Selected core elements of narcissism and how they might be disturbed in pathological narcissism.

Dimensions of narcissism	*Manifestations of pathological narcissism*
Self-perceptions	Characterized by significant over-rating (grandiosity) or under-rating of own self and/or intense instability, fragmentation (vulnerability)
Differentiation of self and others	Psychological and emotional differentiation of self and others is inadequate; projective understanding of others; deficiencies in the acknowledgement of others as independent subjects/actors
Capacity for empathy	Often deficits in emotional empathy
Ability to see beyond the self	Is inadequate, characterized by self-centredness
Self-esteem and self-esteem regulation	Is out of step with reality and/or fragile, highly fluctuating and dependent on mirroring, explicit validation and admiration from others; dysregulated self-esteem
Ability to receive and deal with criticism	Has difficulty handling criticism; gets intensely offended/injured, furious and/or withdraws from contact
Capacity for containing and handling shame, pride; in part also other affects	Is overwhelmed by destructive shame and primitive defences against it, possibly shamelessness, exaggerated pride; emotional dysregulation
Dealing with comparisons of self to others	Is characterized by destructive shame and a persistent inclination to compete with others; intense need for admiration from others; overly focused on the status/value of the self in relation to others
Capacity for psychological and emotional contact	Is deficient, characterized by fear of how contact may threaten the fragile self and self-esteem, because interpersonal contact opens contact with – and activates defensive denial of – parts of the self
Friendliness/antagonism in interpersonal contact	Contact characterized by antagonism (envy) or problems with balancing friendliness/antagonism; dysregulated interpersonal behaviour
Readiness to support/help others	Is limited and/or controlled by own need for admiration, recognition as being 'especially good'
Balancing of own/others' needs and consideration for self/others	Is inadequate; has difficulty seeing beyond their own immediate needs; feels entitled to special treatment – or, alternatively, self-effacing in an attempt to earn others' acceptance
Balancing dominance/submission (control/power) in relation to others	Characterized by a lack of balance; great need for dominance/control or inclination to submission
Handling relationships with ideals/role models	Characterized by unrealistic idealization; recurring disappointment with idealized others and resentment as a result of perceived disappointments
Handling personal goals and ambitions	Tendency towards unrealistically high goals, perfectionism; or, alternatively, pronounced collapse of own goals and ambitions

Dimensions of narcissism	*Manifestations of pathological narcissism*
Ability to handle that others have/ are something that the self would like to have/be	Characterized by envy, perhaps denigration of and attacks on the other; or, alternatively, intense idealization of selected others whom the self identifies with and seeks to be close to
Experience of meaning, authenticity – ability to establish meaningful connections between experiences	Characterized by significant deficiencies; pronounced experience of meaninglessness, emptiness, inauthenticity, sense of being an imposter; attacks/breaks down meaningful connections between experiences

- **Grandiosity:** Varying degrees and manifestations of grandiose self-perceptions, which may range from somewhat realistic perceptions of one's own (in some cases actually) extraordinary abilities and accomplishments (cf. high-functioning narcissism) to obviously inflated self-perceptions that are more or less unrealistic. Furthermore, grandiose perceptions may be more overt (cf. grandiose narcissism) or more covert and largely limited to internal fantasies of own grandeur and uniqueness that only become obvious with more prolonged and close contact with the person (cf. vulnerable narcissism). Grandiose self-perceptions are manifested in implicit or explicit and, to varying degrees, unrealistic perceptions of the self as unique, better and superior compared to others – while others are typically disparaged and devalued as inferior in comparison with the self. Perceived threats to a grandiose self-image and fragile self-esteem may intensify grandiose self-perceptions or lead to aggressive attacks on others who criticize or simply fail to give the self enough attention and admiration. In this sense, grandiosity may to some extent be reactive and dependent on the person's momentary emotional state. Grandiose notions are typically accompanied by remarkably self-centred and self-referential behaviour in interpersonal interactions.
- **Poor empathy:** Poor empathy, particularly with regard to emotional empathy, and an absence of genuine interest in others and their inner lives. While there is often a certain degree of cognitive empathy and an ability to imagine in a purely intellectual or theoretical way how others feel and how one's actions might affect other people, a person with a narcissistic disorder will often lack the ability to feel it at an emotional level (Ritter et al., 2011): 'I know how you feel, but I can't feel it', 'my boyfriend's mother died, and I can tell that he's upset, but I can't feel it, it's a little scary'. The person may show a striking lack of emotionally driven interest in and identification with other people's emotional well-being and balance. This also makes it much easier for the person to act in cynical ways and to ignore how their own actions and decisions may impact others. At worst, emotional empathy deficiencies may result in the narcissistically disordered person to give themself permission to engage in dissocial and abusive acts towards others. Persons with

narcissistic pathology often find it difficult to read other people's needs when these are unrelated to their own narrow interests and needs. Unempathic acts towards others may be driven by a generally egocentric and grandiose approach to the world but may also spring from deficiencies in the capacity for affect regulation. This may cause the self to be easily overwhelmed by powerful affects and cause an otherwise well-developed capacity for empathy to collapse, leading the self to act egocentrically, with no thought for others (Giacomo et al., 2023, p. 8; Baskin-Sommers et al., 2014, p. 328). Poor empathy may cause this important internal brake on dissocial behaviour to fail and thus be a contributing factor in aggressive, intimidating and criminal behaviour – and poorer parenting skills (Hart et al., 2018).

- **Deficits in differentiating between self and other:** Deficits in the ability to recognize others as independent autonomous subjects outside the control of the self, including the urge to control other people's experiences and acts, particularly experiences of – and reactions to – the self (cf. pronounced needs for others' attention and admiration). May be associated with anxious notions related to the awareness that the self is dependent on others over whom it has no control, let alone trusts. Particularly in the case of more severe pathology, the person will experience great difficulties in clearly differentiating between self and others; this may also be associated with a poor ability to differentiate between own and others' subjective experiences. There may also be difficulties in dealing with the existence of multiple possible perspectives on reality, including the possibility of others having a different perception of reality than the self (cf. egocentricity and epistemic narcissism; Baskin-Sommers et al., 2014, p. 324).
- **Fragile self and self-esteem:** The self is fragile and has deficits in the regulation of self-esteem, perhaps concealed behind a sometimes grandiose and self-reliant facade. The person's self-esteem is fragile, unstable and to varying degrees dependent on persistent attention, validation, recognition or even explicit admiration of the self's acts/accomplishments and person from others. The narcissist's grandiose self-image, apparent self-reliance and purported cynical indifference to others may thus be accompanied by what may seem like a paradoxically great need for – and at times aggressively stated demand for – attention and admiration from others, sometimes manifested as intimidating attempts to manipulate and control others. This issue relates to deficits in the establishment of a basic sense of being 'good enough' that is normally established through the internalization of adaptive interactions with significant others early in life. A narcissistically disordered person may attempt to stabilize and enhance their self-esteem through performance (perfectionism), by constructing grandiose perceptions of own merits or by withdrawing from contact with others, because contact is associated with fear/risk of criticism or confrontation with the shameful inadequacy of the self.

- **Difficulty dealing with criticism:** Due to the inherently fragile self-esteem, the self finds it difficult to deal with perceived criticism – or, on some cases, simply the absence of explicit validation and recognition – and may over-react, responding with great intensity to criticism in the form of various fight-or-flight strategies. This may include (counter)attacking the person who criticized the self or, conversely, withdrawing from contact with the person or attempting to entrench itself behind a facade of self-reliance and apparent invulnerability when encountering criticism. This is associated with basic difficulties in regulating self-esteem and affects, including shame.
- **Self-centredness:** Self-referential and egocentric in interpersonal interactions. Generally preoccupied with themself, their own life and their own needs. Limited interest in other people's subjective experiences, needs and inner and external lives. Disinterested in what others say and think, as if the self in its interpersonal communication only has a sender and lacks a receiver. Decidedly self-referential communication style, limited genuine emotional contact with others. Particularly in the case of grandiose narcissism, this may be accompanied by an inclination to meet others with indifference, contempt or one-sided interest in how they might be used to satisfy the person's own needs, including, in particular, how others might be used to stabilize/boost the person's fragile self-esteem. In more severe narcissistic pathology, there may be a parasitic relational style, as others are subjected to severe exploitation and control.
- **Inadequate capacity for engaging in close contact with others:** More pathological narcissism in particular is associated with considerable difficulties in establishing close emotional and psychological closeness with others. This may lead to painful loneliness and a sense of alienation from others, possibly concealed behind a grandiose, emotionally unapproachable and self-reliant facade. The person may attempt to satisfy their need for contact and their dependence on admiration and recognition from others by hiding behind a facade of apparently stoic emotional impassiveness, self-reliance and withdrawal from contact with others. In this case, the person is trapped between lacking the courage or ability to engage in close contact with others and being unable to survive psychologically without doing so (Symington, 1993, p. 52) – and they may struggle with a painful experience of being lifeless and emotionally dead, a sort of inner death and lack of vitality in interactions with others.
- **Interpersonal aggression:** Overt or more discreet/covert aggression and hostility in interpersonal relationships that may be triggered and acutely intensified by perceived narcissistic injury and the resulting narcissistic rage. This may be particularly pronounced in persons who operate in what mentalizing theory calls equivalence mode. In this mode, the self equates the feeling of being overlooked and lacking explicit recognition with not existing, being nothing, a nobody, of no importance to others (Bolm, 2021, p. 661). It is also highly pronounced in the case of

teleological functioning, meaning that the self needs persistent and concrete evidence of other people's interest in and recognition of the self. When this is not forthcoming, it is perceived as narcissistic injury (p. 662). In this narcissistic dynamic, the self perceives the lack of admiration of the self and the failure to have its needs for attention, explicit validation and recognition of its uniqueness met as a sign of disrespect and disrespectful treatment of the self, which may lead to narcissistic rage. Inclination to interpersonal aggression means that narcissistic pathology will typically be associated with varying degrees of relational disturbances – even if the person does not necessarily express this (Ogrodniczuk & Kealy, 2013). Some have argued that narcissistic pathology should be identified not only based on the person's own experiences but also on how others feel and react in contact with the person (cf. also the therapist's countertransference; see Chapter 4.3), which may, for example, become dominated by a feeling of helplessness or a sense of being invaded or violated in response to the narcissistically disordered patient's at times arrogant, invasive, intimidating, controlling and devaluing behaviour (Ogrodniczuk & Kealy, 2013, p. 114).

- **Egocentric sociality:** The expression of interest in and support for others may be primarily motivated by the person's urge to demonstrate their own good qualities, superiority and special abilities and qualities while, in fact, the person may look down upon and feel contempt for others who need and receive this aid and support.
- **Destructive shame, emotional dysregulation:** Difficulties with containing and dealing with powerful affects, particularly destructive shame (Jørgensen, 2023/2024) but also envy, anger and, perhaps, pride. All of these are associated with a fragile self and fragile self-esteem that are activated and may overwhelm the individual when their considerable need for persistent admiration, validation and recognition of the self's unique quality and accomplishments are not met, causing the self to feel wrong, inadequate, overlooked and insignificant. The person may perceive the absence of the expected admiration and recognition as a narcissistic injury, which may lead to either (narcissistic) rage (psychological and/or physical attack on others) or the threat of a collapse of self-esteem with the risk of suicidal ideation and the development of depressive symptoms.
- **Perfectionism:** Strong focus on performance, acting with the purpose of being, becoming or appearing perfect – often in an attempt to escape a painful experience of being inadequate or wrong or, in more severe cases, even a deeply shameful experience of not being worth loving or having the right to exist unless the self persistently earns this right through accomplishments, by taking care of others and adapting to others' needs – at the expense of ignoring its own boundaries and needs. The primary motivation for the self's performance is to achieve others' (in practice, often fleeting and brief) attention, admiration and

recognition. In the case of pathological narcissism, accomplishments are not in themselves associated with internal satisfaction but are instrumental, driven by an urge to escape a sense of inferiority and/or earn others' admiration (Kernberg, 2000, p. 108). Perfectionism is often associated with unrealistically high (grandiose) standards (ego ideals) and a strong competitive streak. Furthermore, an inability to live up to one's own perfectionist ideals may lead to severe self-criticism and destructive self-hatred. Thus, perfectionism may both play a role in attempts to regulate vulnerable self-esteem and, indirectly, be a contributing cause of it.

- **Competitiveness:** The person may feel that they are constantly competing with others for attention, appreciation and recognition and may thus interpret a wide range of different situations as reflective of a persistent struggle for dominance and submission, as the person needs to demonstrate or fight to defend their superiority, social status and exceptional qualities (cf. pride) in order to avoid being humiliated and exposed as inferior, contemptible and not worth loving (cf. shame). Narcissistic imbalance may cause the self to be even more dependent on persistent attention, recognition and admiration from others, at the same time as others are perceived as a constant threat to the self's fragile self-image and self-esteem. This presents a paradoxical situation that may be a considerable source of ambivalence and conflict in interpersonal relations – and (particularly in combination with pronounced perfectionism) of emotional loneliness. Specifically, this may manifest itself as intense preoccupation with own accomplishments and with how the self is perceived (cf. looks, constructed facade), seen and evaluated by others, both in interpersonal relationships and on social media (cf. the notion that the person's worth as a human being is manifested in their ability to gain positive attention and 'sell themself').
- **Entitlement to special treatment:** Given the self's conviction of its own exceptional qualities, accomplishments and significance, it feels only natural and legitimate that the self would be entitled to special treatment and does not have to abide by quite the same laws, rules and social norms as others. The person believes that special rules should apply to unique and extra valuable individuals, such as the self. When this perceived entitlement is not met, the person may feel deeply wronged against and react with anger, resentment and narcissistic rage, bordering on hatred towards the people who fail to recognize and accommodate the self's special status associated entitlement. In specific terms, this may be anything from the partner who is no longer willing to subject to demands for persistently satisfying the self's need for recognition and special treatment, a football coach who puts an underperforming player on the bench, a social worker who refuses to bend the rules in order to meet the self's particular needs or politicians/executives who fail to recognize and accommodate the person's exceptional qualities and special social status by showing the requisite respect and providing the

special treatment that the self believes to be entitled to, simply by virtue of belonging to a particular social category, such as being a White male with a particular nationality. The narcissistic aggression and rage directed at certain other individuals appear clearly out of step with the actual events that outsiders perceive as the cause of the flare-up.

- **Emptiness:** Varying degrees of inner emptiness, boredom and meaninglessness; associated, particularly in more severe pathology, with underlying identity disturbances and deficits in personality structure; identity diffusion characterized by inadequate integration and insufficient balance between positive and negative perceptions of self and others. Lack of access to and contact with inner yearnings, deeper feelings and a 'true self' to make the self feel vital and alive – but in some cases also vulnerable, fragile and exposed, which has led to the person's inner life being shut down, characterized by dissociation and fragmentation, perhaps hidden behind a grandiose and stoic facade. This may also be part of the reason for the person's profound need for persistent positive attention and admiration from others to compensate for inner feelings of emptiness and meaninglessness (cf. the absence of a good internal object).
- **Idealization of others:** In some cases, an inclination to identify with, idealize and lean against individuals or social groups with special qualities and elevated social status. In this situation, the self boosts and stabilizes its fragile self-esteem by cultivating a perceived close attachment to or similarities to idealized individuals or a special social group, for example a political or religious leader or group, a partner or a therapist. Specifically, the narcissistic vulnerable self may try to boost its fragile – and essentially negative – self-image by finding a partner who is celebrated or powerful or otherwise enjoys high social status.
- **Unrealistic ideals:** The person may have obviously unrealistic goals and ideals that they have no reasonable chance of being able to realize. There is a considerable gap between ego ideals and the real self, often related to fantasies of the self's beauty, intelligence, wealth, celebrity, extraordinary accomplishments or strength and power: ego ideals that may, to varying degrees, appear to be primitive and immature. In some cases, this gap is less pronounced in high-functioning narcissism, and we should bear in mind that ego ideals that match the ego's actual characteristics, abilities and potential – and which are flexible and open to modification in light of the ego's actual development – can make a positive contribution to the ego's development and perception of agency.
- **Envy:** Varying degrees of acknowledged or unacknowledged, unconscious, envy directed at individuals who possess qualities or a social status that the self strives for, in vain. Often combined with a pronounced tendency to compare themself and their own accomplishments with others in the hope of earing glory, praise and recognition. An ambition that is doomed to fail, as there will always be others who

> appear more perfect and who outperform the self on various parameters. Envy will often be associated with a more or less unconscious perception of the self as being inferior – perceptions which the person may attempt to handle by disparaging the other or by defining their relative strengths and attained advantages as illegitimate or as the result of some sort of morally dubious injustice. The envy also prevents the person from appreciating, receiving or otherwise benefiting from any positive contributions from others, as this – since the antithesis of envy is gratitude – would require the ability to acknowledge and handle the notion that others who are different from and beyond the self's control might possess or represent something valuable that the self is not or does not possess (Segal & Bell, 1991).

We all possess narcissistic traits, to varying degrees, and in certain situations we may react and act in ways that could be described as narcissistic, for example when we find that our self-image and self-esteem are threatened, if we feel overlooked and insignificant in interactions with others or if we are overwhelmed by pride over something we or someone close to us has done or accomplished. The latter in particular may be viewed as a more mature and adaptive manifestation of narcissism. Similarly, our reactions may be driven by perceived narcissistic injury in situations where we are overwhelmed by unbearable shame, feel unfairly treated or perceive that our self-respect and social status are threatened.

Thus, the concept of narcissism covers a very wide spectrum of possible manifestation forms, just as each of the three previously outlined general manifestation forms have the potential for a high degree of heterogeneity. For example, we should expect to see high-functioning narcissism in generally stable and well-functioning leaders and people who occupy demanding positions in society and who have a reasonably well-developed capacity for critical self-reflection and a fairly realistic assessment of their own actual ability and accomplishments. On the other hand, some individuals may, for short or long periods of time, seem to fall into this category, but beneath a seemingly well-functioning surface they are in fact tormented by inner emptiness, psychological pain and profound doubt about their own abilities. They may collapse if they come under pressure (which may be characterized as a stress reaction, anxiety, depression), if their need for positive attention and admiration from others goes unmet or if they encounter criticism or indifference from others.

In pathological narcissism, particularly in its predominantly grandiose manifestations, deeper self-insight, curiosity about one's own self and the capacity for critical self-reflection will typically be absent or severely compromised. This may further contribute to various forms of shameless and abusive behaviour, given that the person is unable or unwilling to regard their own self and behaviour from someone else's perspective. In this sense, the narcissistically disturbed person is adhering to the blind seer's Tiresias's implicitly stated requirement that Narcissus can only live a long life provided he does not know himself (Colquhoun, 2023, p. 10). Superficially, however, the person may still appear remarkably certain about who they are, what they stand for and what is happening inside them – their inner life – and thus present an image that the person expects others to confirm. This exaggerated, rigid, unfounded and fatal (apparent) certainty about the person's self prevents the narcissistically disturbed person from having new experiences and gaining new insights into themself and others – and from developing a more nuanced and valid understanding of their own and others' inner life and world (Drozek et al., 2023, p. 11).

2.4 Narcissism and destructive shame

Close, genuine and mature psychological and emotional contact with others is only possible when we are able to see and deal with how others are differentiated from our own selves and thus beyond our control. Thus, we need to be able to see and relate to others as independent subjects capable of experiencing, evaluating and reacting to our selves in ways that we recognize as being outside our control. This represents a reality that, fairly obviously, involves the risk that we might be met by perceptions or reactions from others that threaten our established self-image and may cause us to experience shame, inferiority and powerlessness. These are all painful emotions that we may perceive as narcissistic injuries and which may destabilize our self-esteem.

The narcissistically unstable self needs to be able to control others' perceptions of and reactions to the self or, as a minimum, hold onto the (illusory) notion of being able to do so. If not, the object's differentiation from the self may be compromised, and the self may deny the other's existence as an autonomous subject whose subjective experiences and acting are independent of the self. This independence may give rise to painful emotions, including shame, in situations where the self is confronted with the other's objective differentiation from and independence of the self. Another strategy for defending an exposed self and fragile self-esteem may be to avoid recognizing others as equal subjects with their own needs, intentions and perspectives on reality. Instead, the self may attempt to reduce them to inferior and insignificant objects of its own grandiosely superior gaze, rendering their perception and evaluation of the self invalid and irrelevant to the self and allows the self to remain in its own self-reliant universe, independent of others or external recognition. This is, of course, an illusory universe, out of step with reality and our basic human needs for interpersonal contact and recognition from others; a universe in which other people are not seen as ends in their own right but as means of satisfying the needs of the self.

As discussed by the French philosopher Jean-Paul Sartre (1943), among others, the uniquely human emotion of shame is related to our realization of the fact that, in interpersonal interactions, we are reduced to objects of the other's evaluating gaze and that their perception and evaluation of us and our ways of being and acting are beyond our control (see also Jørgensen, 2023/2024). This realization can be challenging to contain and come to terms with and may therefore lead to narcissistic crises. On the other hand, it may also enable forms of interpersonal contact, self-awareness and genuine social recognition that are significant and in fact indispensable if we are to develop into mature and psychological well-functioning individuals.

Normal and constructive shame signals that we may be about to violate someone else's boundaries and social norms or expose ourselves in ways that we would come to regret. This sense of shame supports our awareness of and our ability to comply with normal social norms and conventions. It also helps regulate any grandiose notions and enhance our empathy with and attention to other people's boundaries and needs (Ronningstam, 2005, p. 37; Jørgensen, 2023/2024). Deficits in the capacity for containing and dealing with shame, shamelessness in interpersonal interactions and narcissistic disorders may be closely associated, either in the sense that poor empathy, grandiosity and a poor sense of shame may co-occur, particularly in severe narcissistic personality disorders bordering on psychopathy and antisocial personality disorder (see Chapter 3.1), or in the sense that the fragile self (cf. vulnerable narcissism) may struggle to contain and deal with intense feelings of shame, which are perceived as a serious threat to the person's self-esteem. This latter situation may be perceived as a form of narcissistic and existential crisis, which the person may attempt to handle by means of intensified grandiose notions and an insisting shamelessness in the self's behaviour towards others, who 'better not think they have the right to belittle me or tell me what to do'.

Furthermore, someone who is overwhelmed by destructive shame will often be very self-centred and thus unempathic, because the overwhelmed self will be so preoccupied with its own psychological pain and efforts to escape the shame that it will not be able also to pay attention to others or how its own behaviour might affect them. In addition, strategies aimed at regulating the destructive shame will often involve resentment towards and/or attacks on others (Jørgensen, 2023/2024, p. 101 ff.). More generally, we may imagine that intense emotions and other mental states flooding and threatening to destabilize the self may reduce the person's capacity for paying attention and reacting appropriately to other people's emotions and thus cause (momentaneous or more permanent) a lack of empathy (Baskin-Sommers et al., 2014, p. 326).

Narcissistic crises and reactions to them

Particularly when individuals with more severe narcissistic disorders experience narcissistic injury – perceiving that their grandiose self-image is not confirmed, encountering criticism or simply getting insufficient attention and interest from others – they may experience a narcissistic crisis driven by underlying shame. In individuals with predominantly grandiose narcissism, this will usually manifest itself primarily in the form of anger (narcissistic rage) and potentially shameless behaviour directed at the person(s) seen as causing the perceived (but typically more or less repressed/denied) shame.

In the case of predominantly vulnerable narcissism, the more likely response will be more overt shame, sadness, tendency to withdraw or heightened sensitivity to any indication that others might criticize, ridicule, ignore or otherwise act in ways that might cause shame and reduced self-esteem. As pointed out by the self-psychologist and psychoanalyst Andrew Morrison (1986, p. 357), the most intense levels of destructive shame and narcissistic rage typically occur in individuals to whom absolute control over others appears as a crucial condition for stabilizing their fragile self-esteem and ensuring continued access to validating mirroring from self-objects who admire the self or can be made to act in ways that allow the self to maintain the illusory perception that its key self-objects genuinely validate, admire and recognize the self and its grandiose self-image. Strategies for achieving control over others not only involve the fairly overt and explicit use of power but also more sophisticated strategies that exploit other people's dependence on the self in the form of threats or leaving or abandoning the other unless they do what the self expects or demands, for example in the form of continued confirmation and admiration of the self.

We may speak of at least two narcissistically organized attempts to deal with, or rather avoid dealing with, the challenges associated with the painful realization that others are differentiated from the self and thus outside its control, which carries the related risk that others will view and evaluate the self in ways that are out of step with the self's grandiose self-image and may thus cause shame and other painful emotions threatening to destabilize the individual's identity and self-esteem. One is to deny others' de facto differentiation from the self, including denying their existence or status as independent and equal subjects who see and evaluate the self in ways that are beyond the self's control and to do everything in one's power to monitor and control how others view and react to the self. This may be particularly pronounced in relation to the person's partner, children, workplace co-workers (including any subordinates) or members of social groups that the self also belongs to.

Another approach is the persistent effort to trumpet one's own exceptional qualities (cf. grandiosity and omnipotence), in comparison to which everyone else appears inferior, lesser and insignificant. This also lets the self temporarily escape their own conscious self-perceptions of being worthless, inferior and defective, with the shame and humiliation that this implies. This disparagement of, contempt for and devaluation of others lets the person shrug off any critical perceptions of the self as irrelevant, since they come from inferior beings who are reduced to simple objects of the self's own superior gaze. This approach thus represents the two-pronged strategy of stripping other people's view of the self of any authority or significance by viewing them as clearly inferior in comparison to one's own (grandiose) self and simultaneously (nevertheless) doing everything possible to control their perceptions and behaviour – as if part of the self actually acknowledged that other people's perception of the self does matter and may even have a profound impact on one's own identity and self-esteem.

In addition, the self may identify particularly significant others who are idealized and held up as exceptionally insightful, powerful or successful. The self may then identify with and lean on these strong (idealized) others. This may, for example, be an older family member, a prominent political or business leader, a divine being or a therapist. In its more primitive forms, this identification involves an inadequate differentiation of self and object, in which 'identification has appeared instead of object-choice' (Freud, 1921/1940, p. 106); instead of attaching to and striving to become like an external object that is recognized as clearly differentiated from the self, 'the ego assumes the characteristics of the object' (p. 107), the ego introjects the object into itself, replacing the attachment to the external object (p. 114).

Another narcissistically organized strategy for dealing with fear of others' potentially critical and shaming view of the self, which is outside the control of the self, is to withdraw from contact with others, seeking refuge in one's own inner world and fantasizing or daydreaming about one's own importance, including grandiose self-images that the self protects, as much as possible, from confrontation with reality (see Chapter 3.6 about psychic retreats). Very simply put, the former 'solution' is associated with predominantly grandiose manifestations of narcissism, while the latter is closer to vulnerable narcissism. A common feature is that narcissism, particularly pathological narcissism, is closely associated with destructive shame, which is regarded as a significant affect and driving force behind narcissistic disorders and strategies for stabilizing a fragile self and fragile self-esteem.

Pathological narcissism driven by destructive shame

In terms of pathological narcissism and narcissistic personality disorders, all three aforementioned manifestations of narcissism – grandiose, vulnerable and high-functioning – are, to varying degrees, characterized by underlying shame, including a pronounced preoccupation with being seen and, not least, with how one is seen and evaluated by others. This involves an internal deficit bordering on emptiness and fear of being humiliated or revealed as being inadequate (Crisp & Gabbard, 2020, p. 10). More specifically, it could be argued that the narcissistically disordered person's grandiosity, arrogance and disparagement of others represent attempts to regulate and deal with intense and painful feelings of inadequacy, helplessness and shame (Lecours et al., 2013, p. 130), given that (excessive) pride may be seen as an antidote to (destructive) shame. Arrogant behaviour towards others may thus be seen as a form of preventive attack intended to protect the self from being humiliated and exposed as shamefully inferior (p. 136).

Kohut (1971, p. 64) even pointed to severe shame – associated, in part, with fear of losing others' love – as a core element of severe narcissistic disorders. 'Narcissistic personalities are in general not predominantly swayed by guilt feelings [...]. Their predominant tendency is to be overwhelmed by shame' (p. 232).

Similarly, the psychoanalyst Léon Wurmser (1981) calls shame the essential narcissistic affect, while Andrew Morrison (1989) refers to shame as the underside or underlying affect of narcissism. This internal dynamic relationship stems from the fact that both pathological narcissism and destructive shame spring from the lack of intersubjective recognition of the self from significant others beginning during the earliest years of life (Brauner et al., 2021, p. 319). Kernberg's key focus on aggression, envy and splitting as key factors in the development of identity diffusion and pathological narcissism (see Chapter 3.4) probably helps to explain why he and the field of object relations psychology did not develop a similar awareness of the central role of destructive shame (Broucek, 1982, p. 374).

Pathological narcissism, perhaps vulnerable narcissism in particular, can thus be related to a core self characterized by extensive and destructive shame, which is a key dynamic driver of the maladaptive self-regulation strategies and the destructive interpersonal behaviour that are commonly seen in narcissistic disorders (Sasso et al., 2021). Similarly, exaggerated pride, grandiosity and narcissistic rage may represent attempts to escape or compensate for overwhelming and painful feelings of shame (Russ & Shedler, 2013, p. 31). Both narcissistic grandiosity and vulnerability may be seen as manifestations of deficits in self-esteem regulation with possible connections to destructive shame. Because it is inextricably associated with an experience of the self as defective, inadequate and with no right to exist, destructive shame is both psychologically painful and contributes to the destabilization of self-esteem. Manifestations of narcissism have also been viewed as attempts to regulate dissociated or feared shame. Thus, therapists will need to be at least as attentive to underlying feelings of shame as they are to more overtly manifested affects and behaviours when working with patients with pathological narcissism (Wright et al., 1989, p. 227).

Studies of shame and narcissism

There are still very few empirical studies of possible correlations between shame and the different manifestations of narcissism. However, in a systematic literature review of 25 studies of varying quality, Kesman et al. (under review, 2024) conclude that shame is primarily associated with vulnerable manifestations of narcissism, while grandiose manifestations of narcissism should rather be understood as defences against perceived threats to the self, including attempts to escape destructive shame. A study based on a non-clinical population of young people found a correlation between higher levels of vulnerable narcissism and more intense perceived shame, while it found no correlation between levels of (non-pathological) grandiose narcissism and shame. Other studies similarly found a correlation between the level of vulnerable narcissism and the severity of perceived shame as well as indications that higher levels of grandiose narcissism (in non-clinical populations) may be associated with less perceived shame (Hibbard, 1992; Di Sarno et al., 2020, p. 6). Studies also found that correlations between the degree of vulnerable narcissism and insecure attachment are mediated by shame (Van Schie et al., 2021, p. 5). Thus, vulnerable narcissism is associated with various forms of insecure attachment, with the level of shame as a significant mediating factor for this connection in the sense that higher levels of perceived shame strengthens the correlation.

A related study based on patients in psychotherapy, most of them diagnosed with depression, a smaller share (10%) with borderline personality disorder and none with NPD (despite relatively high levels of NPD-related traits), found that self-reported narcissistic traits show a relatively strong (r=.26) correlation with more frequent experiences of painful shame. Participants with higher levels of narcissistic traits showed even higher levels of painful shame (Bouizegarene & Lecours, 2017, p. 286). In extension of this observation, we might consider whether an inability to understand the effect of one's own behaviour on others, which is common in NPD, may be related to an inability to contain and process (mentalize) painful shame that is triggered by violating other persons' shame boundaries and personal integrity (Bouizegarene & Lecours, 2017, p. 287). Furthermore, more frequent experiences of shame are associated with antagonism towards and contempt for the person's own self, which are typical manifestations and consequences of destructive shame (Jørgensen, 2023/2024). However, since Bouizegarene and Lecours's study is relatively small, mainly explorative and not based on patients diagnosed with NPD, we should be cautious about drawing very far-reaching conclusions about significant causal relations between destructive shame and narcissistic pathology on this basis alone.

A few empirical studies support the possibility that, in particular, unconscious or implicit (denied, repressed) shame may be a defining characteristic and a central underlying driver in narcissistic personality disorders (Ritter et al., 2014); a driver that is often hidden behind a grandiose facade or grandiose defensive strategies, including narcissistic rage as a reaction to perceived injuries of a fragile self. Here, all things being equal, the severity of consciously perceived shame (Wright et al., 1989, p. 219) – and shame that may be reported in simple questionnaire studies – will be significantly lower. Instead, the shame will be dissociated, denied and concealed behind a mask of grandiosity (cf. the mask model). Conversely, we should expect intense and conscious destructive shame to be far more pronounced in more vulnerable manifestations of NPD, where grandiose elements, on the other hand, are less overt and, at times, dissociated.

Alternatively, the person may attempt to regulate or shut down destructive shame by avoiding or withdrawing from the interpersonal contacts that are associated with a risk that the shamefully fragile and inferior self becomes visible, exposed and revealed to others. Overt shame also generally seems more pronounced in patients with BPD, compared to NPD (see also Jørgensen & Bøye, 2024), although this is, so far, based on small empirical studies involving relatively few patients with NPD (Ritter et al., 2014). Conversely, there are indications that implicit manifestations of (underlying) shame is more pronounced in patients med NPD compared with patients with PBD (Ritter et al., 2014). Finally, in a few studies, shame has been identified as the key affect in the development of depressive symptoms in patients with NPD (Fjermestad-Noll et al., 2020b, p. 24), which also lends support to notion of destructive shame as a core affect in pathological narcissism.

References

Ackerman, R. A., Hands, A. J., Donnellan, M. B., Hopwood, C. J., & Witt, E. A. (2017). Experts' views regarding the conceptualization of narcissism. *Journal of Personality Disorders*, 31, 346–361.

Altmeyer, M. (2000). *Narzissmus und Objekt: Ein intersubjektives Verständnis der Selbstbezogenheit* [Narcissism and object: An intersubjective understanding of self-sufficiency]. Vandenhoeck & Ruprecht.

American Psychiatric Association (APA) (2013). *Diagnostic and statistical manual of mental disorders (fifth edition; DSM-5)*. American Psychiatric Publishing.

Balint, M. (1968). *The basic fault: Therapeutic aspects of regression*. Northwestern University Press.

Baskin-Sommers, A., Krusemark, E., & Ronningstam, E. (2014). Empathy in narcissistic personality disorder: From clinical and empirical perspectives. *Personality Disorders: Theory, research, and treatment*, 5, 323–333.

Biberdzic, M., Tan, J., & Day, N. J. S. (2023). It's not you, it's me: Identity disturbance as the main contributor to interpersonal problems in pathological narcissism. *Borderline Personality Disorder and Emotional Dysregulation*, 10, 1–12.

Blasco-Belled, A., Tejeda-Gallardi, C., Alsinet, C., & Rogoza, R. (2023). The links of subjective and psychological well-being with the dark triad traits: A meta-analysis. *Journal of Personality*, 00, 1–17.

Blatt, S. J. (2008). *Polarities of experience: Relatedness and self-definition in personality development, psychopathology, and the therapeutic process*. American Psychological Association.

Bolm, T. (2021). Mentalisierungsbasierte Therapie für Patienten mit narzisstischer Persönlichkeitsstörung [Mentalization-based therapy for patients with narcissistic personality disorder]. In S. Doering, H.-P. Hartmann, & O. F. Kernberg (Eds.), *Narzisssmus: Grundlagen, Störungsbilder, Therapie* (2nd ed., pp. 658–668). Schattauer Verlag.

Bosson, J. K., Lakey, C. E., Campbell, W. K., Zeigler-Hill, V., Jordan, C. H., & Kernis, M. H. (2008). Understanding the links between narcissism and self-esteem: A theoretical and empirical review. *Social and Personality Psychology Compass*, 2, 1415–1439.

Bouizegarene, N., & Lecours, S. (2017). Verbal elaboration of distinct affect categories and narcissistic personality disorder features. *Psychoanalytic Psychology*, 34, 279–289.

Britton, R. (1998). *Belief and Imagination: Explorations in psychoanalysis*. Routledge.

Britton, R. (2003). *Sex, death, and the superego: Experiences in psychoanalysis*. Karnac.

Broucek, F. J. (1982). Shame and its relationship to early narcissistic developments. *International Journal of Psychoanalysis*, 63, 369–378.
Cain, N. M., Pincus, A. L., & Ansell, E. B. (2008). Narcissism at the crossroads: Phenotypic description of pathological narcissism across clinical theory, social/ personality psychology, and psychiatric diagnosis. *Clinical Psychology Review*, 28, 638–656.
Caligor, E. (2013). Narcissism in psychodynamic diagnostic manual. In J. S. Ogrodniczuk (Ed.), *Understanding and treating Pathological Narcissism* (pp. 63–79). American Psychological Association.
Caligor, E., Levy, K. N., & Yeomans, F. E. (2015). Narcissistic personality disorders: Diagnostic and clinical challenges. *American Journal of Psychiatry*, 172, 415–422.
Caligor, E., & Stern, B. L. (2020). Diagnosis, classification, and assessment of narcissistic personality disorder within the framework of object relations theory. *Journal of Personality Disorders*, 34, 104–121.
Charim, I. (2022). *Die Qualen des Narzissmus: Über freiwillige Unterwerfung* [The torments of narcissism: On voluntary submission]. Zsolnay.
Choi-Kain, L. (2020). Narcissistic personality disorder: A coming of age. *Journal of Personality Disorders*, 34, 210–213.
Colquhoun, M. (2023). *Narcissism in Bloom: An alternative story of the selfie*. Repeater Books.
Crisp, H., & Gabbard, G. O. (2020). Principles of psychodynamic treatment for patients with narcissistic personality disorder. *Journal of Personality Disorders*, 34, 143–158.
Crowe, M. L., Lyman, D. R., Campbell, W. K., & Miller, J. D. (2019). Exploring the structure of narcissism: Toward an integrated solution. *Journal of Personality*, 87, 1151–1169.
Dashineau, S. C., Edershile, E. A., Simms, L. J., & Wright, A. G. C. (2019). Pathological narcissism and psychosocial functioning. *Personality Disorders; Theory, Research, and Treatment*, 10, 473–478.
Day, N. J. S., Green, A., Denmeade, G., Bach, B., & Grenyer, B.F.S. (2023). Narcissistic personality disorder in the ICD-11: Severity and trait profiles of grandiosity and vulnerability. *Journal of clinical psychology*, 80, 1917–1936.
Di Sarno, M., Zimmermann, J., Madeddu, F., Casini, E., & Di Pierro, R. (2020). Shame behind the corner? A daily diary investigation of pathological narcissism. *Journal of Research in Personality*, 85, 1–13.
Diamond, D., Yeomans, F. E., Stern, B. L., & Kernberg, O. F. (2022). *Treating pathological narcissism with transference-focused psychotherapy*. Guilford.
Drozek, R. P., Unruh, B. T., & Bateman, A. (2023). *Mentalization-based treatment of pathological narcissism*. Oxford University Press.
Edershile, E.A. & Wright, A.G.C. (2021b). Fluctiations in grandiose and vulnerable narcissistic states.: A momentary perspective. *Journal of Personality and Social Psychology*, 67, 1386–1414.
Ermann, M. (2020). *Narzissmus: Vom Mythos zur Psychoanalyses des Selbst* [Narcissism: From myth to psychoanalysis of the self]. Kohlhammer.
Fiscalini, J. (2004). *Coparticipant psychoanalysis*. Columbia University Press.
Fjermestad-Noll, J., Ronningstam, E., Bach, B., Storebø, O.J., Rosenbaum, B., & Simonsen, E. (2020b). Psychotherapeutic treatment of depressive symptoms in patients with narcissistic disturbances: A review. *Journal of Contemporary Psychotherapy*, 50, 21–28.

Fossati, A., Feeney, J., Pincus, A., Borroni, S., & Maffei, C. (2015). The structure of pathological narcissism and its relationship with adult attachment styles. *Psychoanalytic Psychology*, 32, 403–431.

Freud, S. (1940). Group psychology and the analysis of the ego. In J. Strachey (Ed. & Trans.), *The standard edition of the complete psychological works of Sigmund Freud* (Vol. 18, pp. 65–144). Hogarth. (Original work published 1921)

Freud, S. (1949). Three essays on the theory of sexuality. In J. Strachey (Ed. & Trans.), *The standard edition of the complete psychological works of Sigmund Freud* (Vol. 7, pp. 123–246). Hogarth. (Original work published in 1905)

Freud, S. (1957a). Libidinal types. In J. Strachey (Ed. & Trans.), *The standard edition of the complete psychological works of Sigmund Freud* (Vol. 21, pp. 215–220). Hogarth. (Original work published in 1931)

Freud, S. (1957b). On narcissism: An introduction. In J. Strachey (Ed. & Trans.), *The standard edition of the complete psychological works of Sigmund Freud* (Vol. 14, pp. 67–102). Hogarth. (Original work published 1914)

Freud, S. (1958). The case of Schreber: Psycho-Analytic Notes on an Autobiographical Account of a Case of Paranoia (Dementia Paranoides). In J. Strachey (Ed. & Trans.), *The standard edition of the complete psychological works of Sigmund Freud* (Vol. 12, pp. 3–84). Hogarth. (Original work published in 1911)

Freud, S. (1963). Introductory lectures on psycho-analysis. In J. Strachey (Ed. & Trans.), *The standard edition of the complete psychological works of Sigmund Freud* (Vol. 16). Hogarth. (Original work published in 1917)

Freud, S. (1990). *The ego and the id*. Norton. (Original work published in 1923)

Gabbard, G. O., & Crisp, H. (2018). *Narcissism and its discontents: Diagnostic dilemmas and treatment strategies with narcissistic patients*. American Psychiatric Publishing.

Giacomo, E., Andreini, E., Lurusso, O., & Clerici, M. (2023). The dark side of empathy in narcissistic personality disorder. *Frontiers in Psychiatry*. doi:10.3389/fpsyt.2023.1074558.

Green, A. (2004). *Die tote Mutter: Psychoanalytische Studien zu Lebensnarzissmus und Todesnarzissmus* [The dead mother: Psychoanalytic studies on life narcissism and death narcissism] (E. Wolff & E. Kittler, Trans). Psychosozial Verlag.

GreB, H., Achilles, P., Seel, D. (2002). Von Wandlungen und Anpassungen: Ausdrucksformen des NarziBmus in Individuum und Gesellschaft [Of transformations and adaptations: expressions of narcissism in the individual and society]. In G. Seidler (Ed.). *Das Ich und das Fremde: Klinische und sozialpsychologische Analysen des destruktiven Narzissmus* (pp. 93–113). Psychosozial Verlag.

Grijalva, E., Harms, P.D., Newman, D.A., Gaddis, B.H., & Fraley, R.C. (2015b). Narcissism and leadership: A meta-analytic review of linear and nonlinear relationships. *Personnel Psychology*, 68, 1–47.

Horney, K. (1939). *New ways in psychoanalysis*. Norton.

Huprich, S. K., & Malone, B. C. (2022). Malignant self-regard: Overview and future directions. *Harvard Review of Psychiatry*, 30, 226–237.

Huprich, S. K., Nelson, S., Sohnleitner, A., Lengu, K., Shankar, S., & Rexer, K. (2018). Are malignant self-regard and vulnerable narcissism different constructs? *Journal of Clinical Psychology*, 74, 1556–1569.

Jauk, E., Ulbrich, L., Jorschick, P., Höfler, M., Kaufman, S. B., & Kanske, P. (2022). The nonlinear association between grandiose and vulnerable narcissism: An induvial data meta-analysis. *Journal of Personality*, 90, 703–726.

Jørgensen, C. R. (2019). *The psychotherapeutic stance* (D. Silver, Trans.). Springer. (Original work published 2018).

Jørgensen, C. R. (2024). *Understanding and working with shame: Psychotherapeutic, cultural and philosophical perspectives* (D. Silver, Trans.). Routledge. (Original work published 2023)

Jørgensen, C. R., & Bøye, R. (2024). 'I am ashamed that I exist. I feel like apologizing for existing': The phenomenology of shame in patients with borderline personality disorder: A qualitative study. *Personality Disorders: Theory, Research, and Treatment*, 15, 181–192. doi:10.1037/per0000655.

Jørgensen, C. R., & Bøye, R. (in preparation). *The phenomenology of disturbed self-concept and self-esteem in pathological narcissism: A qualitative study.*

Kernberg, O. F. (1975). *Borderline conditions and pathological narcissism*. Jason Aronson.

Kernberg, O. F. (2004a). *Aggressivity, narcissism, and self-destructiveness in the psychotherapeutic relationship*. Yale University Press.

Kernberg, P. (2000). Developmental aspects of normal and pathological narcissism. In E. F. Ronningstam (Ed.), *Disorders of narcissism: Diagnostic, clinical, and empirical implications*. American Psychiatric Press, 103–120.

Kesman, E., De Amicis, M., Mucci, C., & Scalabrini, A. (under review). The vulnerability of shame for the narcissistic self: A systematic review. *Journal of Clinical Psychology*. https://doi:10.22541/au.172115029.90350833/v1.

Kohut, H. (1971). *The analysis of the self*. The University of Chicago Press.

Krizan, Z., & Herlache, A. D. (2018). The narcissism spectrum model: A synthetic view of narcissistic personality. *Personality and Social Psychology Review*, 22, 3–31.

Küchenhoff, J. (2003). Zur Einführung des Narzißmus: Eine Relektüre [On Narcissism: A Rereading]. *Psyche*, 58, 150–169.

Kuchynka, S. L., & Bosson, J. K. (2018). The psychodynamic mask model of narcissism: Where is it now? In A. D. Hermann, A. B. Brunell, & J. D. Foster (Eds.). *Handbook of Trait Narcissism*. Springer Nature, 89–94.

Lacan, J. (1988). *The seminar of Jacques Lacan. Book 1: Freud's papers on technique, 1953–1954*. (J. Forrester, Trans.). Norton. (Original work published 1975)

Lasch, C. (1979). *The culture of narcissism: American life in an age of diminishing expectations*. Norton.

Lear, J. (2024). Gratitude, freedom and refusal. *International Journal of Psychoanalysis*, 105, 127–141.

Lecours, S., Briand-Malenfant, R., & Descheneaux, E. (2013). Affect regulation and mentalization in narcissistic personality disorder. In J. S. Ogrodniczuk (Ed.), *Understanding and Treating Pathological Narcissism*. American Psychological Association, 129–145.

Levy, K. N. (2012). Subtypes, dimensions, levels, and mental states in narcissism and narcissistic personality disorder. *Journal of Clinical Psychology: In session*, 68, 886–897.

McWilliams, N. (2011). *Psychoanalytic diagnosis* (2nd Ed.). Guilford.

Miller, J. D., & Campbell, W. K. (2008). Comparing clinical and social-personality conceptualizations of narcissism. *Journal of Personality*, 76, 450–476.

Miller, J. D., Campbell, W. K., & Pilkonis, P. A. (2007). Narcissistic personality disorder: relations with distress and functional impairment. *Comprehensive Psychiatry*, 48, 170–177.

Miller, J. D., Crowe, M. L., & Sharpe, B. M. (2022). Narcissism and the DSM-5 alternative model of personality disorder. *Personality Disorders: Theory, Research and Treatment*, 13, 407–411.

Miller, J. D., Lynam, D. R., Hyatt, C. S., & Campbell, W. K. (2017). Controversies in narcissism. *Annual Review of Clinical Psychology*, 13, 291–315.

Miller, J. D., Lynam, D. R., Vize, C., Crowe, M., Sleep, C., Maples-Keller, J. L., Few, L. R., & Campbell, W. K. (2018). Vulnerable narcissism is (mostly) a disorder of neuroticism. *Journal of Personality*, 86, 186–199.

Miller, J. D., & Maples, J. (2011). Trait personality models of narcissistic personality disorder, grandiose narcissism, and vulnerable narcissism. In W. K. Campbell & J. D. Miller (Eds.), *The handbook of narcissism and narcissistic personality disorder. Theoretical approaches, empirical findings, and treatments* (pp. 71–88). John Wiley.

Morrison, A. P. (1986). Shame, ideal self, and narcissism. In A. P. Morrison (Ed.), *Essential papers on narcissism* (pp. 348–371). New York University Press.

Morrison, A. P. (1989). *Shame: The underside of narcissism*. Analytic Press.

Morrison, A. P. (2008). The analyst's shame. *Contemporary Psychoanalysis*, 44, 65–82.

Morrison, A. P., & Stolorow, R.D. (1997). Shame, narcissism, and intersubjectivity. In M. R. Lansky & A. P. Morrison (Eds.), *The widening scope of shame* (pp. 63–87). Psychology Press.

Mortensen, E. L., Jensen, H. H., & Flensborg-Madsen, T. (2017). Big five personlighedstræk som risikofaktorer for psykiske og fysiske sygdomme [Big five personality traits as risk factors for mental and somatic illnesses]. In E. Simonsen & B. B. Mathiesen (Eds.), *Personlighed og personlighedsforstyrrelser: En grundbog* (pp. 141–174). Hans Reitzels Forlag.

Ogrodniczuk, J. S., & Kealy, D. (2013). Interpersonal problems of narcissistic patients. In J. S. Ogrodniczuk (Ed.), *Understanding and treating pathological narcissism* (pp. 113–127). American Psychological Association.

O'Shaughnessy, E. (2008). On gratitude. In G. Lemma & P. Roth (Eds.). *Envy and gratitude revisited* (pp. 79–91). Routledge.

Ovid (2004). *Metamorphoses* (D. Raeburn, Trans.). Penguin. (Original work published ca. 10 BCE)

Pedone, R., Huprich, S. K., Colle, L., Barbarulo, A. M., & Semerari, A. (2023). Exploring guilt differences in grandiose narcissism, vulnerable narcissism, and malignant self-regard. *Journal of Personality Disorders*, 37, 285–303.

Pincus, A. L. (2023). Narcissistic personality disorder and pathological narcissism. In R. F. Krueger & P. H. Blaney (Eds.), *Oxford textbook of psychopathology* (4th ed., pp. 628–649). Oxford University Press.

Pincus, A. L., Ansell, E. B., Pimentel, C. A., Wright, A. G. C., & Levy, K. N. (2009). Initial construction and validation of the pathological narcissism inventory. *Psychological Assessment*, 21, 365–379.

Pincus, A. L., & Lukowitsky, M. R. (2010). Pathological narcissism and narcissistic personality disorder. *Annual Review of Clinical Psychology*, 6, 421–446.

Pincus, A. L., & Roche, M. J. (2011). Narcissistic grandiosity and narcissistic vulnerability. In W. K. Campbell & J. D. Miller (Eds.), *The handbook of narcissism and narcissistic personality disorder: Theoretical approaches, empirical findings, and treatments* (pp. 31–40). John Wiley.

Pulver, S. E. (1986 [1970]). Narcissism: The term and the concept. In A. P. Morrison (Ed.), *Essential papers on narcissism* (pp. 91–111). New York University Press.

Rank, O. (1911). Ein beitrag zum Narzissmus [A contribution to Narcissism]. *Jahrbuch für psychoanalytische Forschungen*, 401–426.

Raskin, R., & Hall, C. S. (1979). A narcissistic personality inventory. *Psychological Reports*, 40, 590.

Raskin, R., & Terry, H. (1988). A principal-component analysis of the narcissistic personality inventory and further evidence of its construct validity. *Journal of Personality and Social Psychology*, 54, 890–902.

Reich, W. (1949). *Character analysis* (3rd Ed.), Farrar, Straus & Giroux. (Original work published 1933)

Ritter, K., Dziobek, I., PreiBler, S., Rüter, A., Vater, A., Fydrich, T., Lammers, C. H., Heekeren, H. R., & Roepke, S. (2011). Lack of empathy in patients with narcissistic personality disorder. *Psychiatry Research*, 187, 241–247.

Ritter, K., Vater, A., Rüsch, N., Schröder-Abé, M., Schütz, A., Fydrich, T., Lammers, C. H., Roepke, S. (2014). Shame in patients with narcissistic personality disorder. *Psychiatry Research*, 215, 429–437.

Rohmann, E., Neumann, E., Herner, M. J., & Bierhof, H.-W. (2012). Grandiose and vulnerable narcissism: Self-construal, attachment, and love in romantic relationships. *European Psychologist*, 17, 279–290.

Ronningstam, E. (2005). *Identifying and understanding the narcissistic personality*. Oxford University Press.

Ronningstam, E. (2012). Alliance building and narcissistic personality disorder. *Journal of Clinical Psychology: In session*, 68, 943–953.

Ronningstam, E. (2021). *NPD Basic: A brief overview of identifying, diagnosing and treating narcissistic personality disorder* (4th Ed.), McLean Hospital, Harvard Medical School.

Rosenfeld, H. (1971). A clinical approach to the psychoanalytic theory of life and death instincts: An investigation into the aggressive aspects of narcissism. *International Journal of Psychoanalysis*, 52, 169–181.

Rosenfeld, H. (1987). *Sackgassen und Deutungen: Therapeutische und antitherapeutische Faktoren bei der psychoanalytischen Behandlung von psychotischen, Borderline und neurotischen Patienten* [Dead ends and interpretations: Therapeutic and antitherapeutic factors in the psychoanalytic treatment of psychotic, borderline, and neurotic patients]. Verlag Internationale Psychoanalyse.

Roth, P. (2008). Introduction. In Lemma, G., & P. Roth (Eds.), *Envy and gratitude revisited* (pp. 1–18). Routledge.

Russ, E., & Shedler, J. (2013). Defing narcissistic subtypes. In J. S. Ogrodniczuk (Ed.), *Understanding and treating pathological narcissism* (pp. 29–43). American Psychological Association.

Russ, E., Shedler, J., Bradley, R., & Westen, D. (2008). Refining the construct of narcissistic personality disorder: Diagnostic criteria and subtypes. *American Journal of Psychiatry*, 165, 1473–1481.

Samuel, D. B., & Widiger, T. A. (2004). Clinicians' personality descriptions of prototypic personality disorders. *Journal of Personality Disorders*, 18, 286–308.

Samuel, D. B., & Widiger, T. A. (2008). A meta-analytic view of the relationship between the five-factor model and DSM-IV-TR personality disorders: A facet level analysis. *Clinical Psychology Review*, 28, 1326–1342.

Sartre, J.-P. (1943). *Being and nothingness*. Routledge.

Sasso, S., Cain, N. M., Meehan, K. B., Zeng, R., & Wong, P. S. (2021). The impact of pathological narcissism on affect following social rejection. *Journal of Personality Disorders*, 35, 691–707.

Saulsman, L. M., & Page, A. C. (2004). The five-factor model and personality disorder empirical literature: A meta-analytic review. *Clinical Psychology Review*, 23, 1055–1085.

Schmidt-Hellerau, C. (2021). Freuds Narzissmus-Theorie [Freud's theory of narcissism]. In S. Doering, H.-P. Hartmann, & O. F. Kernberg (Eds.), *Narzissmus: Grundlagen, Störungsbilder, Therapie* (2nd ed., pp. 16–23). Schattauer Verlag.

Segal, H., & Bell, D. (1991). The theory of narcissism in the works of Freud and Klein. In J. Sandler, E. S. Person, & P. Fonagy (Eds.), *Freud's 'On narcissism: An introduction'*. Routledge.

Shoshani, B., Soshani, M., & Becker, M. (2006). From lifegiver to mutual nurturance: A relational perspective on Symington's monadic view of narcissism. *Psychoanalytic Dialogues*, 16, 499–517.

Steiner, J. (1993). *Psychic retreats: Pathological organizations in psychotic, neurotic and borderline patients*. Routledge.

Stern, D. (1985). *The interpersonal world of the infant*. Basic Books.

Symington, N. (1993). *Narcissism: A new theory*. Karnac.

Van Schie, C. C., Jarmen, H. L., Reis, S., & Grenyer, B. F. S. (2021). Narcissistic traits in young people and how experiencing shame relates to current attachment challenges. *BMC Psychiatry*, 21, 246. doi:10.1186/s12888–021–033249–4.

Verhaeghe, P. (2017). *Narziss in Trauer: Das verschwinden des Patriarchats* [Narcissus in mourning: The disappearance of the patriarchy]. Turia + Kant.

Walter, M., & Bilke-Hentsch, O. (2020). *Narzissmus: Grundlagen, Formen, Interventionen* [Narcissism: Foundations, forms, interventions]. Kohlhammer.

Watts, A.L., Lilienfiled, S.O., Smith, S.F., Miller, J.D., Campbell, W.K., Waldman, I. D., Rubenzer, S.J., & Fascingbauer, T.J. (2013). The double-edged sword of grandiose narcissism: Implications for successful and unsuccessful leadership among U. S. presidents. *Psychological Science*, 24, 2379–2389.

Westen, D. (1990). The relations among narcissism, egocentrism, self-concept, and self-esteem: Experimental, clinical, and theoretical considerations. *Psychoanalysis and Contemporary Thought*, 13, 183–239.

Wilde, O. (2022). *The Picture of Dorian Gray*. Ryerson University. https://pressbooks.library.torontomu.ca/thepictureofdoriangray/ (Original work published in 1891)

Wink, P. (1991). Two faces of narcissism. *Journal of Personality and Social Psychology*, 61, 590–597.

Wolf, E. S. (1996). *Theorie und Praxis der psychoanalytischen Selbstpsychologie* (Theory and practice of psychoanalytic self psychology). Suhrkamp Verlag.

Wright, F., O'Leary, J., & Balkin, J. (1989). Shame, guilt, narcissism and depression: Correlates and sex differences. *Psychoanalytic Psychology*, 6, 217–230.

Zabel, L. (2019). *Narzisstische Depression: Theorie und Konzepte in Psychiatrie und Psychoanalyse* [Narcissistic depression: Theory and concepts in psychiatry and psychoanalysis]. Psychosozial-Verlag.

3 Pathological narcissism

Making and, not least, communicating a diagnosis of narcissistic personality disorder (NPD) presents certain challenges. It is a diagnosis that many associate with a wide range of negative connotations, in the sense that someone who is diagnosed with NPD must be a 'bad' and 'morally dubious' person, who will be marginalized by others, and many of the specific aspects of the diagnosis may be clearly incompatible with the affected person's self-perception. Thus, to some people and in certain (sub)cultures, a diagnosis of narcissism may be deeply stigmatizing. The person who receives the diagnosis may feel profoundly misunderstood, humiliated and shameful and narcissistically injured, a target of attack and criticism. The self may become destabilized, causing the patient to withdraw and reject any further contact with the therapist who reached the diagnosis. Or they may become furious and (counter)attack the therapist (Ronningstam, 2012, p. 943).

Particularly individuals with predominantly grandiose narcissism may have a strong need to place the full responsibility for their possible perceived difficulties outside themselves – in others. Moreover, it may be a source of unbearable anxiety and insecurity and feelings of inferiority and incompetence to have to engage with genuine curiosity in a process of reflecting on oneself and one's possible inner life – an inner life that the person will often try to shut down or treat with (self-)contempt. For these reasons alone, the patient may feel massively challenged when a therapist makes a diagnosis that situates pathological processes in the patient (Drozek et al., 2023, p. 38). Persons with grandiose narcissism may experience the situation of seeking help and being the object of another person's diagnostic assessment as an exceptionally intense threat and a narcissistic injury.

Thus, communicating a diagnosis of NPD takes tact and a well-developed capacity for empathy. It is important for the therapist to focus on the specific problems and challenges that the person has described and demonstrated, in various ways, during the diagnostic process. This may, for example, include problems with establishing and maintaining relationships, recurring interpersonal conflicts and intense anger/rage which the individual struggles to understand and control. Or the patient may have hinted at a painful and perhaps diffuse sense of loneliness, emptiness and alienation in relation to

DOI: 10.4324/9781003744962-3

others and themself, including a sense of lacking contact with themself and having fragile self-esteem, perhaps concealed behind an arrogant and grandiose facade. Some patients with pathological narcissism struggle with the confusion of fluctuating between feelings of superiority and inferiority in relation to others, and, for varying reasons, are so afraid of being humiliated by or becoming dependent on others that they do not dare to establish close contact with others, despite missing exactly that, more or less consciously (Diamond et al., 2022, p. 147).

3.1 Narcissistic personality disorder (NPD): Diagnostic criteria

There are two authorized and widely recognized systems for diagnosing psychological disorders: the World Health Organization's (WHO) International Classification of Diseases (ICD) system and the American Psychiatric Association's (APA) *Diagnostic and Statistical Manual of Mental Disorders* (*DSM*) system. The *DSM* system is by far the most widely used in research, while it has somewhat less of a role in clinical practice, where the ICD system is more widely applied. The transition from the *ICD-10* to the *ICD-11*, between 2015 and 2026, marks a significant shift in the approach to diagnosing personality disorders (PDs): from purely categorical diagnostics, based on about ten different, relatively well-described and (theoretically) quite distinct categories of personality disorders, to a largely – and in some regards much simpler – dimensional approach. Neither the *ICD-10* nor the *ICD-11* operates with a specific diagnosis of narcissistic personality disorder, although the *ICD-10* does mention 'narcissistic personality structure' as one among several possible diagnoses under the category F60.8: 'Other specific personality disorders' (World Health Organization [WHO], 1992, p. 207). However, it offers no detailed description of narcissistic personality disorder. At the time of publication during the early 1990s, the diagnosis was still considered inadequately described, so the only further reference was to the diagnostic criteria for NPD in the APA's diagnostic system *DSM-IV*.

The DSM-5

The APA's diagnostic system the *DSM-5* (American Psychiatric Association [APA], 2013) contains two fundamentally different approaches to diagnosing personality disorders: 1) a categorical model that is still considered the authorized approach and which is used in the American healthcare sector and 2) a much more dimensional approach – also known as the Alternative Model for Personality Disorders (AMPD) – which so far is only intended for research and clinical practice trials. There is reason to assume that this alternative model will at some point be elevated, at least, to applications in formalized personality diagnostics in clinical practice.

A diagnosis of a personality disorder based on the categorical *DSM* system – like the *ICD-10* – is based on a number of general criteria. This involves identifying certain enduring patterns in the person's behaviour and internal experiences that deviate markedly from what would normally be expected in light of the person's culture within at least two of the following four areas:

- **Cognition**: ways of perceiving and interpreting self, others and events
- **Affectivity**: intensity and stability of emotional experiences and reactions as well as how wide a spectrum of emotional experiences and reactions the person has access to and to what degree these may be regarded as 'appropriate' or 'normal' in relation to the context where they occur
- **Interpersonal functioning**: ability to establish and engage in normal and age-appropriate interpersonal relationships and interactions
- **Impulse control**: ability to contain and regulate impulses, including anger and other immediate action urges.

The patterns in question should be enduring, inflexible and manifest themselves across a wide spectrum of areas and social situations; furthermore, they should give rise to clinically significant difficulties (symptoms, subjective distress) and restrictions in the person's social and occupational functioning and other important areas of the person's life. The patterns should date back to at least the person's youth or early adulthood and should not be the likely result of substance abuse (drugs, alcohol, prescription medicine) or other medical conditions, for example head trauma.

According to the *DSM-5*, individuals with a narcissistic personality disorder are characterized by an enduring pattern of grandiosity in cognition (fantasies) and behaviour, a pronounced need for admiration from others and poor empathy. As in most personality disorders, these patterns will typically be ego-syntonic, in the sense that persons with NPD do not perceive these narcissistically organized patterns, experiences and behaviours as deviant or problematic but as a completely natural way of being and acting in the world. Thus, they do not in themselves cause the affected individuals to seek help. Persons with high-functioning NPD in particular will often develop strategies to compensate for their emotional and interpersonal difficulties, as long as they can make others admire and confirm their fragile grandiose selves.

More specifically, in addition to meeting the above-mentioned criteria for a personality disorder, the person should meet at least five of the following criteria (APA, 2013, p. 669 ff.) to be diagnosed with narcissistic personality disorder (NPD):

- Has a grandiose sense of *self-importance*; excessively positive sense of own abilities and achievements – and an expectation of being recognized as superior without any connection to actual achievements; often appears boastful, pretentious; often assumes that others see the self as special and extraordinarily important – and they may be surprised or insulted if/when this is not the case; often accompanied by an inclination to devalue the qualities and achievements of others; in some cases, this may manifest itself in the feeling that only the most gifted therapists would be able to understand and help them and thus insist on seeing the therapist with the highest professional status and authority

- Is preoccupied with *fantasies* of their own unlimited success, power, uniqueness, beauty and ideal love; may tend to compare themself to famous and highly privileged people
- Feels that *the self is absolutely special*, unique and can only be understood by – and should only associate with – other people or institutions that are special or high status; may attempt to prop up/stabilize their own fragile self-esteem by associating with idealized others
- Expects excessive *admiration* from others; because the person's self-esteem will often be very fragile, they will be intensely preoccupied with how favourably they are regarded by others; often has a need for constant attention and recognition from others
- Has a sense of *entitlement to special treatment*; expects others to cater to them and may be puzzled or furious when this does not happen
- Tends to *exploit others*; uses others to meet their own needs; expects to get what the self wants or believes to need and is entitled to, with no regard for the impact on others
- *Lacks empathy*; disinclined to acknowledge or identify with the feelings, subjective experiences or needs of others (that is, primarily lacks emotional rather than purely cognitive empathic capacity); assumes that others are very concerned about their welfare and feelings; tends to place great emphasis on their own needs and experiences in relationships and social settings with no awareness of the experiences and needs of others
- Is often *envious* of others or assumes that others are envious of them; convinced that the self in fact deserved the attention and recognition that others receive; inclination to devalue the achievements of others
- Attitudes and behaviours characterized by *arrogance and haughtiness* towards others.

As mentioned earlier, it is a significant problem that the formalized diagnostic criteria for NPD in the *DSM* system, as described above, focus almost exclusively on manifestations of narcissistic pathology related to grandiosity and obvious antagonism in interactions with others, while the diagnostic criteria have very limited attention on the manifestations of the often very fragile self-esteem and psychological vulnerability of people with a narcissistic personality disorder. In practice, this means that the formal diagnostic criteria and the formalized diagnostic category of NPD do not reflect the clinical reality, or only do so to a limited degree (Pincus, 2023, p. 632). Furthermore, it could be argued that the diagnostic criteria have a moralistic undertone, in the sense that most of them refer to behaviours that most people would consider unlikable and socially exclusive, while the stated criteria show little empathy for the possible underlying reasons of this behaviour.

The comments to the formal diagnostic criteria do mention that fragile self-esteem in persons with NPD often makes them highly sensitive to criticism, perceived defeat and situations where they may feel hurt – situations where they may feel deeply humiliated, devalued and empty. They also mention that when this happens, persons with NPD may react with intense contempt, rage (cf. narcissistic rage) and (counter)attacks on the person(s) who criticized or simply failed to give the self the positive attention and admiration that the person believes to deserve or require. Alternatively, the person may withdraw from social contact and appear humble in an attempt to mask and protect their grandiose self-image (APA, 2013, p. 671).

However, the core vulnerable elements of NPD are not, or only indirectly, included in the formal diagnostic criteria. The aim is to clarify the distinctions between NPD on the one hand and paranoid and borderline personality disorders on the other (South et al., 2011, p. 23). In practice, however, this means that the *DSM* system does not capture the full spectrum of NPD and can thus be expected to contribute to underdiagnosing NPD or underestimating the extent to which people with psychological difficulties are impacted by pathological narcissism and narcissistic issues. Thus, the manual should arguably include, at least, a formalized and somewhat accurately described variant of NPD that is primarily – or also – characterized by more vulnerable manifestations of NPD. Many have pointed out that patients with predominantly vulnerable manifestations of NPD probably often have more pronounced symptoms and may thus appear more overtly tormented and disturbed, while grandiose manifestations of NPD, particularly the more severe forms, are often associated with more severe structural disturbances or personality organization deficits. Thus, even though they may appear more coherent and stable, due to their grandiose facade, which may, to a superficial observer, compensate for and cover up more severe deficits in personality functioning, they will often be more difficult to treat in a psychotherapeutic framework. In relation to this point, the comorbid presence of antisocial or psychopathic traits will further worsen the treatment prognosis (Hörz-Sagstetter & Kampe, 2021, p. 216).

The DSM-5*'s AMPD*

The key strength of the *DSM* system's Alternative Model for Personality Disorders is that it is centred on a predominantly dimensional understanding of personality disorders that allows for both describing the central elements of the individual's personality functioning or personality pathology and assessing the degree of personality disturbance. This model is related to the psychoanalyst Otto Kernberg's (1984) description of different levels of personality organization, ranging from normal and neurotic organization, characterized by, at most, a slight personality disturbance; to borderline personality organization, where the degree of personality disturbance is considerably more pervasive and typically requires long-term treatment from specially trained psychotherapists; to psychotic personality organization, which describes very severe personality disturbances and represents a sort of border zone to the schizophrenic disorders.

Assessing personality functioning and mapping a potential personality pathology using the alternative model of the *DSM* system involves a series of steps. First, the individual's personality functioning and any degree of pathology are assessed in four central functioning areas centred on the self and the ability to handle interpersonal interactions. Next, the assessment addresses whether the person has one or more of 25 specified pathological personality traits within five general domains: 1) dominance of negative affectivity, 2) detachment, lack of contact with others and thus with the person's own inner emotions 3) interpersonal antagonism, 4) disinhibition, lack of impulse control and an urge for immediate gratification and 5) psychoticism (eccentric, near psychotic subjective experiences and behaviours). These aspects will not be discussed here (for elaboration, see APA, 2013, p. 770, 779 ff.). Finally, it is possible to diagnose one or more of six possible more specific personality disorders: antisocial, evasive (avoidant), borderline, narcissistic, obsessive-compulsive or schizotypal PD. A person who is characterized by at least moderate (or more severe) disturbances in one or more of the four domains of personality functioning – and who is characterized by at least one pathological personality trait – has a personality disorder.

According to the AMPD, the core of any form of personality disorder is dysfunction in the person's self and their interpersonal functioning. Thus, more specifically, the individual's personality functioning and possible degree of pathology is assessed on the four dimensions: identity, self-direction, empathy and intimacy. For each dimension, the rating involves five levels or degrees of dysfunction, ranging from little or no dysfunction (healthy, adaptive functioning) to moderate to severe to extremely impaired personality functioning (for elaboration, see APA, 2013, p. 775 ff.).

The AMPD describes NPD as a personality disorder characterized by variable and vulnerable self-esteem which the person attempts to regulate through attention and approval from others and more overt or predominantly covert grandiosity. More specifically, the criterion for a narcissistic PD diagnosis is moderate or greater impairment in psychological functioning in two or more of the following four areas (APA, 2013, p. 767):

- **Identity:** Pronounced dependence on others for self-definition and self-esteem regulation, including exaggerated tendency for comparisons between self and others (Doering et al., 2021, p. 230). Self-perception and self-regard are excessively positive (inflated, grandiose) or negative (devaluing the self), or there are pronounced fluctuations between these two extremes. Any difficulties in affect regulation are associated with fluctuations in self-esteem.
- **Self-direction:** Personal goals are centred on and based on the desire to gain approval from others. Personal goals and standards are either unrealistically high and associated with (attempts to) see oneself as

exceptional (cf. grandiosity) or remarkably low – and associated with a sense of entitlement (justified solely by being a self-perceived 'special person'). Often unaware of own motivations and drivers behind own behaviour.

- **Empathy:** Impaired capacity for (emotionally) understanding the feelings and needs of others. Strongly preoccupied with other people's reactions but only if these are perceived as relevant to the self. Overestimates or underestimates own effect on others.
- **Intimacy:** Relationships are largely superficial and serve own self-esteem regulation. Mutuality in relationships is constrained due to limited genuine interest in others' experiences and a strong need for satisfying own needs and gaining personal benefits.

In addition, the following two pathological personality traits should be present for a diagnosis of NPD according to the AMPD, both associated with interpersonal antagonism:

- **Grandiosity**: An aspect of antagonism. Overt or more covert feeling of entitlement. The person is self-centred (egocentric) with a firm belief that the self is superior to others. Condescending towards others
- **Attention seeking**: An aspect of antagonism. Strong inclination to seek and demand others' attention and admiration.

The model also allows for the possibility that more vulnerable manifestations of NPD may involve several pronounced and negative affects, such as depressiveness and anxiety, just as intense antagonism in interpersonal interactions can be a prominent trait that needs to be specified in connection with the diagnostic assessment, particularly in the case of more malignant narcissism (APA, 2013, p. 768). As pointed out by Miller et al. (2022), among others, of the six specific personality disorders in the AMPD, NPD is clearly associated with the fewest pathological personality traits, which is not necessarily unproblematic.

In order to minimize the overlap between NPD and antisocial PD – two personality disorders that potentially have shared or closely related elements – the description of NPD has thus been narrowed, at the risk of reducing the clinical validity of the diagnosis and the clinical usefulness of the AMPD, because the described diagnosis fails to sufficiently include and describe the pathological traits we typically see in people with NPD (Miller et al., 2022, p. 407). In particular, this applies to concrete manifestations of interpersonal hostility, such as callousness and manipulative and deceitful behaviour (cf. Miller et al., 2022, p. 408). Meta-analyses of the clinical application of the AMPD's NPD diagnosis further suggest that it correlates much more closely with the typical profile for grandiose manifestations of narcissism than with more vulnerable manifestations (Miller et al., 2022, p. 408).

Thus, it seems that the AMPD has limited usefulness when it comes to addressing the poor ability of our most widespread diagnostic systems to capture vulnerable manifestations of narcissism. We still have the problem of how to arrive at a well-defined diagnostic category for capturing vulnerable manifestations of NPD that is also clearly delineated from a more general description of degrees of psychopathology/personality pathology and dominance of negative affectivity, such as depressiveness, anxiousness and manifestations of low self-esteem (cf. measures of neuroticism). This is not particularly surprising, given that the AMPD also cannot make an NPD diagnosis in the absence of two criteria for predominantly grandiose narcissism: grandiose antagonism and attention seeking.

Differential diagnostics and comorbidity

Comorbidity refers to the phenomenon that a person who meets the diagnostic criteria for a psychological disorder also meets the criteria for one or more other psychological disorders. Often, there may be reason to consider possible dynamic relations between these coinciding psychological disorders – although the phenomenon of comorbidity may also sometimes indicate problems in the delimitation of the various categorical diagnoses. In some cases, it may be difficult to determine which of several parallel psychological disorders should be considered the primary one and should perhaps be given top priority in relation to treatment offers. However, the latter consideration will be of less concern to clinicians working with dynamic relational psychotherapy, as this approach focuses more on the individual and on the dynamic-relational processes underlying the presented symptoms. In this case, specific diagnoses have less influence – and only at a general level – on the psychotherapeutic treatment provided, although qualified diagnostic work is always an important aspect of the assessment and intake process and the referral to different formats and settings of psychotherapy and specific therapists with specialized qualifications for treating more specific disorders, for example cluster B personality disorders (see Jørgensen, 2018/2019).

Often, comorbidity may be seen as an indication that the two (or more) diagnosed disorders in the affected person have a shared aetiology (causal factors, such as an attachment disorder or early neglect) or are driven by the same underlying pathological processes (such as a fragile mentalizing capacity, destructive shame or impulsivity). Alternatively, apparent comorbidity may reflect an overlap between diagnosed disorders (such as grandiosity in NPD and manic states) or stem from the fact that one of the diagnosed disorders (for example NPD) has over time been a contributing factor in the development of other disorders (for example depression and drug abuse). In some cases, it can be difficult to determine, for example, whether NPD or substance abuse is the primary or the secondary disorder (Jurist, 2021, p. 375). These considerations do not question the importance of being aware of the features that generally differentiate NPD from several related personality disorders and symptom disorders.

According to the *DSM-5* (APA, 2013, p. 672), the main challenge will lie in differentiating NPD from histrionic (HPD), dissocial (ASPD) and borderline (BPD) personality disorders: the other three PDs in what the *DSM* system categorizes as cluster B personality disorders and which have certain commonalities and will typically be organized at borderline level in Kernberg's (1984) model for assessing personality functioning. The key point to note is that while the former two are characterized by, in one case (HPD), a seductive interpersonal style, in the other (ASPD), a callous one, individuals with BPD will often be much more variable in their way of relating to others, with a persistent and overt need for contact and a pronounced fear of abandonment. In NPD (cf. the dominant focus of the NPD diagnosis on grandiose manifestations), the identity diffusion that is characteristic of the borderline personality organization is often hidden behind and held in check by grandiose self-perceptions, which also mean that people with NPD often have a greater capacity for tolerating aloneness (Akhtar, 1992, p. 74). In a sense, we could say that the grandiose self stabilizes and compensates for the fragile personality organization and disordered identity – but at the expense, for example, of the capacity for close contact with others and parts of the self.

Conversely, grandiosity and the tendency to be arrogant towards others are particularly characteristic of the *DSM* system's (overly narrow) definition of NPD, just as individuals with NPD are often aloof and detached in contact with others. In some cases, they appear indifferent towards others (cf. a facade of self-reliance and pronounced independence of – or fear of dependence for on – others). Behind the self-reliant facade, however, there is typically a strong need for self-objects (see Chapter 3.3) to mirror and admire the self and serve as idealized external objects to boost the self and, not least, stabilize the person's fragile self-esteem. In this sense, both NPD and BPD are structurally associated with a great need for others; a need that is far more overt in BPD – and in more severe manifestations of vulnerable NPD (see Table 3.1 below). Any insistence on including more vulnerable manifestations of pathological narcissism in diagnosing NPD will lead to a greater overlap with BPD – and, to some extent, social anxiety – which may make it more challenging to distinguish clearly between NPD and BPD (Stanton & Zimmerman, 2018).

Borderline personality disorder

At first glance, individuals with BPD appear clearly dependent on others, while individuals with NPD, particularly predominantly grandiose NPD, deny any form of dependence on or need for contact with others. It could be argued that individuals with (in particular, grandiose) NPD are unable to become truly dependent on others as independent and equal subjects, as this would require their recognition of others as autonomous persons who are clearly differentiated from the self (and beyond the self's control) as well as a certain measure of trust in others – both factors that are typically absent in severe NPD (Kernberg, 1975, p. 240; 2014, p. 867). Conversely, individuals

Table 3.1 Selected criteria for differentiating NPD from BPD. In NPD, the primary focus is on individuals with a slightly better personality organization who mostly have grandiose manifestations of NPD (cf. diagnostic criteria in the DSM system), while BPD is focused on individuals with a poorer personality organization. In terms of personality organization, malignant narcissism and NPD with pronounced dyssocial traits and, to some extent, patients with predominantly vulnerable manifestations of NPD, may be close to BPD, while specific symptoms may in some regards deviate significantly from BPD, particularly for malignant NPD and NPD with pronounced psychopathic traits.

	Narcissistic PD *Organized at low NPO or high to medium or lower BPO level*	*Borderline PD* *Organized at medium or lower BPO level*
Contact with therapist	Often distant, aloof, characterized by arrogance, devaluing, indifference – the therapist is treated as an object, not as an equal subject	Often open to both emotional and psychological contact with therapist – including close contact; but struggles to regulate the balance between closeness and distance – contact may overwhelm the self
Need for others, including the therapist	As a self-object for stabilizing self-esteem via empathic mirroring and/or closeness to an idealized other, including the therapist – may be concealed behind a self-reliant and arrogant facade	For stabilizing self and identity, maintaining coherent identity; in attempts to escape painful feeling of abandonment, aloneness, emptiness
Identity integration	Superficially often relatively stable and integrated identity; identity diffusion covered up by relatively stable grandiose self	Often overtly unstable and poorly integrated identity (identity diffusion); significant fluctuations between very positive (idealized) and negative (devalued) self-regard
Emotional stability	Often relatively high emotional stability; may fail in face of perceived criticism or if expected positive mirroring/admiration from others fails to occur	Great emotional fluctuations, mostly triggered by interpersonal interactions
Impulse control	Often relatively good impulse control; may fail in connection with perceived narcissistic injury (cf. narcissistic rage)	Often problems with impulse control; in the form of both weak and overly rigid impulse control (blocking any form of anger and other impulses)
Capacity for aloneness	Superficially no problems with aloneness; need for others often covered up by arrogant, self-reliant facade – behind it, there may be profound loneliness and alienation from others	Often central problem area; overt and insatiable need for others, yearning for care, contact – but also fear of intimacy, of losing oneself, feeling exposed, defenceless and at risk when opening to close contact; in addition, fear of betrayal, abandonment, rejection

	Narcissistic PD Organized at low NPO or high to medium or lower BPO level	*Borderline PD Organized at medium or lower BPO level*
Self-destructive behaviour	Overt self-harming behaviour is rare	Often different forms of self-harming behaviour; often used as a means of self-regulation and affect regulation
Grandiose self-regard	Often pronounced, an element in regulating self-image and self-esteem – in some cases more 'discreet'	Rare; more prone to unrealistically negative self-regard
Sense of entitlement	Associated with grandiose self-regard; 'I am entitled to special treatment due to my unique qualities'	When it occurs, it is typically driven by a prominent sense of a betrayed, unjustly treated self (victim) that is now entitled to the things it previously missed/ did not receive
Reactions when the therapist fails to show empathy	May destabilize self-esteem and lead to anger, narcissistic rage	May trigger severe regression; fragmentation of self and identity, fear of (psychotic) 'breakdown'; may become overwhelmed by a painful sense of aloneness and fear of destruction of the self

with grandiose narcissism are highly dependent on others in the sense that they typically have a great need for others' attention (uncritical) mirroring and admiration to support their often fragile self-image, self-esteem and apparent autonomy: a facade characterized by arrogant self-sufficiency and what often proves to be pseudo-autonomy. However, this dependence will often be unconscious or denied, while others are not seen and recognized as subjects equal to the self, or it will be dependence on an overtly unrealistic idealized other, who is placed in the position of role model or ideal for the self. In a sense, the need for – or dependence on – others' attention, mirroring and admiration is so intense that the person is unable to contain, let alone acknowledge others' differentiation from and independence of the self.

As mentioned earlier, individuals with NPD often have more stable self-perception. Their identity may appear to be better integrated, although NPD is typically organized at borderline level and thus associated with inadequate integration of the ego-identity (Jørgensen, 2018/2019; Jørgensen et al., 2023). Individuals with mild or moderate NPD (without comorbid BPD) will also not be similarly characterized by impulsive and self-defeating behaviour or by the same overt fear of abandonment and aloneness; the grandiose self is typically more stable than the self in borderline PD and vulnerable manifestations of NPD. Furthermore, anger and hatred in BPD are typically directed more at the person's own self, in the form of self-hatred and overtly self-destructive behaviour, which is why it is often easier to establish emotional contact with a patient with BPD than with individuals with (primarily grandiose) NPD, who are more likely to direct their anger and hatred persistently at others, which can make it more difficult to establish close contact with the patient (cf. Daws, 2024, p. 106).

Compared to persons with BDP, individuals with NPD typically have better impulse control and greater anxiety tolerance, just as they are more emotionally stable (Ronningstam, 2005, p. 116). In NPD, self-injury is not normally used as a method for self-regulation and affect regulation (Vater et al., 2013b, p. 605). Finally, like persons with BPD, individuals with NPD may struggle with feelings of emptiness and perceived meaninglessness, but grandiose feelings about their own self and importance will often keep these symptoms of borderline personality organization (BPO) in check (Ronningstam, 2005, p. 111), particularly if we do not include the most severe NPD disorders. Both NPD and BPD may include a sense of entitlement; however, in NPD, this is primarily associated with a sense of the self's superior and unique qualities, while in BPD, it is more closely associated with a sense that the self is the aggrieved victim of an unjust world and thus now has a particularly great and legitimate need for and right to extraordinary care and attention (Ronningstam & Gunderson, 1991, p. 230).

In extension of this point, several writers have argued that individuals with BPD typically have a more clearly traumatic history and upbringing with severe neglect and abuse, while individuals with NPD are more likely to describe being met with cold indifference and lack of empathy from significant others but also, in some cases, being seen and treated as 'very special', albeit in a manner more mechanical and instrumental than emotional and loving and perhaps accompanied by high expectations of achieving and making something special of themselves that are incongruent with the self's actual abilities and characteristics (Akhtar, 1992, p. 73). However, there is no basis for a clear-cut distinction between NPD and BPD based on whether the individual reports traumatic events in their personal history or particular disturbances in attachment relationships.

Evasive personality disorder

Many experts dealing with evasive personality disorder draw comparisons to vulnerable manifestations of NPD, in particular (Nørgaard & Simonsen, 2019, p. 20 ff.; Simonsen & Euler, 2019). Some (Maria et al., 2021) have pointed to the difficulty of reaching a more precise delimitation of predominantly vulnerable manifestations of NPD and evasive PD – in some contexts referred to as anxious self-insecure personality disorder. Because the more vulnerable manifestations of NPD have such limited representation in the diagnostic criteria for NPD in the *DSM-5*, this issue has been relatively understudied, both in discussions of the diagnostic criteria and in study of differential-diagnostic challenges.

Common features of more vulnerable NPD and evasive PD include clearly fragile self-esteem, tendency to withdraw from or avoid close contact with others, shyness or tendency to appear timid in social settings and high sensitivity to others' gaze on and feelings about the self, including a pronounced tendency to react with and be dominated by destructive shame (cf. Jørgensen, 2023/2024).

It could be argued that the evasive behaviour and tendency to withdraw from contact that is seen in both (particularly vulnerable) NPD and evasive PD are highly driven by unbearable shame. Studies of personality traits in university students, based on simple self-report measures, suggest a certain relationship between higher scores on ratings of narcissistic vulnerability and evasive personality traits, while higher scores on ratings of grandiose narcissism are associated with personality traits related to dissocial and histrionic PD (Dickenson & Pincus, 2003). However, precisely because these findings are based on university students and simple self-report measures, we should be cautious about generalizing them to NPD.

The single factor that decisively differentiates the two disorders is the grandiose sense of self in NPD – a sense of own importance and an expectation of others' admiration of the self as well as a sense of entitlement – that is typically more internal, more concealed and, in some cases, less pronounced in more vulnerable manifestations of NPD but which will manifest itself through longer, closer contact with the person. Furthermore, we should expect that withdrawal to a psychic retreat (see Chapter 3.6) characterized by a grandiose and omnipotent sense of own independence and self-reliance is primarily seen in individuals with vulnerable narcissism, rather than in evasive PD: a withdrawal from close contact with others to imaginary relationships or an absence of any form of interpersonal contact in an attempt to deal with dysregulated self-esteem. Moreover, individuals with vulnerable narcissism will avoid close contact with others in order to protect the self from disappointments and shame over having their expectations of being seen and admired dashed, while individuals with evasive PD primarily withdraw from contact out of fear of rejection or ridicule (Dickenson & Pincus, 2003, p. 190). In addition, there will be greater fluctuations in self-regard in NPD, while the self-perception is often more constantly negative in evasive PD; individuals with evasive PD are generally convinced that the self is inadequate and inherently unattractive to others and thus expect criticism and rejection from others, considering it a natural occurrence.

Individuals with NPD may also be more likely to react to perceived criticism by (counter)attacking the person or persons criticizing the self, while individuals with evasive PD will typically perceive criticism as yet more proof of the defectiveness and inadequacy of the self and react with shame, withdrawal and depressive symptoms (Maria et al., 2021). However, this should be expected to be more common in individuals with predominantly grandiose manifestations of NPD. Finally, the personality will normally be better organized – and with much less identity diffusion – in evasive PD compared with NPD and pathological narcissism. Conversely, evasive PD may also include clear elements of narcissistic imbalances in the form of dysregulated self-esteem and destructive shame, among other traits. Overall, however, the distinction between predominantly vulnerable manifestations of NPD and evasive PD is not clear-cut, and there will be cases in between the two where it may be difficult to determine which diagnosis is the more appropriate.

Histrionic and dissocial PD, malignant narcissism

Considering the differentiation of histrionic (HPD) and narcissistic personality disorder (NPD), one of the main features that set apart (primarily grandiose) NPD is the often pronounced pride of own achievements, the relative absence of deep emotional expressions and the lack of concern for others' feelings. Great susceptibility to others (a variant on great emotional dependence) and a tendency to perceive relationships as being closer than they really are is more characteristic of HPD than of NPD. Conversely, pronounced self-centredness, need for attention and a strong dependence on external sources for propping up fragile self-esteem are characteristic of both HPD and (in particular, vulnerable) NPD, but individuals with HPD have greater tolerance for being dependent on others and are also not nearly as explicitly dismissive and devaluing of others in interactions (Caligor et al., 2015, p. 419). HPD is characterized by greater warmth and does not involve the same narcissistic rage when the person's needs are not met (Akhtar, 1992, p. 72).

Several writers have argued that dissocial or antisocial personality disorder (ASPD) should basically be viewed as a narcissistic disorder and thus as part of a broader spectrum of narcissistic pathology (Walter & Bilke-Hentsch, 2020, p. 18 ff.). This view is related to Kernberg's distinction between different degrees of narcissistic pathology and includes individuals with what he describes as malignant narcissism, which, in addition to NPD includes significant antisocial traits, pronounced egosyntonic aggression or even sadism and a paranoid orientation (Kernberg, 2004a, p. 56 ff.). Kernberg's (2018, p. 201 ff.) concept of malignant narcissism thus describes a (presumably fairly small) group of patients who fall between severe narcissistic and antisocial PD and psychopathy, which also challenges the differentiation of these concepts and diagnostic categories. Notwithstanding, individuals with malignant narcissism and antisocial behaviour will typically have a higher overall interpersonal functioning level than seen in ASPD.

However, if we stick to the formalized diagnostic criteria in the *DSM-5*, individuals with NPD will not be characterized by nearly the same degree of interpersonal aggressivity, impulsivity and inclination to deceive others (moral collapse, severe superego deficits) compared to people with ASPD. Furthermore, persons with ASPD typically do not have the same need for others' admiration to support their own self-esteem, and compared with NPD they are not similarly characterized by envy and overtly grandiose self-regard. Finally, individuals with NPD do not have the same history of conduct disorders during childhood/youth, just as they are also less likely to engage in criminal behaviour (APA, 2013, p. 672), with the possible exception of specific situations driven by narcissistic rage or conflict escalation that are perceived to pose a severe threat to their self-esteem (Ronningstam, 2021, p. 19).

Although aggressivity and lack of empathy are aspects of both ASPD and NPD, conscientiousness and the ability and willingness generally to remain within the boundaries of the law will be somewhat higher in NPD (Widiger, 2011, p. 254 ff.). The degree of superego pathology is lower in NPD, and thus the capacity for self-regulation based on a certain sense of common cultural and societal ethical standards is developed and preserved, to varying degrees, in NPD, which is not the case, or only to a limited degree, in severe ASPD and psychopathy. Kernberg (2004a, p. 56) highlights that individuals with malignant narcissism have preserved or developed a certain capacity for feeling guilt over their own actions and for caring about or considering others, even if their behaviour towards others may sometimes be fierce (sometimes even violent), aggressive, cynical and severely abusive (sadistic). Furthermore, a certain ability to feel shame and to react with shame when the self violates others' boundaries or social norms is a key element in differentiating NPD from psychopathy and antisocial PD (Ritter et al., 2014, p. 435).

Conversely, in several regards, Kernberg's concept of malignant narcissism is quite closely related to psychopathy, just as the most widely used operationalization of psychopathy, Hare's Psychopathy Check List (PCL-R; Hare, 2003), includes a large number of elements that may in practice be difficult to distinguish from NPD, particularly from Kernberg's description of malignant narcissism, including the sense of entitlement, lack of empathy and self-centredness. However, it should be noted that neither psychopathy nor malignant narcissism are recognized diagnostic categories, but both psychopathic and antisocial traits may be prominent in severe (predominantly grandiose) NPD. Generally, researchers working with psychopathy tend to consider severely narcissistic states as an aspect of psychopathy, while researchers working with NPD tend to view psychopathy and psychopathic traits as aspects of severe NPD (Widiger, 2011, p. 252). Several writers have argued that early signs of a narcissistic disorder during childhood may erroneously be diagnosed as ADHD or as various forms of conduct disorders; they point to a high tendency to take offence and an inclination to devalue and show contempt for others in interpersonal conflict situations as particularly significant potential indications of narcissistic development (Walter & Bilke-Hentsch, 2020, p. 24 ff.), perhaps supplemented with an excessive need for attention and admiration as well as high levels of impulsivity, aggressivity and a tendency to violate social norms and rule (Cramer, 2011, p. 20).

Manic states

Grandiosity may also occur in manic and hypomanic states, but in that case, it is much more clearly associated with affective fluctuations while it is more permanent and, in a sense, stable in NPD (APA, 2013, p. 672) – although we should note that grandiosity is often more masked in vulnerable manifestations of NPD. Conversely, temporary hypomanic states also occur in connection with grandiose NDP. In this case, however, mood swings will often be meaningfully related to prior events and interpersonal interactions (Ronning-Ronningstam, 2005, p. 121 ff.). The main feature separating (particularly grandiose) NPD from manic states in bipolar disorders is the self's clear need for positive attention and admiration from others, tendency to devalue others and, often, explicit envy of others (Simonsen & Simonsen, 2011, p. 241) as well as the persistence of grandiose perceptions over time. In bipolar disorders, fluctuations in self-regard and self-esteem are much more dependent on neurobiological swings in the self's basic emotional state; cf. shifts between depressive and manic states, relatively independently of more psychological processes and interpersonal interactions (Ronningstam, 2021, p. 19 ff.). The differentiation of NPD and bipolar disorder is clinically significant, as the two disorders will typically be approached with fundamentally different treatment approaches, given that medical treatment is often a key element in relation to bipolar disorder, while it typically has no effect on NPD.

3.2 Empirical studies of pathological narcissism and related challenges

Until a certain – relatively high – level, 'narcissism' (primarily in the sense of high self-esteem and a positive self-image) does not seem to be associated with subjectively perceived psychological distress. In fact, there are indications that (certain) narcissistic traits are related to better mental health and lower perceived symptom loads, including self-reported symptoms of anxiety, depression and loneliness (Sedikides et al., 2004; Egan et al., 2014). This has been taken as an indication that grandiose self-regard in particular – or high self-esteem – may well serve as a defence against psychological distress and stress, just as narcissism is often associated with an inclination to externalize the cause of perceived problems, which are thus perceived to be someone else's fault and responsibility (Hörz-Sagstetter & Kampe, 2021, p. 216). However, these findings should be understood in light of the fact that narcissism has been understood and measured as a normally occurring dimensional personality trait, which is not sufficiently capable of differentiating and considering how these relationships may be significantly different in clearly pathological narcissism (NPD). Also, the vast majority of studies based on populations that, to varying degrees, actually meet the diagnostic criteria for NPD have relied on the diagnostic criteria for the *DSM* system, which focuses almost exclusively on grandiose manifestations of NPD, not on vulnerable manifestations, which, all things being equal, will be much more closely related to psychological suffering (Blasco-Belled et al., 2024). This point should be borne in mind in relation to the discussion of selected empirical findings in relation to pathological narcissism in the subsequent sections.

Prevalence: How common is NPD?

Normally, it is estimated that about 10% of the population meet the diagnostic criteria for a personality disorder (Morgan & Zimmerman, 2018, p. 186) or perhaps slightly more (cf. Mattia & Zimmerman, 2001, p. 116). NPD is one of the less common personality disorders with a prevalence of about 1% or less. The general consensus is that far more men than women develop a narcissistic personality disorder. The *DSM-5* (APA, 2013, p. 671) estimates that 50–75% of the people who are diagnosed with NPD are men. However, this gender distribution does not necessarily reflect the actual distribution in the general population. The *DSM-5* states prevalences of NPD that vary from 0 to 6.2% (p. 671). The prevalence of NPD in clinical populations is considerably higher. Here, it is estimated at 2–15% (Diamond et al., 2022, p. 27), presumably highest in outpatient clinics (p. 4) and in some settings as high as around 20% (Pincus, 2023, p. 630). One systematic review estimates the prevalence of NPD in clinical populations to be up to 35% (Dhawan et al., 2010, p. 336). This latter level may occur in certain specific clinical populations but is unlikely to reflect the presence of NPD in clinical populations overall. A few slightly older studies, conversely, found a remarkably low prevalence of NPD in clinical populations, as low as around 2% (Zimmerman et al., 2005, p. 1912), although it is somewhat higher in more specific clinical populations, for example close to 6% among patients with alcohol abuse (p. 1915).

However, there are several problems associated with these estimates of the prevalence of NPD. First, there are very few large and high-quality population studies in which researchers with clinical qualifications rated the presence of NPD based on interviews; that is, studies that are not based on self-report questionnaires, which is a notoriously unreliable method for more valid diagnostic assessments. Furthermore, almost all prevalence studies are based on the diagnostic criteria for the *DSM* system, which does not capture vulnerable manifestations of NPD.

The largest single prevalence study of personality disorders was carried out in the United States from 2004 to 2005. In this study, more than 34,000 participants were interviewed in an effort to measure the prevalence of psychological disorders in a fairly representative adult population group (Stinson et al., 2008). The study found a prevalence of NPD of more than 6% – close to 8% among men and under 5% among women. It has been pointed out that these apparent gender differences in the prevalence of NPD may be more reflective of variations among ethnic groups – and thus possible (sub) cultural differences – in this prevalence study (Pulay et al., 2011, p. 174). The highest prevalence was found among men aged 20 to 29 years, of whom 9.4% met the formal diagnostic criteria for NPD. Generally, the share of people who meet the diagnostic criteria for NPD is highest in early adulthood and then tapers off significantly (Hasin & Grant, 2015, p. 1617). Even though this study is methodologically exemplary in many regards, it also presents a few significant problems.

The main problem in relation to the present context was pointed out in connection with a subsequent re-analysis of the data (Trull et al., 2010). The core of the problem is that the researchers initially looked only at the number of people who formally meet the narrow diagnostic criteria for NPD without also addressing whether the individual participants' level of psychosocial functioning was markedly impaired and/or whether they experienced significant subjective distress in relation to the NPD criteria that they met. Furthermore, the diagnostic assessment was conducted by research assistants, rather than experienced clinicians, which is also problematic (Paris, 2014, p. 221). When this aspect is considered – for each diagnostic criterion leading to a fairly conservative interpretation of the diagnostic criteria – the prevalence of NPD drops sharply, to about 1%, with just 0.7% for women and 1.2% for men (Trull et al., 2010; see also Eaton et al., 2018, p. 29).

A special issue in relation to this point is that particularly more grandiose manifestations of NPD may be seen in individuals who in many ways have a high level of functioning with no significant level of perceived subjective distress. These individuals may meet the formal diagnostic criteria for NPD but, due to their high level of functioning and apparent absence of subjective distress, it could be argued that an NPD diagnosis is not appropriate, even though they formally meet the authorized diagnostic criteria. Conversely, it could also be argued that grandiose manifestations of NPD may cover up and serve as attempts to compensate for severe personality pathology but that this pathology is not necessarily overt, let alone captured by more superficial assessments, precisely because of these individuals' grandiose appearance. Further, we might consider whether and, if so, how subjective distress in others caused, for example, by cynical and unempathic actions by a person with grandiose NPD should be included in the diagnostic assessment; a choice that would presumably increase the estimated prevalence of NPD. It is also worth noting that NPD occurs more commonly among individuals who live alone, compared with people who are in a steady relationship (Stinson et al., 2008, p. 1036), which may not be a coincidence.

The relatively few and mainly older existing meta-analyses of population studies of NPD all arrive at a prevalence around 1% (Torgersen et al., 2001; Dhawan et al., 2010; Morgan & Zimmerman, 2018, p. 183), perhaps with a slightly rising trend from the *DSM-III* to the *DSM-IV* (Morgan & Zimmerman, 2018) but still in line with the 'corrected' prevalence (Trull et al., 2010) in the above-mentioned large-scale American study (Stinson et al., 2008). Overall, the most reasonable estimate of the prevalence of the largely grandiose manifestation of NPD is thus around 1% of the adult population. If individuals with predominantly more vulnerable manifestations of NPD are included as well, there is reason to assume that the prevalence is higher but probably not much more than 1.5–2%, corresponding to the prevalence of most of the other personality disorders.

Gender differences

Even though it is estimated, as mentioned above, that a higher share of men, compared with women, meet the diagnostic criteria for NPD, there is reason to consider whether this is in fact correct. As argued by leading researchers in the field (Diamond et al., 2022, p. 26; Levy et al., 2021, p. 191), based on the existing prevalence studies, it is difficult to determine the true gender distribution of NPD, in part because most formalized methods that are used in diagnostic assessments of NPD focus mainly on the more grandiose manifestations of narcissism. To the extent that women with NPD might be characterized more by predominantly vulnerable manifestations of NPD, such diagnostic practice would skew the gender distribution of NPD and result in underdiagnosis among women. A few studies support the assumption that more vulnerable manifestations of pathological narcissism in women are underdiagnosed (Riegel et al., 2022). In addition, there is also reason to assume that there may be considerable cross-cultural variation in the specific manifestations of NPD (Ronningstam, 2005, p. 63), just as we may presume the influence of cultural variation in, for example, when a given behaviour is considered to be so grandiose and so out of step with 'reality' – which to some extent is determined based on social norms and conventions of what is considered normal socially acceptable being and acting – that it is regarded as pathological and thus included in diagnosing a psychiatric disorder such as NPD.

A comprehensive meta-analysis of narcissistic traits (not NPD) based on 350 studies totalling more than half a million participants, primarily studies of university students and other non-clinical populations and mostly in North America, found that men on average have more pronounced narcissistic traits than women (Grijalva et al., 2015a). This gender difference is primarily driven by men typically getting higher scores on self-report measures for tendency to exploit others, sense of entitlement due to their uniqueness, and urge to assume positions of leadership and authority. The observed gender differences occur less for measures of so-called self-absorption and exhibitionism, although men do have marginally higher scores here, while no gender differences have been observed for more vulnerable manifestations of narcissism.

Thus, overall, this meta-analysis finds that men on average have higher scores for what might broadly be described as non-pathological grandiosity, while there do not appear to be discernible gender differences for more vulnerable manifestations of narcissism. However, it should be noted that the vast majority of studies included in this meta-analysis focus mainly on more grandiose manifestations of narcissism, which somewhat weakens the basis for assessing the true gender variation in the prevalence of vulnerable narcissistic traits. Furthermore, there may be reason to consider how the methods that were used to operationalize key narcissistic traits are associated with prevailing stereotypical perceptions of (possibly toxic) masculinity in modern

Western culture (cf. physical manifestations of anger and aggressivity, need for power, tendency to assume authority, lack of empathy and so forth).

A more recent meta-analysis confirms the impression that men generally have higher scores on measures of narcissistic traits (Weidmann et al., 2023). In line with earlier analysis, it also found that the level of narcissism is higher among young adults and then tapers off over the course of life. Here too, the observed gender differences seem to be attributable to predominantly grandiose narcissistic traits: the variation is highest for measures of what this study calls self-centred antagonism and agentic extroversion (p. 1292), both of which are associated with manifestations of more grandiose traits and have higher scores among men. The authors also note that the studies used a wide range of self-report questionnaires, which do not all measure the same factors, let alone rely on the same definition and understanding of narcissism. This is not unproblematic and raises the question that should always be asked of meta-analyses: do they conflate things that are in fact different in a laudable attempt to summarize existing findings?

Comorbidity: NPD and other psychological disorders

Because narcissistic disorders, particularly their more grandiose manifestations, are associated with a tendency for inflated self-perception and an urge for self-reliance (cf. also fear of dependence and of revealing one's own vulnerability), individuals with NPD will typically come into contact with therapists at a stage when more vulnerable manifestations of NPD are dominant or when the narcissistic disorder is overshadowed by other, comorbid disorders, such as depression, anxiety or substance abuse or in connection with attempted suicide, which serve as the initial basis of referral to various forms of treatment. In this situation, it is crucial to be able to uncover any underlying narcissistic personality pathology and to make this a key focus of the treatment.

Some of the above-mentioned issues with empirical studies of NPD also apply to the available studies of comorbid disorders in relation to NPD. Because the formal diagnostic criteria for NPD that are used in these studies (typically the *DSM*) focus overwhelmingly on – and capture only – more grandiose manifestations of NPD, more vulnerable manifestations of NPD will typically be overlooked. This may also lead us not just to underestimate the prevalence of vulnerable NPD but also of comorbid disorders that are primarily associated with more vulnerable manifestations of NPD.

The above-mentioned large-scale prevalence study in the United States (Stinson et al., 2008) also looked at the prevalence of comorbid disorders with NPD and at how often NPD appears as a comorbid disorder in connection with some of the most common psychological disorders. The study of both these topics looked primarily at lifetime prevalence to identify how big a share of the study participants who at some point in their life met the diagnostic criteria for NPD also, at some point, had another psychological disorder and, vice versa, how many of the participants who at some point in life met the diagnostic criteria for a given psychological disorder also met the diagnostic criteria for NPD sometime in their life.

Depression and other symptom disorders

In relation to the Stinson study's assessment of comorbidity with some of the most common psychological disorders, it is worth noting that almost half of the individuals with NPD have or previously had an affective disorder; 29% within the past year (Stinson et al., 2008, p. 1037). Close to two-thirds have or previously had substance abuse issues; 40% within the past year (see also Ritter et al., 2010). Also, more than half the people with NPD have or previously had an anxiety disorder; 40% within the past year (Stinson et al., 2008, p. 1037).

Conversely, the prevalence of NPD among individuals with anxiety or affective disorders is relatively low, which should be understood in light of the generally fairly low prevalence of NPD in the population at large. Furthermore, the relatively low prevalence of NPD among people with depression may also be related to the fact that the assessment is based on the *DSM* system's diagnostic criteria for NPD. Studies thus suggest that vulnerable manifestations of narcissism are far more closely associated with depression than are grandiose manifestations, which are the predominant variant captured by the diagnostic criteria for NPD in the *DSM* system (Marcinko et al., 2014; see also Russ et al., 2008, p. 1478; Zabel, 2019). One study found perfectionism to be a significant mediator of the relationship between vulnerable narcissism and depression (Marcinko et al., 2014). Finally, it should be noted that the prevalence of NPD among individuals with drug abuse/dependence is relatively high; Stinson et al. (2008, p. 1038) find that as many as 26% of men with drug addiction meet the diagnostic criteria for NPD.

Compared with other (typically far smaller) studies, there are some indications that the Stinson et al. (2008) study may somewhat overestimate the comorbidity levels, perhaps apart from the sometimes relatively close relationship between NPD and depression (Ritter et al., 2010; Simonsen & Simonsen, 2011). Other, relatively small studies based on clinical populations thus found a somewhat lower comorbidity of, for example, anxiety disorders in individuals with NPD (29% within the past year; Ritter et al., 2010, p. 19).

Depression and various forms of substance abuse are relatively common in persons with NPD, and in the individual case, it may be relevant to consider whether the development of depression and abuse might be associated with a collapse of grandiose self-regard or underlying destructive shame, with substance abuse offering a form of escape from a painful reality and an attempt to stabilize fragile self-esteem. In extension of this point, several authors have argued that depression and depressive symptoms in NPD should, in many cases, be regarded as a sequela or as a manifestation of underlying destructive shame, with despair, emptiness and meaninglessness as prominent symptoms (Ronningstam, 2005, p. 124). Individuals with NPD may also develop a depression later in life, as they inevitably come face to face with the finite nature of life and their own beginning decay and the resulting difficulties with continuing to achieve the same positive attention and admiration from others that they were able to secure earlier in life. Often, the grandiose self is unstable and dependent on persistent confirmation from others.

More generally, it is debatable whether it is meaningful to distinguish as sharply and categorically between certain psychological disorders, including NPD and depression, as our diagnostic systems clearly suggest (cf. the close dynamic psychological relationship between the breakdown of grandiose self-regard and the development of depression-like symptoms). As stated by several authors (Diamond et al., 2022, p. 27), depression in NPD will often be characterized more by emptiness, meaninglessness and anhedonia than by extensive sadness, guilt and a sense that the self is worthless; cf. the close relationship between NPD, identity diffusion and borderline personality organization (see Chapter 3.4) and Kohut's (1977, p. 126) concept of 'empty depression', which he associates with pathological narcissism. This also means that clinicians diagnosing and treating depression need to bear in mind that a symptom picture characterized by depressive symptoms, destructive shame and perhaps pronounced perfectionism could be a manifestation of vulnerable narcissism, which may not really become evident until the patient also shows signs of grandiose feelings or (narcissistic) anger/rage (Kealy & Ogrodniczuk, 2011, p. 293; Fjermestad-Noll et al., 2020a, p. 26 ff.).

Conversely, comorbid depression or depressive symptoms may also be a positive prognostic factor in individuals with severe and predominantly grandiose manifestations of NPD, since they may indicate a certain ability to grieve, emotional sensitivity beyond outward aggression and cracks in the grandiose armour; all of these are psychological processes that are important for the ability to establish emotional contact with a therapist and maintain more persistent motivation for psychotherapeutic work; cf. also Melanie Klein's concept of the depressive position and related depressive affects as signs of a certain integration of the personality (Klein, 1952/1975, p. 64 ff.; Jørgensen, 2009, p. 262 ff.).

As mentioned earlier, the most significant criticism of Stinson et al.'s (2008) otherwise very convincing population study is that it does not give nearly enough consideration to subjectively perceived distress and clearly reduced functioning levels in assessing whether the diagnostic criteria for NPD have been met (see above). Specifically, this means that the study includes a considerable group of people who, although they meet the formal diagnostic criteria for NPD, are unlikely to seek treatment, given that they do not experience significant subjective distress, let alone markedly impaired functioning, and that individuals with high-functioning narcissism may in some cases meet the diagnostic criteria for NPD. If they were to seek treatment at some point, this is likely to be because they have developed secondary symptom disorders, substance abuse or other forms of self-harming behaviour, and the underlying NPD may go undetected. In relation to everyday clinical practice, this may mean that the comorbid disorders seen here do not necessarily fully correspond to what Stinson et al. (2008) presented, based on their study of the general population.

As several researchers and clinicians have noted, there is generally reason to assume that grandiose manifestations of NPD are more likely to be associated with more externalizing comorbid disorders, such as substance abuse, bipolar disorder, antisocial and perhaps histrionic and paranoid personality disorders, while more vulnerable manifestations of NPD will be more likely to co-occur with more internalizing disorders, such as anxiety and affective disorders, perhaps also borderline, evasive (avoidant) and dependent PD (Dickinson & Pincus, 2003; Russ et al., 2008, p. 1478; Caligor et al., 2015, p. 417; Kaufman et al., 2020; Hörz-Sagstetter & Kampe, 2021, p. 217). However, these relationships still lack sufficient empirical support, mostly because empirical studies of NPD, as mentioned earlier, focus exclusively on grandiose manifestations of NPD. Generally, there is reason to assume that if more vulnerable manifestations of NPD were included in studies of comorbid symptom disorders, one would find significantly higher levels of comorbidity between NPD and several more internalizing symptom disorders (Simonsen & Simonsen, 2011, p. 243; Marcinko et al., 2014, p. 342; Zabel, 2019, p. 109). Conversely, particularly mild and moderate grandiose narcissistic traits may offer some protection against the development of certain internalizing symptom disorders and diminished psychological well-being (Kaufman et al., 2020, p. 122 ff.).

Other personality disorders

As many as two-thirds of the people who meet the diagnostic criteria for NPD at some time in their lives will also have met criteria for at least one other PD (lifetime prevalence), usually BPD, which occurs in more than one third (37%) of the people who meet the criteria for NPD, followed by schizotypal PD (StPD), with about one quarter (27%). In relation to this, Stinson et al. (2008) found that 39% of the individuals who meet the diagnostic criteria for BPD at some time in their life also met the criteria for NPD at some point; the similar share for StPD is as high as 43%. Taken together, these findings suggest a considerable overlap between NPD and, in particular, BPD as well as, to some extent, schizotypal and histrionic PD. We should also expect a significant overlap between NPD and evasive PD, perhaps also dependent PD, if the diagnostic assessment sufficiently takes into account the predominantly vulnerable manifestations of narcissistic personality pathology. Individuals with comorbid NPD and BPD will often be among the most challenging PD patients to treat (Diamond et al., 2022, p. 328), in part because they will often have very low anxiety tolerance, severe identity diffusion, poor impulse control, very fragile self-esteem, severely disturbed relationships, primitive defences, a history of traumatic experience, and a grandiose self that is both rigid and fragile. Conversely, comorbid BPD may make the patient's poor functioning and need for help more obvious and thus enhance the patient's treatment motivation (Ronningstam & Weinberg, 2023, p. 350).

It should also be noted that some older studies found somewhat higher levels of comorbidity between NPD and the other cluster B personality disorders than were found in Stinson et al. (2008). This includes findings that 40% of individuals who meet *DSM-III-R* criteria for NPD also meet criteria for antisocial PD, and 40% meet the criteria for histrionic PD (HPD), while as many as 60% of individuals who meet *DSM-III-R* criteria for HPD also meet the diagnostic criteria for NPD (Widiger, 2011, p. 249).

Gender variations

The comorbidity between NPD and other psychological disorders shows some degree of gender variation. Simply put, NPD is considerably more common among men with various types of substance abuse than among women with substance abuse issues. NPD is also considerably more common among men with affective disorders. For several affective disorders, the prevalence of comorbid NPD is about twice as high among men than among women; for example, Stinson et al. (2008, p. 1038) found that 17% of men with severe depression meet the diagnostic criteria for NPD, while the same is only true of 9% of women with severe depression. In several anxiety disorders, the prevalence of comorbid NPD is also clearly higher among men than among women; for example, about one in four men with PTSD meets the diagnostic criteria for NPD (26%), while the same was only found for 13% of women with PTSD.

As for gender variations in the prevalence of other comorbid disorders in persons with NPD, there are a few striking patterns. One is that all types of substance abuse are much more common among men with NPD. For example Stinson et al. (2008, p. 1038) found that 63% of men with NPD have some form of alcohol abuse, while the same was only found for 34% of women with NPD. Conversely, more internalizing symptom disorders – affective and anxiety disorders – are generally somewhat more common among women with NPD than among men; for example, 25% of women with NPD had a depression at some time in their lives, while the same was only found for 17% of men with NPD. Also, 34% of women with NPD were diagnosed with PTSD at some point in life, which was only found for 20% of men with NPD.

Looking at the prevalence of comorbid NPD in individuals with other personality disorders, it is particularly noteworthy that comorbid NPD is clearly more common in men with borderline, histrionic or dependent PD than in women with the same personality disorders. Generally, it is only among individuals with antisocial PD that the prevalence of comorbid NPD is not considerably higher for men than for women (Stinson et al., 2008, p. 1038). Similarly, antisocial PD is almost twice a common among men with NPD (14%) than among women (8%) who meet the diagnostic criteria for NPD (p. 1038).

Naturally, all comorbidity findings should be viewed and understood in light of the fact that NPD, as it is defined in the *DSM* system, is generally considerably more common among men than among women (see the section on prevalence above). Thus, we should expect NPD to appear more often as a comorbid disorder in men with various other psychological disorders. Unfortunately, we still have little insight into the prevalence and comorbidity of various psychological disorders in individuals with a non-binary gender identity. This is problematic and marks an important future research topic, not least with a view to understanding possible dynamic psychological interactions between gender identity, sexual orientation, perceived social inclusion/exclusion and the development of psychological disorders.

Arguably, studies of comorbidity are in themselves relatively uninteresting expressions of the zealous classification of people into various diagnostic categories with related statistical analyses of which diagnoses are likely to occur or co-occur in these individuals. From a clinical perspective, however, it is meaningful to have a sense of the possible relationship and, not least, dynamic psychological connection between NPD and substance abuse – perhaps as an attempt to stabilize fragile self-esteem – and depression – perhaps in reaction to or as a result of the breakdown of a grandiose and omnipotent sense of self. It is also meaningful to understand how a grandiose sense of self may be an attempt (perhaps in combination with a form of substance abuse) to deal with anxiety and past traumas (PTSD).

Furthermore, studies of comorbidity may help indicate overlaps between specific disorders that differ in key regards – especially with regard to treatment – which makes careful diagnostics particularly crucial. This includes the border zone between NPD and bipolar disorders (particularly bipolar I), given that medication is often a central element in the treatment of bipolar disorders and is ineffective in NPD. Finally, the high level of comorbidity between certain personality disorders, such as NPD and BPD – and in some cases, NPD and schizotypal PD – among others, is seen as an indication of serious problems in the way our authorized diagnostic systems delimit some of the categorical PD diagnoses. These problems may be viewed as an argument both for the need to operate with fewer specific PD diagnoses and for replacing the purely categorical PD diagnostic approach with a more (but not exclusively) dimensional understanding and diagnosis of PDs, including narcissistic pathology.

Suicide risk

There is reason to assume that individuals with a combination of affective dysregulation (including impulsivity), a grandiose sense of self as an attempt to deal with fragile self-esteem, and narcissistic vulnerability have a heightened risk of suicidal behaviour, particularly in association with relational difficulties, including painful loneliness, experiences of exclusion or abandonment and escalating interpersonal conflicts (Blasco-Fontecilla et al., 2009, p. 1583). Acute narcissistic injury to a fragile narcissistic self may result in overwhelming shame and humiliation and thus a significantly increased risk of suicide (Gabbard & Crisp, 2018, p. 133). The same is presumably true of self-harming behaviour without suicidal intentions (Dawood et al., 2018). In dynamic psychological terms, both may be viewed as attempts to escape or regulate overwhelming mental states and may be associated with an urge for self-punishment and aggression directed at the self.

Several studies have found that manifestations of pathological narcissism, particularly vulnerable ones, are associated with a higher occurrence of suicidal ideation and increased risk of attempted suicide (Giner et al., 2013; Ansell et al., 2015; Jaksic et al., 2017). A few of these studies suggest that NPD is associated with increased risk of attempted suicide in connection with interpersonal conflict, negative life events (job loss) and stressful life circumstances (health issues, financial worries) (Blasco-Fontecilla et al., 2010). Furthermore, a few studies found that NPD, as the only PD, is associated with a growing number of suicide attempts over time (Ansell et al., 2015) and that attempted suicide in individuals with NPD is less impulsive and, not least, associated with greater risk of completed suicide, compared with suicide attempts in individuals with other personality disorders (Blasco-Fontecilla et al., 2009).

In extension of this point, a study comparing individuals who attempted suicide (n=446) to individuals who completed suicide (n=190) found that individuals in latter group were 20 times more likely to have NPD and other health issues – and 10 times more likely to be male – compared to the former group. More than 20% of individuals in the latter group had NPD (Giner et al., 2013). Studies also suggest that NPD in itself is associated with a heightened risk of suicidal behaviour in connection with stressful experiences and negative life events, such as serious conflicts with a partner, job loss or financial problems, that are generally associated with a heightened risk of suicidal behaviour (Blasco-Fontecilla et al., 2010).

The role of destructive shame

Researchers have suggested that there may be a close relationship between destructive shame and suicidal behaviour in individuals with narcissistic disturbances, particularly severe NPD (Ansell et al., 2015, p. 165). Severe emotional crises and suicidal behaviour in persons with NPD may thus be understood in connection with destructive shame triggered by a sense of failure or humiliation (Links, 2013, p. 176), just as severe destructive shame may cause the narcissistically disordered person to withdraw from contact and choose not to share their suicidal ideation with anyone, which may in itself increase the risk of acting out the suicidal ideation in the form of attempted suicide and ultimately complete suicide, given that destructive shame should be viewed as an antitherapeutic affect that it is important for the therapist to be able to capture and address in psychotherapy (Jørgensen, 2023/2024). Conversely, suicidal ideation and attempted suicide may also put persons with NPD into contact with the mental healthcare system (Links, 2013, p. 167), where they may – ideally – receive an offer of qualified psychotherapeutic treatment.

In a study based on individuals in outpatient psychiatric treatment found that vulnerable narcissism (as a personality trait) in particular is associated with an increased occurrence of suicidal ideation (Jaksic et al., 2017). Although the study also found a certain relationship between grandiose narcissistic personality traits and suicidal ideation, it was much less pronounced. It also found that the relationship between narcissistic vulnerability and suicidal ideation is mediated by perceived shame, which supports the assumption that destructive shame is a potentially highly significant driver of suicidal behaviour, possibly not only in individuals with NPD but generally. The authors point to perceived narcissistic injury and the absence of positive feedback or mirroring from others – mirroring that would serve to support a fragile self-image and fragile self-esteem – as contributing factors in causing a breakdown of grandiose self-regard in individuals with a narcissistic disorder in combination with overwhelming destructive shame, which may subsequently be a driver of suicidal behaviour (Jaksic et al., 2017, p. 1672).

For a person with grandiose self-regard, threats to a fragile self-image may be an extraordinarily shameful and humiliating experience that may lead to narcissistic rage; a rage that may, in some cases, be directed at the self, perhaps in the form of suicidal behaviour (Ronningstam & Maltsberger, 1998, p. 267). Conversely, grandiose self-regard and manipulation of others to achieve support for fragile self-esteem can often help regulate (reduce) suicidal behaviour (Jaksic et al., 2017, p. 1676). This will presumably be particularly likely as long as these grandiose feelings do not become so severely challenged by actual setbacks or absence of confirmation from others that they break down and in persons who are not characterized by a high degree of impulsivity. Similarly, outward aggression or rage in response to narcissistic injury or perceived unjust treatment of the self, perhaps indignation that the (grandiose) self does not receive the expected and demanded special treatment, may presumably reduce the risk of suicidal behaviour – provided the self is able to act out this defence strategy without being met by firm social sanctions, including social exclusion, which in some cases may contribute to the collapse of the grandiose sense of self.

Suicidal behaviour as an attempt to regulate the threatened self

An older qualitative interview study of NPD patients who attempted suicide found that grandiosity may be associated with attempted suicide (Ronning-Ronningstam & Maltsberger, 1998). It described how attempted suicide may be related to illusory ideas that this will give the self control (agency) and thus confirms its grandiose fantasies of the self as unique. This may, for example, include notions that suicide would allow the self to explore life after death or demonstrate its ability to overcome death – but also massive denial of the risk of serious self-injury and death. The danger that the person subjects itself to is dissociated or trivialized: 'I fear nothing, not even death' (p. 262). In addition to using impulsive suicide as an illusory way out, in an attempt to escape unbearable subjective experiences of defeat, humiliation, having failed, being a failure and feeling trapped in an unbearable situation, glorification of death and grandiose (perhaps near psychotic) fantasies of the self's life after death may also play a role in connection with attempted suicide in persons with NPD (Ronningstam et al., 2018).

Suicidal ideation and suicidal behaviour may thus also be understood as manifestations of dysfunctional and potentially fatal strategies for regulating unbearable emotional states, perhaps associated with grandiose fantasies that the self may thus demonstrate its superiority and ability to overcome any form of pain and even death, in a dissociation of the potential real consequences (death) of one's own actions (Ronningstam & Maltsberger, 1998, p. 268). Suicidal behaviour may be a desperate attempt to escape passive humiliation or protect the self from an anticipated or dreaded narcissistic injury or humiliation, as the person, so to speak, prefers death to such deep humiliation (Ronningstam, 2005, p. 161 ff.).

Particularly in the case of severely malignant narcissism, serious self-harm and suicidal behaviour may represent attempts to achieve some degree of control over others and demonstrate one's own power or superiority in relation to others; a severely disturbed and desperate attempt to demonstrate that one is not afraid of pain, disease or death and is in control of one's own existence (Diamond et al., 2022, p. 360). If the world is not going to live up to what the self perceives as its completely legitimate needs and expectations, the self prefers to leave (through suicide), rather than suffering the humiliation of submitting itself to a cold and cynical world that does not understand and is unwilling to meet the needs of the self (Diamond et al., 2022, p. 360). Finally, in some cases, we may understand suicidal behaviour as an attempt to demonstrate one's own superiority and take revenge on the people around the self who have tried to help the person who has malignant narcissism. In this case, the urge for omnipotent control over others or 'reality' in general and destructive aggression are both important drivers (p. 360).

Tolstoy's (1878/2010) description of the internal and external events leading to Anna Karenina's suicide may be seen as an illustration of how suicide may be both an attempt to reclaim agency, take revenge on others, and escape unbearable mental states, particularly perceived narcissistic injury and unbearable shame. All of this is further embedded in grandiose fantasies about how the self stands to benefit from and be rehabilitated after death. After yet another row and an escalating conflict with her lover, officer Vronsky, that left her feeling humiliated and overwhelmed by shame, Anna thinks,

> Yes, that was the thought that would solve everything. 'Yes, to die! Alexis Alexandrovich's shame and disgrace, and Serezha's, and my own – terrible shame – all will be saved by my death. If I die he too will repent, will pity me, will love me and will suffer on my account!'
>
> (pp. 876 ff.)

Anna Karenina sees death

> as the sole means of reviving love for herself in his heart, of punishing him, and of gaining the victory in that contest which an evil spirit in her heart was waging against him, presented itself clearly and vividly to her. [...] [She] began thinking with pleasure of how he would suffer, repent, and love her memory when it was too late.
>
> (p. 884)

Just before she throws herself under the enormous cast-iron wheels of the passing train, she thinks, 'There, into the very middle [between the wheels of the moving train], and I shall punish him and escape from everybody and from myself!' (p. 904).

Together, the findings outlined above suggest that NPD is associated with a considerably heightened risk of suicidal behaviour and underscores the importance of continually considering the risk of suicide in contact with individuals with NPD. Similarly, when assessing the risk of suicide in general, it is important to screen for NPD or signs of pathological narcissism. Another reason for the increased risk of suicide in NPD is that suicidal behaviour may be more difficult to determine in persons with NPD and that we may typically associate suicide risk with depression, while increased suicidal behaviour in NPD is not associated with depressive symptoms (Pincus, 2023, p. 614). Furthermore, disinclination and a poor ability to articulate and share painful emotions and thoughts with others may intensify feelings such as loneliness, hopelessness, abandonment, social isolation and self-hatred, and thus increase the risk of suicidal behaviour in individuals with NPD (Ronningstam et al., 2018, p. 497). Moreover, this may further exacerbate a painful – but in some cases also ambivalent – feeling of not being seen, of being invisible, and a resulting tendency to seek refuge in an inner world where no one else has access. Here, the self may have constructed its own imaginary universe and, in a sense, feel safe, but it may also be a very lonesome place, where suicidal ideation can escalate without being shared with and moderated by others. In extension of this point, it is also important to be aware that destructive shame may cause the NPD patient to withdraw and intensify an existing reluctance to share difficult experiences with others, including therapists, which may further raise the risk of suicidal behaviour (Jaksic et al., 2017, p. 1678).

Relational difficulties

Narcissism, grandiose narcissism in particular, is associated with certain other personality traits and behaviours in interactions with others that will often lead to considerable problems with establishing and maintaining well-functioning relationships. As mentioned above, individuals with pathological narcissism will typically try to use others to stabilize their fundamentally vulnerable self and unstable self-esteem. To the extent that others are thus used as self-objects for the satisfaction of the self's own needs and are not, or only partially, recognized as differentiated and autonomous subjects, it becomes difficult to establish more mature relationships characterized by reciprocity and equality. In pathological narcissism, grandiose self-regard develops in an attempt to stabilize the self, as parts of reality that do not support or which threaten to undermine these grandiose self-fantasies will have to be denied (Caligor et al., 2015, p. 417 ff.). Close and genuine contact with others may confront the self with these denied and dissociated aspects of itself and with characteristics in others that it lacks, which may also lead to toxic envy, feelings of inferiority and shameful inadequacy. For this reason too, these individuals may withdraw from and avoid contact with others in an attempt to protect a vulnerable self from humiliation and other forms of harm. Alternatively, the other may be reduced to a one-dimensional mirror that is perceived solely as an extension of the person's own self and be used to mirror and support the person's own fragile – perhaps superficially grandiose – self. The other is not seen and recognized as an independent subject in their own right, which will pose an obstacle to the establishment of mature and equal relationships.

To varying degrees, the person's approach to others is instrumental and characterized by attempts to make others admire and recognize the self as special and thus accept their entitlement to special treatment. When persons with pathological narcissism, for various reasons, are self-referential, self-aggrandizing, intrusive and intimidating in their interactions with others, this may in many ways be detrimental to the development of close emotional contact, resonance and well-functioning relationships (Gabbard & Crisp, 2018, p. 35; Diamond et al., 2022, p. 124 ff.; Kealy & Ogrodniczuk, 2011). The same applies to tendencies to appear blunt, unempathic, vindictive, dominant and controlling and to constantly compare themself to – and act as if the self is in a constant competition with – others. This said, it is important to bear in mind that there may be considerable variation and fluctuations in the interpersonal functioning of individuals with pathological narcissism, with some individuals mostly appearing charming and friendly, while others are far more likely to appear shy, vulnerable and quiet, and yet others will appear arrogant, domineering, aggressive, manoeuvring and intimidating (Ronningstam, 2021, p. 10). Finally, there may be significant swings between grandiose self-reliance and vulnerable inferiority accompanied by a pronounced need for others to prop up and stabilize the self.

In an encounter with someone who has a strong need to control others, driven by narcissistic pathological processes, it is important to preserve one's ability to have nuanced thoughts about how to understand this powerful urge for control, being on top and appearing arrogant and implicitly or very explicitly degrading towards others. In one case, a male patient, large and powerful of stature, who has a personality disorder with clear pathological narcissistic traits and who generally appears resolute and often describes himself solving various problems for others, mentions that he always needs to stay ten steps ahead of everyone else. Gradually, it becomes clear that, above all, he has to avoid being surprised, caught unawares and overwhelmed by other people's reactions, which to him is associated with being humiliated and in danger. The same applies in the therapeutic space, where he clearly becomes nervous and requests a short break whenever the therapist approaches areas that are sensitive for him, and when the therapist asks questions or articulates impressions or reflections that had not occurred to the patient himself. Over the course of the therapy, it becomes clear that this grandiose defence is driven by experiences during his upbringing when he and his mother always had to be alert and ready to flee at a moment's notice if his father had an outburst and threatened to kill the whole family. From an early time in his life, he had had to develop physical strength and rely on his own ability to predict and handle other people's reactions in order to protect himself, his mother and his younger sister from a seemingly severely dissocial and violent father.

Several have argued that grandiose narcissism in particular is associated with disturbances in the capacity for loving attachment to others, including difficulties with balancing one's own needs and those of significant others and to strike an appropriate balance between closeness and distance in interpersonal contact (Akhtar, 2021, p. 456). The ability to engage in a mature and complex loving relationship will often be damaged or underdeveloped. One consequence of this is that sexual arousal is not associated with erotic desire, or only to a limited degree, and that the ability to identify and empathize with and respect the other as a subject with a related gender and sexual identity may be deficient, just as sensuousness is not sufficiently superior to more aggressive elements of human sexuality (p. 456). More specifically, perceptions of own superiority and entitlement may mean that individuals with largely grandiose manifestations of pathological narcissism tend to overlook or actively ignore sex partners' signals of sexual desire and to force through the satisfaction of their own sexual – and other, non-sexual – needs with no consideration for the other (p. 457). More generally, they may struggle to give up their own total autonomy and control, which is a precondition for accepting the other's independent mental life and for a relationship to work (Akhtar, 2009, p. 102).

Sexual difficulties

Sexual intercourse may be characterized by a lack of reciprocity, as sex is primarily or exclusively seen as a source of the person's own sexual satisfaction or the satisfaction of other, non-sexual needs. The other becomes instrumentalized as a simple object for the satisfaction of the person's own needs. The compulsive repetition of sexualized rituals may be a dominant feature, just as sexual arousal may come to serve as a replacement for love and the establishment of a loving relationship (Schalkwijk et al., 2021, p. 8) and intimate emotional contact in general. Furthermore, the self may seek sex partners who support and enhance their own grandiose and egocentric self-images, which may lead to problematic sadomasochistic relationships (Akhtar, 2021, p. 463), sexualized violence and sexual abuse. This may occur, for example, if a person with severe grandiose narcissism forms a relationship with a person with vulnerable narcissism who is ready to do and accept almost anything in order to be allowed to exist and achieve some form of acceptance and contact.

As pointed out by several authors, this risk is particularly pronounced when aggression and violence fuses with sexual desire and is expressed in severely disordered sexual behaviour. However, this is mainly seen in severe pathological narcissism in combination with comorbid psychopathic and sadistic traits (Ronningstam, 2005, p. 106). This constitutes paraphilia (Møhl et al., 2019) or perversion in a clinical – not a moral – sense, as the sexual activity does not primarily serve a sexual purpose but should be seen in relation to the person's psychopathology (Binswanger, 2024, p. 28). In this regard, a distinction is drawn between sexual fantasies and acts driven primarily by an urge for sexual satisfaction versus fantasies and acts with a predominantly non-sexual purpose, which should be seen primarily as attempts to satisfy non-sexual urges, for example to act out aggression, stabilize a narcissistic vulnerable self, dealing with internal or external (interpersonal) conflicts, seeking to escape painful loneliness, emptiness and sadness, processing traumatic experiences or achieving some sort of contact as a way of dampening inner anxiety or feelings of abandonment (p. 23). The latter may also be understood as attempts to compensate for deficiencies in personality structure and a fragile self-esteem via sexual fantasies and acts. This is not a rigid or categorical either–or distinction between sexual acts driven solely by sexual versus other, non-sexual urges, and in some cases, it can be difficult to determine whether sexual or other, non-sexual urges are dominant or have primacy in the specific individual's sexual fantasies and acts.

Studies of narcissism and relational functioning

A large meta-analysis of empirical studies (n=127) of correlations between dimensional measures of the various *DSM* personality disorders and interpersonal style in relation to relational dysfunction found that higher scores on dimensional measures of grandiose manifestations of NPD are associated with a higher inclination to be dominant, intimidating, invasive, vindictive and cold in interpersonal interactions (Wilson et al., 2017, p. 689 ff.). These correlations are stronger among women and in non-clinical populations (p. 706 ff.), which may indicate that they mainly reflect associations between non-pathological grandiose manifestations of NPD and dimensional measures of the above-mentioned interpersonally problematic traits and behaviours. In our interpretation of this meta-analysis, we should note that it is based on studies that have used *DSM* criteria for NPD to assess degrees of narcissism. Thus, we should assume that it only captured grandiose aspects of narcissism. Furthermore, the included studies are almost exclusively based on women from non-clinical populations, just as the assessments of NPD traits rely mainly on self-reporting; thus, their validity seems questionable.

Several studies have found a connection between vulnerable narcissism in particular and relational difficulties, including avoidant behaviour (tendency to withdraw from contact) and heightened sensitivity to others' view of the self, while grandiose narcissism up to a certain – non-pathological – level seems to be associated with lower levels of self-reported interpersonal problems, including less avoidance and higher scores for social-cognitive skills (Bogaerts & Jankovic, 2024, p. 3916). For example, a study among male forensic psychiatric outpatients (n=64) and a somewhat larger, non-clinical group (n=157) found that higher scores on measures of self-reported grandiose narcissism were associated with better relational capacity – defined, in part, as the ability to sincerely care for and connect with others and to communicate personal experiences to others – while higher scores for vulnerable narcissism, on the other hand, were associated with poorer relational functioning (p. 3921). However, subsequent analyses of mediating factors found that the degree of identity integration is the key factor for the participants' reported relational difficulties, not the degree of vulnerable versus grandiose narcissism in itself.

A related study among individuals who had received some form of psychiatric treatment within the past two years found that higher scores on measures of grandiose narcissism tend to be associated with fewer relational difficulties, while vulnerable narcissism was associated with greater relational difficulties and interpersonal dysfunction (Dashineau et al., 2019, p. 475). Studies based on student populations – and, in many cases, somewhat dubious measures of narcissism – found that higher scores on measures of vulnerable narcissistic traits relate to higher self-reported levels of being cold, socially avoidant and overly nurturant towards others – the latter presumably in an attempt to compensate for the self's perceived deficiencies – while higher scores on measures of narcissistic grandiosity were associated with a higher self-reported tendency to be hostile-dominant towards others (Dickenson & Pincus, 2003, p. 199 ff.).

As mentioned earlier (see Chapter 2.3), pathological narcissism is associated with deficiencies in particularly the more emotional aspects of empathy, while more cognitive elements of empathy may be normally developed, such as the capacity for cognitively registering and thinking about other people's emotions and other inner states, given a motivation to do so. Having deficiencies in emotional empathy means that the person cannot sense how others feel, what is going on inside others, and how they are affected by what the person says and does. This hampers relational functioning and may lead to relational difficulties when the person acts cynically, is intimidating or otherwise hurts others or fails to react with an empathic response when others are clearly emotionally affected, given that empathy normally promotes social behaviour and inhibits dissocial behaviour. A meta-analysis of empirical studies of correlations between the degree of self-reported narcissistic traits and various measures of empathy – based on 97 studies with more than 32,000 participants – found that both grandiose and vulnerable narcissism are associated with a lower level of self-reported cognitive and emotional empathy (Urbonaviciute & Hepper, 2020). Unfortunately, many of the underlying studies included in this meta-analysis are weakened by somewhat dubious methods for measuring empathy; thus, there is reason to assume that the self-reported empathic capacity does not necessarily reflect the respondent's actual capacity for empathy but rather a degree of readiness or motivation to do so. In relation to this point, the correlation between self-reported empathy and empathy as assessed in various behavioural tests has been found to be remarkably poor b (*r*=.1) (Urbonavi-Urbonaviciute & Hepper, 2020, p. 2). This indicates the need to develop more complex and valid methods for measuring empathic capacity.

If we look at more behavioural measures of empathy, based on various tests, lower levels of emotional empathy are only associated with higher levels of grandiose narcissism, while there is no correlation with cognitive empathy. However, it should be noted that there are very few studies of this; nearly 90% of the available studies are based on self-reported level of empathy. Furthermore, the correlation between grandiose narcissism and lower levels of emotional empathy is stronger for experimentally tested empathy than for self-reported empathy (*r*=.251 vs *r*=.145), which could indicate that grandiose narcissism is in fact associated with significantly impaired emotional empathy (Urbonaviciute & Hepper, 2020, p. 9 ff.). Studies using behavioural measures of empathy show no correlation between level of vulnerable narcissism and cognitive empathy (level of emotional empathy was not studied). This might indicate that correlations between narcissism and impaired empathy are largely or solely driven by more grandiose elements of pathological narcissism and that empathic capacity is normally developed in individuals with predominantly vulnerable manifestations of narcissism.

Overall, existing empirical studies thus suggest that while manifestations of vulnerable narcissism are associated with relational difficulties, grandiose narcissism – up to a certain level below actual pathological narcissism – is associated with a lower level of self-reported relational difficulties. On the other hand, we should assume that clearly pathological levels of grandiose narcissism also lead to significant relational difficulties, although there is insufficient empirical data on this. In addition to the usual problems stemming from the fact that most of the available studies, in this area too, involved individuals without a diagnosis of pathological narcissism, there is reason to ask whether relational difficulties should be measured through self-reporting alone, given that grandiose narcissism may be associated with interpersonal behaviour that is distressing for others, while the person self-reporting relational difficulties may not have acknowledged or is particularly interested in the impact of their behaviour on others.

Consequences for partners and family members

In relation to this discussion, two studies based on relatives of individuals with predominantly grandiose narcissistic traits are interesting. The participants in these studies were recruited in part via support groups for partners and family members of persons with narcissism, although 'narcissism' was somewhat vaguely defined. One of these studies (Day et al., 2020) involved a large group of partners/family members (n=683) of persons who, based on the relatives' description of them, were deemed to have clearly exalted – predominantly grandiose – narcissistic personality traits. Most of the participants (78%) were former or current partners of someone with 'narcissism'; the rest were mothers or other close relatives. The vast majority of the participants were women (94%), while the supposedly narcissistic person was almost always a man (77%). The designation of narcissistic traits must be considered somewhat uncertain, at best. Generally, the participants reported that their relationship with the person with narcissism was associated with significant emotional, psychological and practical distress (the latter including money and time, among other issues), and many (70–80%) reported a level of psychological difficulties matching the diagnostic criteria for an affective or anxiety disorder (Day et al., 2020, p. 806). However, there is no basis for determining whether there is a causal link between these symptoms of psychological distress and their relationship with a person with narcissism.

Unsurprisingly, there is considerable indication that emotional over-involvement and generally maladaptive strategies for dealing with someone with narcissism affect the participants' reported level of psychological distress (Day et al., 2020, p. 807), which also points to various focus areas of potential support for partners and family members. With regard to the different manifestations of narcissism, it is notable that partners or family members of persons with predominantly vulnerable manifestations of narcissism are more likely to express sorrow over what is happening in their relationship, while predominantly grandiose manifestations of narcissism are more likely to be associated with practical (money and time) and personal burdens (p. 807). Generally, current partners of persons with narcissism report a significantly greater emotional burden in their relationship than other relatives (p. 809).

A related study with a fairly similar design (n=436) and a similar gender distribution included brief interviews asking the participants to describe the person with 'narcissism' and their mutual relationship. Subsequently, the researchers carried out thematic analyses of the interview material with a view to identifying specific areas that the participants find especially distressing in their relationship (Day et al., 2022). Close to half the participants (44%) spontaneously describe various forms of abusive behaviour by the person with narcissism (p. 208), including emotional (21%), physical (17%), verbal (17%) and sexual (6%) abuse. When asked about the person's specific behaviour, a third of the participants (32%) describe economically irresponsible behaviour (takes on debt, steals, is controlling) and a third (34%) speak of unwanted sexual behaviour. The latter involves sexual abuse or unacceptable sexual transgressions, including perverted sexual behaviour, infidelity, sex addiction, a one-sided focus on own sexual needs, using sex to achieve or demonstrate power and violating normal sexual boundaries in interactions with the couple's children (p. 208 ff.). Finally, just under a third of the participants describe emotional challenges stemming from the narcissistic person's tendency to alternate between idealization and devaluation (p. 209 ff.). A few studies suggest that sexual narcissism is associated with increased risk of infidelity (McNulty & Widman, 2018, p. 329). Furthermore, narcissistic traits have been associated with a tendency to underestimate the distressing impact of own abusive behaviour on one's partner, sense of entitlement to sex in return for being 'generosity' to others, greater acceptance of domestic violence and rape-supportive beliefs, and a general tendency to be manipulative and act in ways that cause painful jealousy in the partner, among other aspects (Foster & Brunelli, 2018, p. 320).

The studies outlined above point to the potentially severe relational and psychological consequences to family members and partners of persons with pathological narcissism. There is reason to assume that partners and relatives of persons with predominantly grandiose pathological narcissism face greater challenges and distress, compared to partners and relatives of persons with predominantly vulnerable manifestations of pathological narcissism, although the real picture is more complex than this rather categorical distinction. For example, smaller studies of perceived challenges related to physical abuse in partners of persons with 'narcissism' suggest that persons with both vulnerable and grandiose narcissistic traits may use physical violence against their partners but that this physical abuse may be driven by different psychological dynamics (see also Littlebear et al., 2024). They appear to be driven by perceived threats to the person's self-esteem and grandiose self-image in persons with predominantly grandiose narcissism versus fear of abandonment in persons with predominantly vulnerable narcissism (Green & Charles, 2019). See also Chapters 4.2 and 4.3 on relational manifestations of pathological narcissism in the psychotherapeutic relationship (cf. transference and countertransference).

Studies of narcissism and aggression

For decades, psychoanalysis and clinical practice have linked higher levels of narcissism and, not least, pathological narcissism with heightened sensibility to narcissistic injury and a tendency to react to these injuries with various forms of aggression and narcissistic rage. There is reason to assume that heightened sensitivity to narcissistic injury in combination with a sense of entitlement, poor emotional empathy – including empathy with the targets of the self's aggression – and impaired impulse control/self-regulation is associated with greater risk of acting out anger/rage, aggression and violence on others. A person with pathological narcissism who has developed a grandiose self-image – and, perhaps, a high level of perfectionism, in an attempt to keep their perceived vulnerability and feelings of inferiority in check – will be more likely to perceive external criticism or perhaps merely the absence of admiration and explicit recognition as narcissistic injury. When this happens, the person may be overwhelmed by destructive shame and react with anger, including by counterattacking anyone who criticizes or simply fails to admire the self (Fjermestad-Noll et al., 2020a, p. 38).

Narcissistic rage triggered by perceived narcissistic injury may be expressed in many different ways, all driven by an urge to avenge perceived injustice, an illegitimate offence to the self and its self-image (Kohut, 1985, p. 143), and escape a position of passive victimhood and claim active agency. Resentment, outrage and anger over being wronged against and a strong urge to restore justice may be drivers of intense thirst for revenge. This resentment further helps to alleviate the self's painful experience of helplessness and impotence (Wurmser, 2002, p. 116).

Narcissistic rage may be intensified by feelings of shame and inferiority and perceived devaluation, disparagement, ridicule and exposure of the self as inadequate or inferior. In this situation, the self's rage may be directed at the specific other who is exposing the self's vulnerability and inadequacy (Bogaerts et al., 2021; Krizan & Johar, 2015, p. 716). In case of more persistent narcissistic rage, this may in itself give rise to additional shame, which needs to be warded off via aggression towards others in a self-fuelling cycle of shame and rage (Krizan & Johar, 2015, p. 716). When the person's actions are driven by narcissistic rage, the other – the object of the rage – is no longer perceived as an equal and autonomous subject with their own goals and motives. In practice, the person turns into an aggressor, an avenger who is convinced that they are restoring justice with acts that are driven by seething rage (Kohut, 1985, p. 148; Krizan & Johar, 2015, p. 785 ff.). Narcissistic rage is immature anger that is out of proportion, unfocused, out of control and often directed at someone other than the person or persons who initially sparked the anger and which is not integrated with more mature and rational goals (Krizan & Johar, 2015).

Most of the existing empirical evidence on the possible connections between narcissism and aggression, resentment and vindictiveness, is based on non-clinical populations, just as most of it relies on simple self-reporting that only or predominantly capture non-pathological manifestations of grandiose narcissism and relatively trivial forms of aggression/aggressive behaviour. Thus, we should be cautious about simply generalizing the presented findings to persons with pathological narcissism (Krizan & Johar,

2015, p. 785; Rasmussen, 2016). Several meta-analyses have sought to summarize the many different studies of links between narcissism and aggression that have been presented in recent decades. One meta-analysis (Kjærvik & Bushman, 2021) of a large number of studies (n=437) representing a very large number of participants (n=123,000) found that many measures of narcissism have a fairly strong correlation with various measures of aggression (r=.26) and violence (r=.23). These correlations are stronger when the self or ego feels threatened or provoked; if the self feels humiliated, shamed or criticized or feels that its social status is jeopardized.

These links apply to both vulnerable and grandiose manifestations of narcissism and in various forms of self-reported aggression, including direct, indirect, displaced, physical and verbal aggression. Another meta-analysis (Du et al., 2022b) found that the greater the emphasis on grandiosity in the applied measures of narcissism, the weaker the link between narcissism and both general and reactive aggression. Conversely, in this case, the correlation is stronger between narcissism and proactive aggression; a more targeted and instrumental aggression. This finding suggests that vulnerable narcissism is associated with a higher risk of reactive aggression – aggression when the self is threatened – but with lower levels of aggression when the self is not threatened. Furthermore, it might suggest that non-pathological grandiosity is associated with increased risk of more or less unprovoked aggression towards others.

One systematic literature review (Lampe et al., 2018) found that six out of seven studies based entirely or partially on patients (and prison inmates) showed a strong correlation between pathological narcissism and heightened risk of violent behaviour. A high score on measures of pathological narcissism is associated with an up to 11-fold increase in violence and is an important predictor of severe violence, including homicide, among prison inmates (p. 209). Among prison inmates, persons with NPD are about seven times more likely to be convicted of violent crimes, including homicide, than persons without NPD (p. 221). One study among forensic psychiatric outpatients similarly found an indirect correlation between higher levels of vulnerable pathological narcissism and criminal behaviour. However, this only applies to persons who also have a poorly integrated identity and poor self-control, which suggests generally poor personality organization; thus, it unlikely to be primarily or solely about pathological narcissism (Bogaerts et al., 2021).

A few studies suggest that generally maladaptive strategies for regulating painful affects, including shame, in connection with narcissism may increase the risk of aggressive and violent behaviour (Kealy et al., 2017a; Velotti et al., 2020). Correlations between vulnerable narcissism and aggressive behaviour are mediated by strategies for regulating shame, in the sense that higher levels of vulnerable narcissism in combination with maladaptive strategies for regulating shame are associated with higher levels of aggressive and violent behaviour directed at others (Velotti et al., 2020, p. 3). Only a small number of studies of clinical populations addressed the significance of gender, but studies that did consider this aspect suggest that the link between pathological narcissism and risk of violence applies to women too and is thus not isolated to men (Lampe et al., 2018, p. 22).

In summary, the existing literature and empirical evidence suggest that narcissism – particularly pathological narcissism – is a significant risk factor for aggression and violence, and that pathological narcissism is an important element in the understanding of interpersonal violence (Lampe et al., 2018, p. 225), probably especially among persons with comorbid psychopathic traits and pronounced problems with impulse control and emotional empathy. Among other factors, it appears that violence may be triggered by narcissistic injuries of persons with fragile and unstable self-esteem (vulnerable narcissism), particularly in connection with perceived threats to the vulnerable self. Acting out anger and rage may temporarily alleviate painful emotions related to a destabilized self-image and create a sense of agency (Kealy et al., 2017a, p. 156). Violence may be the narcissistic vulnerable self's desperate attempt to escape unbearable destructive shame and restore threatened and destabilized self-esteem and a form of pride (Lampe et al., 2018, p. 209; Fonagy, 2021, p. 118). Thus, there is reason to believe that it is relevant to devote considerable attention to pathological narcissism in our understanding and treatment of persons who behave aggressively and violently towards others in various ways.

Aetiology: Possible causes of pathological narcissism

There are few empirical studies to shed light on any specific causes of the development of pathological narcissism. Over time, clinical psychology has built a fairly large knowledge base about key risk and causal factors in the development of psychological disorders in general, while we have much less empirically based knowledge about more specific causal factors that increase the likelihood of specific disorders, such as NPD. Childhood neglect, various types of abuse, dysfunctional family interactions, psychological difficulties in the parents and deficiencies in the parent–child relationship are some of the fairly unambiguous risk factors for the development of psychological illness in general and are likely to be contributing factors in the development of pathological narcissism as well. However, none of these factors are specific in the sense that its presence indicates a certain likelihood that a child or young person develops NPD rather than any other psychological disorder.

Psychological disorders are generally the result of a complex developmental process that unfolds over many years as individual vulnerability factors, to varying degrees, interact with conditions during the child's upbringing, particularly interactions with significant others during childhood and youth and the general emotional atmosphere in the childhood home. Additional factors include any traumatic experiences, such as the loss of emotionally significant others, life-threatening or debilitating somatic illness, various forms of physical, sexual or verbal abuse or persistent neglect and deficiencies in significant others' empathic and loving mirroring of the self. Most of our models for understanding the causal factors behind psychological disorders have a rather limited empirical research base. Most of them are more heuristic models based on a combination of psychological theory, clinical experience and empirical studies of individual isolated causal factors.

Few causal factors are specific, in the sense that if a particular event or factor is present, the person is certain to develop a particular psychological disorder (such as NPD) rather than another one (such as BPD or depression) – or any psychological disorder at all. The vast majority of causal factors are nonspecific and probabilistic. This means 1) that no single causal factor is in itself sufficient to lead to the development of a psychological disorder, 2) no psychological disorder is always caused by one particular factor, and 3) any given causal factor will rarely be implicated in just one specific psychological disorder. Thus, we are dealing with a wide range of risk factors that in combination increase the likelihood of an individual developing, not one specific psychological disorder but any of a wide range of related disorders. This applies very much also to pathological narcissism.

Theoretical aetiological models

Our empirically based knowledge about the causes of pathological narcissism are limited, and it appears that pathological narcissism develops via complex individual combinations of a very large and diverse selection of causal factors. Thus, we cannot point to one or a few specific causal factors behind the development of narcissistic disorders. Nevertheless, the prevailing models for understanding the basis of pathological narcissism are largely concentrated around a number of general factors in the family that the child grew up in, traumatic experiences (see below) and, not least, relational disorders, especially attachment disorders (see below). A small number of studies have focused on hereditary factors. A fairly large (n=1386) study of twins in Norway estimates heredity to account for just 24% of the development of personality traits related to NPD. Furthermore, hereditary factors are fairly common across cluster B personality disorders (Torgersen et al., 2008, p. 1622; see also Torgersen et al., 2000), which again points to the absence of specific causal factors for pathological narcissism. Most empirical studies of aetiological factors for NPD focus on parental behaviour (Yakeley, 2018, p. 309).

Theoretically, there is reason to assume that excessive and undifferentiated praise and admiration of the self from significant others, perhaps especially during childhood and youth, may contribute to the development of an inflated positive, grandiose and omnipotent self-image. In some cases, this may be accompanied by negative and devaluing perceptions of others, who are primarily perceived as inferior in comparison to the person's own – at least superficially – grandiose self. Others may also be reduced to a somewhat desubjectified audience, expected to admire, praise and be very interested in the self, and the self may become puzzled, offended and furious when others fail to admire, or even notice, the self as expected.

Distorted praise and admiration

If the parents are excessively preoccupied with and overestimate certain traits and characteristics in their child, this may contribute to the child internalizing an unrealistic, distorted and idealized image of self and what is expected of the self. Meanwhile, the child's real or true self may be neglected, just as their need for basic nurture, dependence and empathic mirroring of the true self may be overlooked (Diamond et al., 2022, p. 97). The child experiences a form of selective appreciation or even idealization of certain traits, while other aspects – including core emotional needs – are neglected or perhaps even met by the parents with rejection, devaluation and contempt (Diamond et al., 2022, p. 44). This may give the child – and, later the young person and the adult – a sense of being appreciated for certain abilities, traits or qualities but not for their true self, with their whole person and subjectivity (Fiscalini, 2004, p. 82). These are all experiences that may contribute to the development of narcissistic imbalances and pathology.

Parents who generally overestimate and admire their child far beyond what is objectively justified fail to see the real child. Instead, perhaps, they see who they wish and expect the child to be, which is a form of invalidation of the child or, at least, constitutes incongruent mirroring and lack of recognition of the child (Vater et al., 2013a, p. 38; Gabbard & Crisp, 2018, p. 44). Both the lack of empathic support and mirroring and over-involvement, coddling and excessive support can inhibit the development of healthy self-esteem and the ability to function as a balanced autonomous subject without inhibiting narcissistic imbalances (Pincus, 2023, p. 633). Some authors also see these distinct imbalances in the parent–child relationship as an indication that the parents are using their child as a narcissistic object, an extension of themselves, expecting the child to realize the parents' own ambitions and primarily showing affection when the child's way of being and acting confirms and lives out the parents projections (Rus-Russell, 1985, p. 142 ff.).

A child growing up in this sort of relational dynamic will find it harder to develop healthy self-esteem, as the child is not seen, recognized, appreciated or loved as 'themself' but primarily for behaving in certain ways, playing certain roles, performing on certain parameters or, generally, satisfying others' needs and expectations (McWilliams, 2011, p. 183; Ronningstam, 2021, p. 6). As one of the earliest narcissism scholars, the feminist psychoanalyst Karen Horney (1939, p. 91), put it, the child feels that 'he has no rights of his own and should live only for the parents' sake; parents who transfer their own ambitions to the child and regard the boy as an embryonic genius and the girl as a princess, thereby developing in the child the feeling that he is loved for imaginary qualities rather than for his true self'. The child's true self is not seen and mirrored, and the child may develop a false self in a desperate attempt to gain the parents' recognition and love.

Neglect, unpredictability and abuse

There is reason to assume that an upbringing characterized by repeated rejections, neglect and various forms of abuse and unpredictability by and in significant others may contribute to the development of negative, painful and shameful perceptions of the self as being insignificant, invisible, uninteresting and of no importance in the eyes of significant others. These are all notions that must be regarded as reflective of varying degrees of narcissistic pathology, given that the person's self-image and self-esteem have been destabilized and are unrealistically negative. Furthermore, the self may develop the impression that others are not interested in the self, are unreliable and are generally distant and detached in relation to the self (Meyer & Pilkonis, 2011, p. 435 ff.). In some cases, the child or young person will protect themself from these negative self-perceptions by means of a grandiose self-image or by constantly clinging to others and doing everything possible to avoid being abandoned and thus losing access to a form of self-validation. Perhaps the self may try to control others in an attempt to make sure that these others are always available to prop up this fragile self-image and self-esteem.

Alternatively, the child will have learned from a young age that caregivers (self-objects) are unreliable, erratic, dismissive or (in concrete or emotional terms) absent, and that the child therefore has to rely on themself and cannot trust anyone. This survival strategy may result in an air of narcissistic self-reliance (Ronningstam, 2021, p. 6). Children and young people who, for various reasons, have a greater need for attention and explicit validation and recognition from others – whether this need stems from their innate temperament or has developed as a result of earlier stressful experiences – may handle interpersonal interactions in a way that causes others to withdraw or otherwise react in ways that enhance the self's need for being contained, validated and approved, perhaps by an idealized other who needs to be able to handle being idealized without withdrawing. This may create a self-fuelling negative cycle driven by the self's narcissistic imbalances or disorder.

Deficiencies in empathic mirroring

Parents who struggle to contain their child's idealization and who, for various reasons, are unable to meet the child's self and varying narcissistic needs with empathic mirroring may inadvertently contribute to the development of narcissistic imbalances and disturbances, particularly if they use their child to satisfy their own narcissistic needs (Kohut, 1977, p. 274). Poor empathy and a poor ability to decode and satisfy the child's age-appropriate needs may interfere with the normal development process (Kernberg, 2000, p. 117). The child needs to be contained and to meet themself in the parents' eyes. With a focus on psychological development during infancy, Winnicott (1971, p. 112) rhetorically asks what happens if this parent-infant process is disturbed – 'the case of the baby whose mother reflects her own mood or, worse still, the rigidity of her own defences. In such a case what does the baby see?' Winnicott's reply: 'Many babies […] do have to have a long experience of not getting back what they are giving. They look and they do not see themselves. There are consequences.' (p. 112). The child – and, later, the young person – may learn to adapt to others' desires, needs and moods, abandoning their own true self, which is covered up and remains underdeveloped. Instead, the person develops a false self, and behind this superficial adaptation to the needs of the parents and others, the person may feel inauthentic, fake, empty and alienated from others (Diamond et al., 2022, p. 97 ff.). Alternatively, the person may withdraw from intimate contact with others in an attempt to protect their – perhaps particularly sensitive and vulnerable – self. Psychological processes such as these may well be playing out behind the facade of a person with symptoms of predominantly grandiose pathological narcissism.

A few authors have proposed more specific possible causal factors behind the development of predominantly vulnerable or grandiose pathological narcissism. This includes the notion that growing up in an environment characterized by cold detachment and excessive emotional control tends to predispose the person more for developing of vulnerable narcissism, while socialization characterized by excessive indulgence and lack of boundary-setting is more likely to contribute to the development of grandiose narcissism (Yakeley, 2018, p. 305), or that a child whose perceptions of grandiosity, extraordinary uniqueness, superiority and entitlement are not challenged (disillusioned) will have a heightened risk of developing grandiose narcissistic traits and disorders (Mollon, 2020, p. 9). Furthermore, children whose parents have divorced may find themselves in a position where they meet the needs of the parent who was abandoned, which may in practice lead to a blurring of intergenerational boundaries. It may also require the child, to varying degrees, to abandon their own developmentally appropriate needs or to attain a special status in relation to one of the parents or in the family as a whole as the empathic, caring, understanding and strong son or daughter. The latter may contribute to the development of fantasies of omnipotence (Kernberg, 2000, p. 117 ff.) but may also cause the self to abandon their own needs for nurture, dependence and an idealized parental figure, given that the other side of the grandiose self may be an emotionally neglected, lonely and narcissistically vulnerable self. Similar dynamics may, of course, develop in families where the parents live together but, for various reasons, have to have certain emotional needs met by the child that would normally be met primarily by the parent's partner or other adults.

Studies of possible causal factors: Distressing childhood experiences

There are few studies of factors occurring during childhood and youth with a possible role in the development of pathological narcissism. Most of the studies that do exist are based on non-clinical populations, including university students. In combination with an often overly narrow understanding of pathological narcissism in the few studies that are based on clinical populations, this makes it difficult to reach any clear-cut conclusions about specific causal factors for NPD. Furthermore, there is reason to assume that factors that may contribute to the development of predominantly grandiose narcissism – perhaps in particular high-functioning grandiose narcissism – are not necessarily the same as the ones that may be involved in the development of predominantly vulnerable manifestations of narcissism. Based on an understanding of pathological narcissism as an essentially fairly delimited disorder that may manifest itself in different ways – predominantly vulnerable versus grandiose narcissism – there is reason to consider whether different events and experiences during childhood and youth may increase the likelihood of an individual developing, for example, a tendency to deal with their fundamental narcissistic imbalance and vulnerability by means of a grandiose facade and behaviour.

The connections found in some studies between individual potential causal factors and pathological narcissism are generally rather weak. This reflects the fact that severe psychological disorders, such as pathological narcissism, are typically a result of a long and complex developmental process, in which individual factors are rarely decisive in themselves. Generally, a range of indicators of the quality of recollected early parent–child relations are associated, to varying degrees, with certain measures of problematic narcissistic traits later in life (Otway & Vignoles, 2006; Maxwell & Huprich, 2014; Huxley & Bizumic, 2017; Nguyen et al., 2020), just as negative recollections of early relations with parents is associated with lower self-esteem (Maxwell & Hubrich, 2014).

Thus, the development of pathological narcissism should normally be understood as the preliminary culmination of an interaction of many causal factors, which often co-occur and mutually enhance each other. In some cases, the co-occurrence of multiple risk factors will lead to an exponentially increased risk of developing psychopathology. For example, physical and sexual abuse rarely occurs in a well-functioning family characterized by empathy and nurture but is more likely in families and subcultures characterized by different conditions, which may also increase the risk of developing pathological narcissism and other psychological disorders. This includes, for example, psychological difficulties and narcissistic imbalances in the parents, economic and cultural deprivation, a weak social network, and poor capacities for empathy, mentalizing, psychological cognition and seeing and understanding what is happening inside self and others. Each of these factors may in itself increase the risk of psychopathology, and together they may be associated with dramatically increased risk.

Early neglect and physical abuse

A meta-analysis of 15 studies of recollected childhood neglect and abuse and subsequent development of more or less pathological narcissistic traits found a statistically significant – albeit relatively weak (r=.2) – correlation between various forms of early neglect and abuse and subsequent development of vulnerable narcissistic traits (Gao et al., 2024, p. 279). In this review, neglect and abuse are defined as acts or omissions by caregivers that result in harm to the child. The same meta-analysis found a similar but even weaker (*r*=.1) connection with grandiose narcissistic traits. Correcting for methodical weaknesses in the studies included in the meta-analysis reduced the already fairly weak statistical correlations by almost half. As for more specific forms of abuse and neglect, there is a much stronger correlation between neglect and the development of vulnerable narcissistic traits (*r*=.3) than between physical abuse and vulnerable narcissism (*r*=.1) (p. 281). Here it should be noted, however, that just one of the 15 studies included in the meta-analysis is based on patients, and in this study, the applied diagnostic standard is unclear, and the study is unlikely to include patients with NPD, while 12 of the included studies are solely based on university students, which limits the usefulness of the review for enhancing our understanding of the aetiology of NPD.

Overall, based on this meta-analysis, we can conclude that there is probably a general connection between distressing childhood experiences and pathological narcissism but that the connection is fairly weak and that no single risk factor in itself appears to play a very big causal role in the development of NPD. Furthermore, the findings of this meta-analysis suggest that the development of vulnerable and grandiose narcissistic traits, to some extent, follows different paths – that is, they do not have a shared aetiology. For example, we may imagine that severe childhood neglect and abuse, which is often accompanied by destructive shame, is more closely related to the risk of developing vulnerable narcissism and generally more severe psychopathology (Gao et al., 2024, p. 284).

More generally, there appears to be some association between, in particular, physical abuse and physical neglect during childhood and youth and subsequent development of vulnerable narcissistic traits, while recollections of parents who were overprotective and excessively indulgent and who admired and overestimated the self undiscriminatingly appear to be associated, to varying degrees, with increased risk of both vulnerable and, perhaps in particular, grandiose narcissistic traits later in life. A study based on a student population found that individuals who were subjected to physical abuse during childhood are angrier and more aggressive and more likely to react with and be overwhelmed by destructive shame, just as they are more narcissistically vulnerable than individuals without such a history (Keene & Epps, 2016).

This latter study also found a correlation between earlier perceived physical abuse and a tendency towards physical aggression in adulthood. To some degree, this tendency was mediated by vulnerable narcissism and feelings of shame. In extension of this point, the authors conclude that a combination of narcissistic vulnerability and shame-proneness – two factors that we must assume are closely related – may be a driver of anger and aggressive behaviour in persons who have been subjected to physical abuse in childhood (Keene & Epps, 2016, p. 281). A related study based on data from a large population survey similarly found that early physical neglect was particularly strongly associated with a dimensional measure of NPD symptoms (Hengartner et al., 2013, p. 479), while many other potential risk factors for the development of psychological illness during childhood was more generally associated with measures of PD symptoms without being more specifically associated with risk of developing NPD symptoms.

A few studies based on various patient populations, including, to varying degrees, patients diagnosed with NPD, found a certain (relatively weak) link between childhood physical neglect or verbal abuse by the parents and later development of NPD symptoms and an elevated level of pathological narcissism but not a full NPD diagnosis (Johnson et al., 2000, p. 179 ff.; Johnson et al., 2001). However, it also found that persons who had been subjected to verbal abuse from the mother during youth and early adulthood had more than three times the risk of developing a narcissistic personality disorder and other PDs (Johnson et al., 2001).

A study among psychiatric patients, including a somewhat larger group diagnosed with NPD (n=59), similarly found that physical abuse was the only negative childhood experience that had a significant association with NPD symptoms, while other forms of childhood maltreatment, such as sexual abuse, emotional abuse and neglect, were not significantly associated with NPD symptoms among adults once other possible risk factors had been factored in (Cohen et al., 2014, p. 196). However, several other studies have found a statistically significant correlation between emotional abuse during childhood – seen in isolation – and later development of NPD traits (Neu-Neumann, 2017, p. 436; Cohen et al., 2014, p. 196). These findings suggest a meaningful association between the two, in which early emotional abuse just is not a significant isolated causal factor. A related study found a similar connection between physical abuse during childhood and NPD symptoms later in life. However, this connection disappears if the co-occurrence of other comorbid PDs is factored in (Lobbestael et al., 2010). This suggests that there is no unique or specific connection between early physical abuse and later development of NPD symptoms rather than, for example, symptoms of other PDs. Several studies point to a more general connection between different forms of childhood abuse and higher levels of a wide range of PD symptoms later in life, including symptoms of NPD (Grover et al., 2007). Unfortunately, like the vast majority of studies in the field, the value of these studies is limited by the fact that even though they are, to varying degrees, based on patients in treatment, the participants' NPD symptoms are measured in accordance with the *DSM*'s criteria, which only capture grandiose aspects of NPD.

Invalidation and rejection of the self

Studies suggest that parental invalidation of the self during childhood is associated with increased risk of both vulnerable and grandiose narcissism later in life (Huxley & Bizumic, 2017, p. 138). Maternal invalidation of the self appears to have a particular impact, but invalidation by the father is also significant. Perceived rejection by the parents appears to be particularly relevant for the development of grandiose narcissism (Huxley & Bizumic, 2017, p. 139), with the absence of emotional warmth from the parents enhancing the connection (Otway & Vignoles, 2006, p. 111). Studies also suggest that parental emotional neglect is associated with higher levels of vulnerable narcissism but lower levels of grandiose narcissism later in life (Nguyen et al., 2020). Furthermore, there are some indications that parental emotional control combined with emotional coldness is associated with increased risk of developing vulnerable narcissism (Horton, 2011a, p. 186). Generally, several studies suggest that an authoritarian parenting style is associated with problematic narcissism in the child but also with many other psychological difficulties and academic underperformance. Authoritarian parenting includes cold, controlling and emotionally invasive behaviour that induces feelings of guilt and shame in the child and the withdrawal of love as an instrument of control or discipline (Horton, 2011b, p. 130). However, as in many other contexts, we should note that these are merely statistical correlations and not necessarily causal links. For example, it is conceivable that certain narcissistic traits in a child may trigger or heighten authoritarian behaviour in certain parents (p. 134 ff.).

Several studies suggest that deficient parental mirroring of the self is associated with higher levels of both vulnerable and grandiose narcissism later in life. Numerous studies, mainly based on university students, thus found that overprotective parenting is associated with higher levels of both grandiose and, in particular, vulnerable narcissism (Otway & Vignoles, 2006; Van Schie et al., 2020), just as parental overestimation and exaggerated admiration of the self correlates in particular with grandiose narcissistic traits (Otway & Vignoles, 2006, p. 114; Nguyen et al., 2020). However, there is reason to consider to what extent these studies – which mainly associate current recollections of the parents' communicated image of and reactions to the self in the past with current non-pathological levels of narcissistic traits – can be taken as generalized indications of the drivers of the development of severe pathological narcissism in young people and adults.

The association between parental overestimation of the self and grandiose traits is particularly pronounced when it is accompanied by lenient or indulgent parenting – parents who are more reluctant to set boundaries and make demands on the child – and a dynamic that might contribute to both grandiose self-overvaluation and entitlement (Van Schie et al., 2020). It is also conceivable that the child or young person may perceive the parents' extreme and undiscriminating overvaluation of the self as fake and inauthentic, just as it may lead to a, possibly vague, sense of not really being seen. The child may find that their true self is overlooked or undesirable. Perhaps the child feels that the parents have certain specific expectations of the self – or would even prefer a very different child from the one they have. This may increase the risk of developing a false self that tries to adapt to the parents' expectations and live up to their unrealistic ideas about the self.

Furthermore, a childhood environment characterized by unrealistically positive perceptions of the child and a lack of boundaries – perhaps combined with overinvolved and overprotective parenting – may prevent the child from learning to deal with demands and boundaries. As a result, the child risks being unprepared for and experiencing failure when encountering the real world outside the family setting (Van Schie et al., 2020). The child or young person does not have a chance to correct their unrealistically grandiose self-image until later, when they encounter the less forgiving world outside the family that is beyond the parents' ability to control or compensate for, as they did earlier. In this sense, an overprotective and overly lenient or indulgent upbringing can undermine the development of robust agency and autonomy in the child, who may experience demands and boundaries outside the family as a narcissistic injury, for example when their sense of entitlement and expectations of unconditional admiration from others are not met.

More generally, deficiencies in parental responsiveness – the parents' ability to match their demands, parenting behaviour and socialization practices to the child's development and maturity – as well as self-centred parents who are more focused on their own needs than on the child's will probably contribute to the development of psychopathology. However, this is in no way specific to the development of pathological narcissism, given that children and young people need clear boundaries as well as freedom ('leniency') but to varying degrees and in varying forms at different stages in their psychological development (Paulsen et al., 2014, p. 36 ff.; Horton, 2011b, p. 128). One longitudinal study that followed a group of children for 20 years from the age of 3 lends some support to the link between parenting behaviour during childhood and later 'narcissism' but mainly in the sense that nurturing and boundary-setting (authoritative but not authoritarian) parenting is associated with the development of 'healthy' or 'autonomous' narcissism during adolescence and early adulthood, while any direct associations between problematic parenting during the early years and later development of pathological narcissism are weak, at best (Cramer, 2011, p. 24).

Studies of attachment style and narcissism

Relatively few empirical studies have been published of possible links between attachment and pathological narcissism. A slightly older meta-analysis of studies on connections between attachment style and narcissism concludes – based almost exclusively on studies of non-clinical populations – that there seems to be a relatively strong statistical correlation between vulnerable narcissism and attachment anxiety, while there also appears to be a – somewhat weaker – association between grandiose narcissism and the defensive avoidance of contact and emotional intimacy (cf. anxious avoidant and, not least, dismissive attachment; Meyer & Pilkonis, 2011, p. 438).

Generally, however, the presented findings about possible links between grandiose narcissism and attachment paint a more mixed picture, in the sense that some studies find some connection between grandiose narcissistic traits and both anxious avoidant and dismissive attachment styles, while others find no link (Biberdzic et al., 2023, p. 3). The link between vulnerable narcissism and both anxious avoidant and ambivalent overinvolved attachment appear clearly more consistent across studies (Biberdzic et al., 2023, p. 3). The above-mentioned meta-analysis associates both vulnerable and grandiose narcissism with insecure attachment in general. It should be noted that these links are merely statistical correlations, meaning that the studies do not offer any clear-cut conclusions about possible causal links between attachment and pathological narcissism.

In more specific findings, a few newer studies based on university students have found, in part, that higher scores on dimensional measures of both vulnerable and grandiose narcissism are associated with higher scores on measures of both anxious avoidant and overinvolved attachment and with lower scores on measures of secure attachment, while only grandiose narcissism is associated with higher scores on measures of dismissive attachment style (Biberdzic et al., 2023). On the other hand, there are also studies that do not lend support to a link between grandiose narcissism and dismissive attachment style (Van Schie et al., 2021, p. 7). This may be related to the fact that the grandiose narcissism that is captured in these studies of student populations must be assumed to be fundamentally different from the pathological grandiosity that is sometimes seen in patients with severe pathological narcissism. This may also be part of the explanation why a small number of studies have found that higher levels of (non-pathological) grandiose narcissism are associated with more secure attachment (Van Schie et al., 2021). It is worth considering whether a certain (no more than moderate) level of grandiose self-perception may sometimes make it easier to be in and, not least, handle conflicts in close relationships in ways that are not immediately distressing to the person's self or self-image. How it might affect others is a different issue.

Studies have associated vulnerable narcissism with less positive and more negative models of self (Van Schie et al., 2021, p. 5), just as the experience of shame appears to be an important mediating factor for the link between vulnerable narcissism, insecure attachment and negative models of self (Van Schie et al., 2021). Furthermore, a few studies suggest that both anxious avoidant and ambivalent-overinvolved attachment are associated with unstable self-esteem and a need for persistent external validation (Biberdzic et al., 2023, p. 5), which may be seen as manifestations of vulnerable narcissism. Finally, it is worth noting that a few studies among university students have found that vulnerable narcissism mediates links between insecure/anxious attachment and self-reported symptoms of anxiety, depression (Set, 2021) and bulimic eating behaviour (Dakanalis et al., 2016). This might indicate that narcissistic vulnerability – which does not necessarily imply pathological narcissism – may play a role in the development of symptom disorders, such as depression and anxiety disorders, as well as eating disorders.

There are a small number of studies based on patients in treatment for personality disorders, including, to varying degrees, patients with NPD. One study among patients in psychiatric treatment for BPD found that persons with comorbid BPD and NPD had anxious avoidant attachment as their primary attachment pattern (Diamond et al., 2014, p. 431). Furthermore, a study of a group of patients seeking treatment for personality pathology found that higher scores on dimensional measures of vulnerable narcissism are strongly associated with higher levels of various manifestations if insecure, anxious-ambivalent and overinvolved attachment, while higher scores on measures of grandiose narcissism are also – but to a lesser degree – associated with overinvolved attachment, including the need for external validation (Fossati et al., 2015, p. 414). Overall, there is thus some empirical evidence of a relatively strong link between, in particular, vulnerable pathological narcissism and disordered attachment, mainly anxious-ambivalent and overinvolved attachment, while there are also studies suggesting that pathological grandiose narcissism is associated with disordered attachment, including in particular – but not exclusively – anxious and dismissive attachment, although the empirical evidence of this latter connection is somewhat weaker.

3.3 Heinz Kohut and self psychology

Unlike many other theories that, simply put, primarily view narcissism as something that is either isolated to the early years and is then normally replaced by mature object love or constitutes some form of immaturity or disorder, Kohut believed that all human beings contain elements of egocentric narcissistic needs and that human psychology has a separate narcissistic line of development, from early archaic to mature narcissism (Altmeyer, 2000, p. 65). Thus, narcissism and narcissistic needs are not necessarily signs of immaturity or psychological disorder, even in adults, just as narcissism does not necessarily present an obstacle to the establishment of object relations and object love. Being preoccupied with oneself and one's own emotional needs may thus be completely legitimate and is not necessarily pathological, provided this does not come to dominate or manifest itself in ways that are obviously destructive to others or the self (Morrison & Stolorow, 1997, p. 72). In this sense, Kohut can be seen as representing a moral rehabilitation of narcissism as a psychological phenomenon by viewing it as a distinct line of development in human psychology that is not necessarily an indication of immaturity or pathology (Altmeyer, 2023, p. 73) and which, in normal cases, culminates in what Kohut describes as a bipolar and coherent – that is, not fragmented – self characterized by healthy and realistic goals and ideals.

With Kohut (1971, p. 26) we can speak of two basic narcissistic structures with related archaic narcissistic needs that, in a normal course of development, are transformed, moderated and integrated into the mature personality: 1) the grandiose self and 2) idealized images of significant others, beginning with the young child's omnipotent perceptions of their own powers and the parents' enormous strength, efficiency and ability to protect the child. Conversely, it is a key issue in persons with pathological narcissism that this normal transformation and maturation of archaic needs and structures have failed, and that archaic needs that are normal early in life persist, appear increasingly immature, are actualized and come to dominate the self's interactions with others. This includes interactions with therapists and determine the patient's transference (see Chapter 4.2). In an attempt to preserve a fragile self that is threatened by internal fragmentation, the person holds onto the archaic grandiose self and idealized perceptions of the parental figures. In a simplified form, this can be summarized into the idea that 'I am perfect' and 'You are perfect, but I am part of you' (Kohut, 1971, p. 27).

Kohut associates the archaic grandiose self with fantasies of the self's omnipotence, omniscience, perfection and deep yearning (hope, expectation) of being admired and loved for being so extraordinary and perfect. The archaic idealized parent imago similarly attributes omniscience, strength and omnipotence to parents (and other significant self-objects), and the self experiences itself as part of or nearly merged with this idealized figure or person (Ermann, 2020, p. 62). The merger causes the self to perceive itself as part of (its own) idealized images – an experience that may help to strengthen and stabilize its self-esteem. Although Kohut does not explicitly describe a particular sequence or stages of normal psychological development, the prominent self-psychologist Andrew Morrison (1989, p. 70) argues that it is possible to speak of a narcissistic development process in Kohut's theory from the grandiose self to an outward search for external objects in the form of idealized parent imagos to the internalization of moderated versions of these imagos, the development of an internal psychological structure and the establishment of increasingly mature ego ideals.

Self-objects

Self-objects occupy a key place in Kohut's theory. In a sense, self-objects belong in both the internal and external worlds and handle important functions in regulating the self and its affects, impulses, behaviour and self-esteem. In a concrete sense, self-objects may be other people, other living beings and physical objects that, from the individual's perspective, are not clearly separated from the self but are subjectively experienced as part of the self. Thus, self-objects are not ordinary objects or subjects, which are clearly separate from the self. To varying degrees, they are experienced as part of the self, while 'true objects' are experienced as being independent of the self and as autonomous subjects (Kohut, 1977, p. 84). They are objects that 'are either used in the service of the self [...] or objects which are themselves experienced as part of the self' (Kohut, 1971, p. xiv). The key is the particular subjective and emotional significance that the individual attributes to the self-object – a significance that matches the individual's unique emotional needs and the particular function it serves in the person's psychology. Often, however, this function only really becomes evident when the self-object, for various reasons, no longer functions as such, and there is a break in the self's relationship with the self-object, often because the self experiences that the self-object does not meet its needs, or because the self-object is perceived to be outside the control of the self and is thus separate from the self (Karterud, 1995, p. 70 ff.). This dynamic will inevitably play out in the therapeutic space when the therapist – inevitably – fails the patient's expectations of being the ideal – empathically mirroring, infinitely nurturing and needs-satisfying – self-object. In these situations, the patient may have an intense emotional reaction, for example by withdrawing from contact, attacking the therapist or being deeply wounded and personally offended by the therapist's inadequate satisfaction of the patient's self-object needs, for example the need for unconditional support, nurture and admiration of the patient's self.

In a normal course of development, the individual's self-objects will be 'good enough' and meet their self-object needs sufficiently to prevent traumatic frustrations or breaches of self-object relations, which is crucial for the above-mentioned transformation and maturation of the grandiose self and the idealized images of significant others. The child's developmentally appropriate needs for empathic mirroring and idealization of significant others are met with sufficient responsiveness and emotional attunement, just as the inevitable breaches and episodes of imperfect responses in central self-object relations are not so intense that they overwhelm and traumatize the developing self (Kohut & Wolf, 1978, p. 416). Meanwhile, a certain measure of frustration and correction of the child's perceptions of the perfect of self-objects is necessary to initiate what Kohut calls transmuting internalizations of self-objects and over time develop a mature and realistic understanding of reality (Kohut, 1977, p. 123).

Generally speaking, the grandiose self is then transmuted to embrace healthy and realistic goals, ambitions, interests and self-respect, while the archaic idealized parent imagos are transmuted into healthy and realistic ideals, strivings to attain these ideals and the development of the self's ability to admire others and to self-soothe and self-regulate (Kohut, 1971, p. 27ff.; Russell, 1985, p. 143). In the normal course of development, through experiences in interactions with others and, not least, with key self-objects, the child/young person thus gradually 'learns to accept his realistic limitations, the grandiose fantasies and the crude exhibitionistic demands [unrealistic ideas about external attention and admiration] are given up, and are *pari passu* replaced by ego-syntonic goals and purposes, by pleasure in his functions and activities and by realistic self-esteem' (Kohut, 1971, p. 107). Similarly, the child will gradually realize and accept that the idealized self-objects and parent imagos are imperfect, like everyone else, with natural but manageable flaws and shortcomings.

Consequences of deficiencies in self-object relations

If, on the other hand, the key self-objects are seriously flawed, and the satisfaction of the individual's archaic self-object needs – which involve both a need for empathic mirroring and a need to be able to idealize and experience emotional intimacy or even merger with the self-object – the result may be severe narcissistic imbalances in the self. Also, over time, the individual may develop narcissistic deficiencies and disturbances in their internal personality structures. Disturbances and deficiencies in the child's interactions with their self-objects may thus lead to fixation at early developmental levels characterized by archaic narcissism and self deficiencies, including fragmentation (lack of integration) of the self and unstable self-esteem, fluctuating between grandiose self-overvaluation and painful feelings of inferiority (Kohut & Wolf, 1978, p. 414).

Perceived deficiencies in the early self-object relations may result in diffuse narcissistic vulnerability (structural weakness) and problems with affect and impulse regulation, including sexual regulation (Kohut, 1971, p. 51). This may result in 'a hypersensitivity to disturbances in the narcissistic equilibrium with a tendency to react to sources of narcissistic disturbance by mixtures of wholesale withdrawal [from contact or even to a psychic retreat] and unforgiving rage' (p. 65). In pathological narcissism, the normal internalization of the good self-object has failed, and the self has not developed the ability to maintain some of the psychological functions of the idealized parent imagos. In the normal course of development, positive experience from the contact with others, especially with self-objects, will drive the development of the internal personality structure via transmuting internalization: a development in which the self gradually becomes able to contain and deal with affects, disappointment and frustrations on their own. Pathological narcissism is characterized by various degrees of deficiencies in this transmuting internalization (Kohut & Wolf, 1978, p. 416).

Archaic fantasies of own omnipotence, invulnerability, independence and self-reliance are not modified but persist in their archaic form. Dynamically, this may be seen as the self's attempt to compensate for deficiencies of the self and its internal organization (Ermann, 2020, p. 63). Similarly, the self's idealized notions have not been transmuted into more realistic and moderate images of significant external objects; the self is stuck in archaic fantasies of unrealistic idealized self-objects and 'the personality will throughout life be dependent on certain objects in what seems to be an intense form of object hunger' (Kohut, 1971, p. 45), an eternal search for self-objects to replace, fill in or compensate for deficits in the self's psychological structure. When the child's need for self-assertion and for showing themself and receiving attention (exhibitionism) is not met by empathically mirroring self-objects, the self may become stuck in archaic (including sexualized) forms of exhibitionism. Furthermore, idealized self-objects who are unable to contain the child's idealization and images of their omnipotence and omniscience and the need for temporary merger may contribute to the child's healthy admiration shutting down in favour of an archaic preoccupation with powerful and authoritarian objects (Kohut, 1977, p. 171 ff.): pathological narcissism that hinges, to a high degree, on disturbance of the self's individuation from and profound dependence on others and ability to engage in equal intersubjective relationships.

In the development of a mature form of narcissism and a coherent self, the self could be said to have two chances. If the development at one end of the two poles of the self – the grandiose self and the idealized parent imago – fails or is disturbed, the person may compensate or make up for this through a particularly successful development at the other pole (Kohut, 1977, p. 134 ff.). Thus, severe pathological narcissism will mainly develop if the development of both poles is characterized by severe deficiencies in the self's relationships with their self-objects. Conversely, deficiencies in the self-objects' empathic mirroring of the child's grandiose self can, to varying degrees, be ameliorated by the self-objects' capacity for containing and dealing with the child's need to idealize and attach closely to their self-objects, and vice versa. In some cases – for example if the child grows up with a single parent who does not have a strong social network – the child may try to have both of these basic needs met by the same self-object, in which case the self-object's deficiencies in dealing with one need may be balanced by their strength in dealing with the other. In some cases, deficiencies in the relationship with the single parent as a self-object may also be balanced by the child's or young person's relationship with another significant person than the single parent. Patients with pathological narcissism will often, to varying degrees, require a therapist who is able to deal with both self-object needs.

Vertical and horizontal splitting of the personality

In pathological narcissism, according to Kohut (1971, p. 176 ff.), the personality, or psyche, may be characterized by two types of splitting, vertical and horizontal. In a vertical split, the self attempts to keep its grandiose and its vulnerable parts separate, often in vain. As a result, the self continually alternates emotionally between, on the one hand, grandiosity, arrogance, the omnipotent denial of needs for recognition and social isolation and, on the other hand, inner emptiness, low self-esteem, destructive shame, helplessness and a strong need for external empathic mirroring and recognition (Cain et al., 2008, p. 640). This internal vertical split of the personality may be the dynamic psychological reason for constant shifts between grandiose and vulnerable manifestations of an underlying pathological narcissism in NPD.

The horizontal split, which Kohut (not entirely aptly) also calls a repression barrier, is characterized by the permanent repression or denial of unacceptable emotions and self-object needs and by a greater tendency for the self to give an impression of emotional coldness, self-reliance and detachment, corresponding to predominantly grandiose manifestations of pathological narcissism. In addition, the self has a strong – often unconscious or denied – need for interpersonal contact, as it will otherwise feel profoundly lonely and socially isolated. In this situation, loud grandiosity may be seen as a desperate attempt to escape emotional pain, including blocking emotions that the self is convinced are unacceptable to others, such as dependence, loneliness (object hunger), anxiety and sadness (Morrison & Stolorow, 1997, p. 81). Alternatively, most of the archaic grandiose self and self-object needs may be barred from consciousness, driven by traumatic deficiencies in self-object responsiveness, particularly early self-objects. As a reaction to severe deficiencies in early self-object relations, the self has blocked out any yearning or hope to ever be met with loving and empathic mirroring (p. 80) and to find a self-object that is able to contain and deal with its idealization. The self then appears largely empty, dead, depressive, paralysed, self-effacing and tormented by destructive shame (Karterud, 1995, p. 82), corresponding to predominantly vulnerable pathological narcissism. This may also be the dynamic motivation when individuals with pathological narcissism withdraw from external reality and seek refuge in their psychic retreat (see Chapter 3.6).

Kohut described this distinction between a vertical and a horizontal personality split several decades before the current distinction between predominantly vulnerable and grandiose manifestations of pathological narcissism was introduced. Hence, parts of his more specific description of the two types of personality split do not appear entirely consistent (see, e.g., Kohut, 1977, p. 176). He does not appear to consider that narcissistic pathological defects in the personality may be evident in the patient's being and acting as, alternately, predominantly vulnerable or grandiose manifestations of narcissism. It is also not clear how Kohut's understanding of these splits of the personality relate to Kernberg's descriptions of borderline personality organization, centred on identity diffusion and a relatively primitive psychological defence organized around the defence mechanism of splitting. However, Kohut would be unlikely to speak of a defence – driven by a fairly coherent ego and organized around splitting – but rather of a personality characterized by internal deficits and fragmentation or poor internal integration. Basically, Kohut views pathological narcissism as a deficit pathology, driven by deficits in the personality organization, while Kernberg tends to view it more in relation to internal conflicts.

Challenging classic psychoanalysis: Guilty man versus tragic man

Particularly in his later writings, Kohut (1977, p. 206 ff.) articulated what may be seen as a break with classic psychoanalysis and an attempt to propose a new and unique form of psychological disorder (see also Ehrenberg, 2004, p. 145 ff.; Ehrenberg, 2011). He posits a contrast between what he calls 'guilty man' versus 'tragic man'. While the guilty person is tormented by internal (oedipal) conflict – between their own ego, superego and external reality – and guilt, the tragic person is troubled much more by narcissistic disturbances centred on (pre-oedipal) themes related to their own identity, the deficits/inadequacies of the self, feelings of shame and low or unstable self-esteem. The mature and well-developed self is stable and coherent, which is normally manifested in a fundamentally healthy (realistic and nuanced) sense of self, healthy self-esteem and general psychological well-being (Wolf, 1996, p. 46).

The tragic person's self is, to varying degrees, defective, characterized by internal fragmentation, deficits in the development of internal structure and narcissistic objects – pathologies of the self that Kohut associates with the above-mentioned deficits in early self-object relations, including the lack of empathic mirroring and significant others that the self could idealize and attach to. These are all psychological processes, which means that the self lacks stable ambitions (goals) and ideals that might provide a foundation for a stable direction and agency in life (Zabel, 2019, p. 80 ff.), corresponding to severe identity disturbances (Jørgensen, 2020). It might be added here that various forms of abuse, neglect and loss of significant others may obviously be key themes in connection with deficits in early self-object relations.

In extension of this point, Kohut describes what might be called symptoms of narcissistic depression or emptiness depression, which is seen mainly in somewhat older persons with pathological narcissism (Zabel, 2019, p. 80 ff.) who have prominent feelings of shame, meaninglessness, inner emptiness, feelings of having failed and being unable to remedy their failure, and anxiety associated with the self's vulnerability and loss of love. When suicidal ideation and self-directed aggression appear in connection with emptiness depression, according to Kohut (1977, p. 241), this should be understood as a reflection of the self's urge to escape unbearable destructive shame over their own inadequacy – not as an urge to punish the self, as is the case for the guilty person struggling with internal conflicts. Thus, it represents a fundamentally narcissistic issue rooted in early (and perhaps current) self-object relations.

Pathological narcissism as a deficit pathology and relational disorder

As outlined above, Kohut basically views pathological narcissism as a deficit pathology, a result of serious deficiencies in early self-object relations and in the development of internal personality structures. In a break with the prevailing understanding of conflict in much of classic psychoanalysis and the psychoanalytic methods that were dominant during his time – primarily ego-psychology and early object relations theory – Kohut (1977, p. 2) writes that narcissistic pathology should not be understood as 'the pathological results of unsatisfactory solutions of conflicts between structures that are in essence intact, but with forms of psychological malfunctioning arising in consequence of the fact that the central structures of the personality – the structures of the self – are defective'.

In some cases, this means that the self is incapable of establishing mature relationships with others who are loved and admired for their real properties. Because interpersonal relationships in connection with pathological narcissism are dominated by the self's need for others to conduct certain psychological functions for the self, a person with a narcissistic disorder will find it difficult to enter into equal relationships with other autonomous subjects who are seen and recognized as clearly separate from and independent of the self and who are perceived as they are, and not deeply coloured by the person's own projective notions and egocentric needs. This may, for example, be a man with pathological narcissism who is in a relationship with a woman that he does not love or even respect as an equal partner but who rather inspires contempt and disgust in him, perhaps because he struggles to deal with intimate contact with her or anyone else. Nevertheless, he stays in the relationship because he needs her in order to feel secure and to fill out a painful inner void. He needs the feeling of control, respect and normality that comes from daily ordering her around and having her handle all the everyday tasks in 'his' (not 'their' shared) home and from her apparent obedience and admiration of his 'masculine strength'.

Even though he speaks of traumatic ruptures in the self-objects' response to the self's basic emotional and relational needs, Kohut (1977, p. 187) in no way claims that pathological narcissism can be understood as a simple consequence of isolated traumatic experiences. Isolated incidents, including various forms of loss and abuse, may always play a key role in complex interaction with many other aetiological factors (see Chapter 3.2) in the development of any form of psychological disorders, including pathological narcissism. However, according to Kohut (p. 187), 'in the great majority of cases it is the specific pathogenic personality of the parent(s) and specific pathogenic features of the atmosphere in which the child grows up that account for' the development of psychopathology, including pathological narcissism.

'The gross events of childhood [isolated traumas] that appear to be the cause of the later disturbances will often turn out to be no more than crystallization points for intermediate memory systems,' while the basic atmosphere and recurring patterns in the contact and interaction between the individual and significant others (self-objects) play a crucial role in the development of pathological narcissism. Behind the individual traumatic incident 'lies the much more important absence of the parents' empathic responses to the child's need to be mirrored and to find a target for his idealization' (p. 187); that is, finding a significant other capable of containing and accepting the self's at times intense idealization and overwhelming need for contact – a need that, in some cases, becomes a psychotherapist's task to respond to with appropriate empathy and an apt sense of boundary-setting (see Chapter 4.2).

Yearning for contact: Object hunger

Kohut associates pathological narcissism with a heightened vulnerability to disappointment, injury and setbacks. He also links pathological narcissism with a generally vulnerable self and self-esteem characterized by inner emptiness, a sense of unreality, alienation and a tendency to play-acting (an inability to be 'themself', an inclination to be inauthentic) and an insatiable need for empathic mirroring and contact with the idealized other (Kohut & Wolf, 1978, p. 413; Russell, 1985, p. 139). People with pathological narcissism are easily hurt and overstimulated and tend to sexualize emotional needs and conflicts, just as anxiety and worries can easily escalate and overwhelm the self (Kohut, 1971, p. 230). Kohut describes categories and degrees of narcissistic pathology that manifest themselves in particular relational dynamics (Kohut & Wolf, 1978, p. 421 ff.); according to Kohut, the last two are unambiguously pathological:

- The mirror-hungry self that **hungers for self-objects** capable of mirroring the self and satisfy its great need for admiration and recognition, including giving the fragile self a form of emotional nourishment, inner peace and organization. This is a self that attempts to escape low self-esteem, destructive shame and an inner sense of worthlessness by evoking external attention – but which at the same time finds it difficult to feel that its needs are satisfied and thus go on trying to seek new self-objects. It should be noted that self-objects are not necessarily only other people but may also include pets, physical objects, a particular piece of music or other forms of art, a building, a city, a nature area or another physical location that, for various reasons, holds particular significance and meaning to the self.
- The **ideal-hungry self**, forever searching for others it can admire for their status, power, beauty, intelligence and moral integrity. This is a fragile self that seeks to stabilize itself and fill its painful sense of emptiness or boredom by experiencing a connection with the idealized self-object, which is attributed ideal qualities that, to varying degrees, are at odds with the self-object's objective characteristics – and the self is repeatedly disappointed. Thus, deficits in personality structures cannot be remediated on a more permanent basis with this mainly internal and imagined connection to idealized objects.
- The **alter-ego-hungry self**, which searches for a self-object that by appearing to be like the self and sharing its being, opinions and values can confirm the self's existence through a form of identification and a perceived community with the self-object. However, the self's internal deficits and emptiness that drive this desperate search for self-objects cannot really be remediated via these alter-ego relationships or twinships. When the self inevitably realizes that the other is not – or is not like – the self but is separate and different from it, the self feels alienated from the former alter-ego self-object and needs to go searching for a replacement, a new alter-ego self-object, a new soulmate, whom the self hopes to be able to engage in deep and everlasting internal connection with.

- **The merger-hungry self** that yearns to be unified with and control mirroring or idealized self-objects in an attempt to create an internal structure and keep together a fragile self structure that is at risk of fragmentation. The boundaries between the self and its self-objects are compromised, and the self has difficulty distinguishing between its own and the self-object's thoughts, feelings, needs and intentions. Specifically, this may mean, for example, that the self is convinced that it has shared thoughts and feelings with the self-object that in fact only the self has been in contact with. Furthermore, the self struggles to deal with being separated from its self-objects and expects or demands them to be permanently accessible, just as the self has difficulty dealing with indications that a self-object might be separate or independent from the self or that it might want to leave the self.
- The **self that avoids any form of intimate contact** and thus superficially appears as the direct opposite of the merger-hungry self. In many ways, however, it is in fact closely related to the merger-hungry self but shuns contact and seeks social isolation out of fear of its own overwhelming need for contact and equally intense fear of rejection and abandonment. The self seeks to deal with this persistent fear and profound vulnerability to abandonment and keep it in check by avoiding emotional and other forms of intimate (physical, psychological) contact with others. This is a self that is terrified by what it perceives as its own greedy need of contact but also by how the self may become swallowed up and disappear or lose itself if the all-encompassing union that it yearns for actually were to happen. Thus, it is also a self that is tormented by profound and troubling ambivalence in relation to potential self-objects – and it may be related to Steiner's (1993, 2014) description of the self that seeks safety in psychic retreats (see Chapter 3.6).

The common quality of these different manifestations of pathological narcissism and its expression in the fragile self's relationship with and search for self-objects is a persistent and insatiable hunger for a self-object – an other – capable of stabilizing and completing a self that is characterized by a diffuse sense of inner emptiness and deficits; a hunger that will also typically be expressed in the relationship with a therapist. Thus, we should be cautious about mindlessly considering any patient's – even very positive – perception of the therapist or others as good and caring (self-)objects as solely an expression of primitive infantile idealization.

Generally, we should take the patient's subjective experience seriously and notice how the patient actually describes and justifies their perception of the other and consider to what extent this is meaningfully related to the described person's actual characteristics, or whether it appears to contain elements of denial of non-ideal characteristics in the other (which everyone, including therapists, obviously possesses). It is important to do this, rather than delegitimizing and invalidating the patient's experience off-hand by categorizing it as primitive idealization. When the patient's self-object needs, for various reasons, are not seen and met with the empathic mirroring and responsiveness that the vulnerable self in particular needs, the reactions may be quite intense. For example, the patient may withdraw from all relationships or be overwhelmed by narcissistic rage, which may be directed both at the self and at others.

According to Kohut, this aggression and anger should be seen as a reaction to the self's perceived disappointments and betrayals, not as a form of constitutional aggression or the self's intrinsic evil. As Kohut (1977, p. 116) puts it:

> In essence then, I believe that man's destructiveness as a psychological phenomenon is secondary; that it arises originally as the result of the failure of the self-object environment to meet the child's need for optimal – not maximal, it should be stressed – empathic responses.

We should view anger as irretrievably connected with natural human self-assertion, while openly destructive anger and aggression are always 'motivated by an injury to the self' (p. 116). Similarly, Kohut (1977, p. 121) believes that when Melanie Klein – in a phenomenologically nuanced and apt description – speaks of the patient in the paranoid-schizoid position, who is convinced that the world is inherently hostile to the self, this also does not spring from any intrinsic human aggression or death urge. It is, instead, a consequence of traumatic deficiencies in early self-objects' empathic responses to the self.

3.4 Otto Kernberg and object relations theory

According to Kernberg, the personality in patients with pathological narcissism is generally organized at borderline level (BPO). Thus, they have a number of traits in common with other relatively severe personality disorders, particularly borderline personality disorder (BPD) and, to a lesser degree, dissocial personality disorder (ASPD), which typically also has a BPO. Kernberg's main focus is on pathological narcissism in patients whose personality structure is at the medium or lower levels of BPO. This will also be the main focus of the following, although later developments of Kernberg's understanding of narcissism to some extent also address higher-functioning and less disordered manifestations of pathological narcissism (Diamond et al., 2022). Patients with malignant narcissism – who in Kernberg's work represent a particularly disordered and treatment-resistant subgroup of pathological narcissism – are somewhat more closely related to ASPD and psychopathy (see Chapter 3.1). However, this will not be discussed further in the present context. According to Kernberg's (1984, p. 12 ff.) general description of the personality with a borderline organization, patients with pathological narcissism will be characterized, in particular, by identity diffusion, disordered object relations and primitive psychological defence mechanisms. In addition, Kernberg (1975, p. 261 ff.) views pathological narcissism as characterized by disordered self-esteem, envy and a pathological grandiose self and a resulting unusual level of self-absorption in interpersonal interactions.

During the early years, the child develops internal mental representations of self, others and normal human interactions based on exchanges with significant others, particularly close family members. The child develops what Kernberg and object relations theory calls internal object relations. Attachment theory similarly speaks of the development of internal working models (Bowlby, 1988, p. 144 ff; Bartholomew et al., 2001, p. 201 ff.; see Chapter 3.2), which in many regards covers the same phenomenon, except that object relations theory has a stronger focus on the affects associated with the developing internal object relations. This includes, for example, the fact that the development of internal object relations characterized by perceptions of the self as extraordinary and admirable (grandiose) and perceptions of others as (potentially inferior) objects who admire and are always available to satisfy the self's needs may be accompanied by pride in the person's own self, discreet or overt contempt of most other people and (narcissistic) rage if others fail to act in accordance with the self's perceptions of others as an attentive and grateful audience that loves and admires the self in everything it does.

These internal object relations with their related perceptions of self, others and interpersonal relationships subsequently lay the foundation for how the self meets, perceives and interacts with others in the external world. They have a significant impact on how the self interprets others' intentions and behaviour in interactions with the self, including how the self imagines that it is perceived and evaluated by others and what others expect of the self. They also play an important role in shaping the self's way of being and acting in interactions with others. For example, the young man who has always been given the impression that he is unique and that extraordinary accomplishments are expected of him – and that normal rules and norms therefore might not fully apply to him – may develop a grandiose self-image. He may develop mental self-representations that support a sense of entitlement. He may also develop the impression that others exist mainly to admire and support his egocentric self-expression and realization of his extraordinary abilities and potential, given his mental representations of others and of interpersonal relationships. These ideas about self and others may, naturally, make it difficult to establish and maintain equal relationships with others. They also carry a considerable risk of defeat in his encounters with the real world, especially as an adult, as only people who actually possess extraordinary abilities may sometimes get away with being and acting in ways that are driven by these grandiose perceptions.

Behind this apparent grandiosity, there may be a very different reality if the parents' high – and in fact unrealistic – expectations of their child are shaped by their own failed dreams. In this case, they are using their child to meet their own narcissistic needs or to deal with their own feelings of inferiority (narcissistic imbalances), expecting the child or young person to be in a certain way and achieve things that are misaligned with who the child or young man is and with his actual abilities and potential. The child is not met and mirrored as he is but as an object that is shaped by the needs of other (the parents) and their projective ideas about who the child is and ought to be. This may contribute to the development of a false self, as the child does not express its true self but adapts to the expectations of the people around them, trying desperately to be and become what significant others want – or even demand – of the child as a condition for admiring and loving the self. This relational dynamic may be a contributing cause of the development of severe identity disorders (identity diffusion).

Similarly, some people have general experience of being met with disinterest, indifference, coldness, contempt and a lack of empathic mirroring, both as children and throughout much of their life. They may have been seen and used as objects, things – perhaps even subjected to physical or sexual abuse – to satisfy the needs of others. This sort of history will often lead to the development of internal object relations centred on perceptions of the self as inferior, shamefully inadequate, worthless, contemptible and unlovable. Based on experiences from their relations with significant others who were emotionally detached, inaccessible, erratic and mainly focused on their own needs, these people will typically develop mental representations of others as being generally emotionally inaccessible and unreliable, disinterested in and dismissive of the self and at best responsive to the self's needs if the self is continually perceptive of and meets their needs and, not least, consistently seeks to meet their expectations (cf. internal object representations). These are all elements that are typically seen in connection with vulnerable manifestations of pathological narcissism.

Identity diffusion

Persons with an upbringing characterized by mainly positive experiences in interactions with significant others will develop internal object relations with a similar emphasis on positive perceptions of self, others and interpersonal relationships. The internalization of these positive experience will lay the foundation for establishing a good internal object defined by a basic belief in self, others and the world at large. Thus, a mature and well-developed identity is associated with realistic, nuanced, integrated and clearly differentiated mental representations – notions – of self and others, as positive and negative perceptions mutually balance and modify each other to form representations of reality that, overall, are mainly positive and valid (Diamond et al., 2022, p. 18).

The identity of persons with pathological narcissism, on the other hand, is characterized by severe deficits in the integration of perceptions of self and others. Their sense of self and, in particular, of others is fundamentally unstable, vague, superficial, generalizing and distorted and tends to divide the world into polarized black-and-white (devalued–idealized) categories

(Caligor et al., 2020, p. 109). In some cases, their descriptions of their own self will be more detailed, specific and, in some aspects, realistic compared to the case for persons with BPD, but they will also be characterized by a sense of emptiness and obvious self-overvaluation in certain areas, particularly in more grandiose manifestations of pathological narcissism (p. 118). Typically, their perceptions and descriptions of the self will be somewhat superficial and focus on accomplishments/victories and comparisons with others, while their perceptions and descriptions of others will be noticeably clichéd, superficial and vague (Caligor, 2013, p. 71).

A few studies of psychiatric patients with reliably diagnosed personality disorders found clear indications of severe identity diffusion in persons with pathological narcissism (NPD) (Jørgensen et al., 2023, p. 8). Some studies based on non-clinical populations (mainly students) found that relational disorders (Bogaerts & Jankovic, 2024) and poor emotional empathy (Di Pierro et al., 2018) in persons with narcissistic traits are mediated by disordered identity, as evaluated via dimensional measures of identity integration and degree of instability in mental representations of self and others. One study among a student population found that the degree of self-reported identity disorder mediates correlations between vulnerable and, in particular, grandiose narcissism and relational difficulties (Biberdzic et al., 2023).

Furthermore, studies based on university students found a fairly strong correlation (r=.62) between measures of pathological narcissism (PNI, Pathological Narcissism Inventory) and subscales for pathological identity diffusion on an instrument for evaluating personality organization (IPO, Inventory Personality Organization) (Pincus et al., 2009b, p. 372). With the significant reservation that none of the latter studies was based on patients with NPD, these findings do suggest a relatively strong link between pathological narcissism and identity diffusion. This lends support to Kernberg's understanding of identity diffusion as a key personality-structural factor in pathological narcissism (see also Jørgensen, 2020; Jørgensen et al., 2023; Jørgensen & Bøye, 2022).

In contrast to patients with BPD, whose painful confusion about their own identity – 'who am I really?' – is typically fairly obvious, these significant disturbances of the self's sense of identity in patients with pathological narcissism may, to varying degrees, be covert or hidden behind fairly coherent and stable – in practice, often quite rigid – grandiose perceptions of self, particularly in patients with NPD with a relatively high level of BPO. These idealized and unrealistically positive self-perceptions may be accompanied by similar – overt or more covert – unrealistic and polarized perceptions of others as inferior and insignificant, perhaps threatening competitors to the self or, conversely, as highly idealizing perceptions of a few others, whom the self identifies with or seeks comfort from through actual or imagined contact.

Initially, the identity of persons with pathological narcissism may thus appear to be relatively well integrated and stable, particularly compared to BPD, but behind the self-assertive, self-referential and grandiose facade, they will often struggle with highly varying and contradictory self-perceptions (Ronningstam, 2021, p. 10). However, Kernberg argues that their representations of others are typically characterized by a striking lack of integration and depth as well as an egocentric tendency to focus on others' similarity or dissimilarity to the self. The latter tendency may be understood in relation to their poor empathy, particularly when it comes to emotional empathy (Kernberg, 1984, p. 193 ff.; Caligor et al., 2015, p. 418). Similarly, their emotions will generally lack depth, just as persons with pathological narcissism may give the impression of not having an inner life and living entirely in the external reality, where they attempt to handle all forms of contact at a purely cognitive-rational level, and the self shows no sign of curiosity or even interest in their own or others' inner life or emotional reactions (Kernberg, 2018, p. 158).

In particular in patients with a poorly organized personality, including patients with a clearly fragile grandiose facade, persistent fluctuations between grandiose and vulnerable manifestations of narcissism may be linked to identity diffusion and the related fluctuations between different ego-states and perceptions of the self as grandiose and self-sufficient versus empty, inferior and in need of – perhaps entitled to – attention, nurture and admiration from others: fluctuations between a self-sufficient self that does not need anybody and who keeps others at a distance versus a self that cannot possible get by on its own and who clings to others in a desperate attempt to keep itself together. Similar fluctuations also occur in connection with disorganized attachment, with confusing and unpredictable fluctuations between anxious avoidant and anxious clingy attachment strategies (see Chapter 3.2).

Grandiose self-structure

In pathological narcissism, the personality is dominated by a grandiose self-structure, in which all perceptions of the real and the ideal self as well as perceptions of ideal objects have fused into one. Ideas about one's own power, wealth and beauty and of ever-giving, ever-loving and accepting objects merge with perceptions of the real self (Russell, 1985, p. 141). These grandiose self-perceptions hamper the development of more realistic perceptions of the self that match the self's actual abilities, potential and characteristics (Diamond et al., 2022, p. 22). In this sense, they are clearly dysfunctional, even if they may momentarily and in the short term help stabilize and keep a fundamentally fragile and unstable self together. The grandiose self-structure may be accompanied by notions that the self contains all the goodness and everything it needs – the self already 'is' its own ideal (Kernberg, 1975, p. 266). As the self does not appear to need others, they fade and appear inferior in comparison to the grandiose self. Furthermore, all the negative, aggressive and devalued parts of the self and perceptions of the self and others may be split off and projected onto others (Kernberg, 2004a, p. 54).

This grandiose internal self-structure is an important part of the dynamic driver of the self-reliance and arrogance of patients with NPD, including their tendency to distance themself from others. It may also contribute to keeping their vulnerability and fear of dependence on others in check. In light of their relational history, we may, with Kernberg's (1984, p. 202) work in mind, view it as an indication that these patients have identified with idealized, grandiose, manipulative, perhaps sadistically frustrating aspects of mental representations of early object relations, while complementary aspects are projected onto others, for example in the form of perceptions of the devalued, humiliated and exploited other. In some patients and at other times, these positions may, so to speak, 'change places', causing them to perceive themselves as shamefully humiliated and exploited in relation to a sadistically exploitative and deliberately frustrating other in a recurring and severely destructive relational pattern of victim-abuser.

Disordered object relations

The patient pays a high price for this apparent – and sometimes ineffective – attempt to stabilize their identity. The self withdraws from and denies parts of reality and becomes unable to be authentically present and in intimate contact with others; a contact that might challenge the grandiose self-perception and cause it to crack and collapse. Thus, when the self avoids intimate contact with others, the purpose is to protect the self's vulnerable and sometimes covert (cf. more vulnerable manifestations of pathological narcissism) perceptions of its own uniqueness. Opening up to and forming attachments to others would be shameful and a threat to the vulnerable self and risk making the self dependent on others (including a therapist) who are outside the self's control. The self has difficulty dealing with any form of real intimacy and would typically be unable to combine emotional and sexual contact (Caligor et al., 2015, p. 416 ff.).

In persons with pathological narcissism, sexuality may furthermore be closely associated with aggression, which makes it even more complicated to combine sexual and real emotional contact (Diamond et al., 2022, p. 363). Even though the capacity for sexual arousal and release (orgasm) is normally intact, the self's sexuality will thus typically be lived out in ways that reflect their highly limited capacity for real emotional contact. Among other consequences, this may involve having several parallel sexual partners without any real engagement or emotional commitment to any of them. Conversely, it may also involve seeking sexual satisfaction via pornography, masturbation, prostitution, online sex or other forums where the self can avoid coming into contact with and developing what it perceives as the frightening prospect of dependence on a concrete sex partner (Kernberg, 2018, p. 241 ff.).

Even though some persons with pathological narcissism may appear highly dependent on others, who can satisfy their need for admiration and control over other's view of the self, they are often fundamentally incapable of developing, containing and dealing with actual authentic dependence: the kind of dependence that implies a certain measure of interpersonal trust, which pathological narcissism makes it very difficult to develop (Kernberg, 1975, p. 271). In cases where they appear to be emotionally dependent on an admired and idealized other, this person is perceived as an extension of the self. The delimitation between self and other has been compromised, and thus, this is not an actual object relation, let alone dependence on a delimited autonomous subject (p. 271). Kernberg (2018, p. 182) also views defence against any form of authentic dependence as one of the most significant manifestations of the grandiose self. Actual dependence thus implies that the self has acknowledged and recognizes the other's great importance for the self; a situation that, among other consequences, may give rise to overwhelming envy, given that the other has something that the self does not possess but needs. The self may attempt to escape this unbearable envy by devaluing or withdrawing from – or, alternatively, trying to gain absolute control over – the other (Kernberg, 1975, p. 302). Dependence may also be associated with unbearable feelings of shameful inferiority, as the need for others creates dangerous cracks in the grandiose self's facade of self-reliance.

In pathological narcissism, both internal and external object relations are disturbed, and according to Kernberg, they are characterized by primitive aggression, envy and categorical divisions of the self's relational universe based on perceptions of idealized good and devalued bad figures – distinctions that are associated with primitive defence mechanisms organized around splitting, which similarly breaks the world up into black-and-white categories. Because of the inadequate integration of internal object relations – perceptions of self and others – persons with pathological narcissism are dependent on continual admiration and recognition from others to stabilize the self and its grandiose defence, which is organized around the perception of the self as being extraordinary (Caligor et al., 2020, p. 107). The grandiose self is rigid, incapable of adapting to different circumstances and thus also quite vulnerable and dependent on others who support its perceptions of uniqueness in various ways (p. 109).

Furthermore, varying degrees of pathology are seen in the development of the superego, with deficient moral standards and dissocial traits as well as immature values with a focus on material wealth, beauty, power and fame and, not least, values centred on the self's own narrow and short-sighted gratification rather than values that go beyond the self's own needs and interests. Some might claim that by making this point, Kernberg is moralizing, applying an inappropriately normative view of persons with pathological narcissism. On the other hand, behaviour that is guided by these immature values will typically have serious consequences for the individual, for the self's ability to engage in well-functioning relationships and communities as well as for the social communities and significant others, who need to try to deal with these individuals. Thus, they are an important part of the reason why people with pathological narcissism often struggle with profound emotional loneliness and are socially ostracized. This makes it relevant to view these immature values, superego pathology and disturbed object relations as important aspects of pathological narcissism.

3.5 Key differences and similarities between Kohut's and Kernberg's understandings

Kohut and Kernberg must be regarded as the two most important figures in the development of our ability to understand and treat pathological narcissism. Although they are both psychoanalysts and originally based their work on parts of Freud's drive theory, with Kohut in particular later distancing himself from it, on crucial points they represent very different perspectives on and approaches to narcissism. As for the purely descriptive understanding of pathological narcissism – the specific manifestations of the narcissistic personality disorder in patients' subjective experiences and behaviour – in many regards, they are in agreement (Kernberg, 1975, p. 302). However, there are significant differences in their more specific understanding of the pathology and their suggestions for the psychotherapeutic treatment of pathological narcissism (see Chapter 5).

Kohut views narcissism as a natural part of children's and adults' psychology; Kernberg, on the other hand, does acknowledge a form of narcissism as part of normal early psychological development, but he also views it as something that is overcome and left behind in the normal psychological maturation process; he mainly views narcissism in adults as indication of psychological immaturity or disturbance. According to Kernberg (1975, p. 311 ff.), in several key regards, pathological narcissism in adult patients with NPD differs fundamentally from what could be called normal childhood narcissism. This also implies that Kernberg rejects Kohut's idea that the (pathological) narcissism that is actualized in the transference in psychotherapeutic work with patients with NPD (see Chapter 4.2) should be considered a normal or, at least, empathically understandable actualization of archaic childhood narcissism in the therapeutic space. According to Kernberg, the two forms of narcissism have the following key differences, among others:

1. Children's grandiose fantasies and urge for attention and to control others is much more aligned with their current reality than in pathological narcissism.
2. In addition to the strong reactions to criticism, defeat and guilt (which should probably rather be understood as feelings of shame; cf. Jørgensen, 2023/2024), which relate both to childhood narcissism and to pathological narcissism, children will also show genuine love, gratitude, capacity to depend on others and authentic interest in others, which are largely absent in pathological narcissism.
3. While children's demands and sense of entitlement reflect real needs, in pathological narcissism, these are often obviously overblown and, in practice, impossible to satisfy.

4 Pathological narcissism is accompanied by emotional coldness, ruthlessness, destructiveness, disregard for and contempt of others as well as a striking absence of emotional warmth and attachment to others that are not similarly seen in connection with normal narcissism in children.
5 The child's fantasies of power, wealth and beauty are not accompanied by the megalomaniacal fantasies of possessing all that is valuable and enviable in the world that characterize the pathological grandiose self.(Kernberg, 1975, p. 272 ff.)

Kohut and Kernberg disagree on what constitutes the central dynamic processes underlying the different manifestations of pathological narcissism and also represent fairly different positions as to what are the most significant causal factors in the development of pathological narcissism. According to Kohut, defects in early self-objects and self-object relations, including deficiencies in the empathic mirroring of the self and capacity to contain the self's idealization, are crucial aetiologal factors, deficits that lead to deficits in the normal integration and moderation of the grandiose self and idealized perceptions of parents and significant others. Kernberg also points to disturbances of early object relations, including the internalization of these early relations and, thus, the development of internal mental representations of the self and others, as key causal factors, but he also argues that constitutional aggression (stemming from innate drives) play a decisive role in the development of pathological narcissism, just as he is far more focused on internal conflicts than on deficits in the self and its internal structures.

In principle, the two authors represent two different understandings of human psychology, in the sense that Kohut views pathological narcissism as a result of the encounter between an inherently good and innocent self and a 'bad' or inadequate world – a deficient self-object environment – that distorts the self's psychological development, while Kernberg attributes a form of original aggression to the self (cf. his original adherence to Freud's drive theory) and views internal conflicts, envy and self-other conflicts as basic aspects of the human psyche and, thus, not as challenges that only arise in the encounter with a bad or inadequate external world. For a very brief outline of some of the most significant differences between Kohut's and Kernberg's understanding of narcissism, see Table 3.2 overleaf.

Effective factors in psychotherapeutic treatment: Contact and/or technique?

In natural extension of their specific understandings of what constitutes the core of pathological narcissism, to some extent, they also offer fairly different suggestions for how the therapist should meet persons with pathological narcissism. This includes the extent to which the therapist should be containing, offer empathic understanding and strive for optimal frustration of the patient (Kohut) versus being more confronting and attentive to how the

Table 3.2 Selected elements in Kohut's and Kernberg's perspectives on pathological narcissism (see also Ermann, 2020, p. 117 ff.; Ronningstam, 2011, p. 50).

	Kohut	*Kernberg*
General understanding of narcissism	Part of normal psychological development process; has separate development line	Part of early psychological development that is normally overcome; distinguishes categorically between normal and pathological narcissism
Main focus in the understanding of pathological narcissism	Deficits in the self, fragile/low self-esteem, perceptions of the self as inadequate and empty	Grandiose and aggressive aspects of self-perception and envy – grandiose aspects are viewed as possible compensation for or concealment of fragile self-esteem and associated with biologically driven aggression
Basic understanding of causes of pathological narcissism	Manifestation of deficits (fixation) in self development; result of empathic failures/deficiencies in self-objects – normally grandiose and exhibitionist self was not neutralized and integrated; deficits in transmuting internalization of experiences with self-objects	Result of internal conflicts; lack of integration and modification of archaic anger, splitting and development of pathological grandiose self as defence
Emotional core	Shame, anxiety, reactive anger/rage	Constitutional anger/rage, envy
Understanding of the source of aggression	Secondary consequence of deficiencies in early (and later) relationships and in the ability of significant others to function as self-objects; related to fear of revenge from others or loss of the self-object	Driven by constitutional aggression, envy – and, possibly, unsatisfied archaic longing for object
Understanding of relationship between narcissistic and borderline pathology	Views narcissistic pathology as fairly distinct from borderline states	Views moderate and severe narcissistic pathology as being organized at borderline level and thus structurally close to BPD
Central transference constellations	Need for mirroring (admiration), for idealized object, for 'twinship'/alter ego	Regressive/immature devaluation versus idealization of the therapist
Aggression, greed, sexualization in the transference	Viewed as secondary consequences or manifestations of vulnerable, threatened or fragmented self	Viewed as (drive-based) primary motivation factors in the interaction with the therapist

	Kohut	*Kernberg*
Understanding of idealization of the therapist	Expresses the activation of idealized parent imagos, expression of hope and a part of normal narcissistic development process	Expresses that the patient is projecting their own grandiose self-perceptions onto the therapist
Dealing with transference	The therapist should contain, accept and empathically mirror the patient's needs and yearnings in the transference	The therapist should confront and interpret the patient's needs in the transference as regressive and as expressions of narcissistic defences against, in particular, envy and greed
Central elements in the therapeutic process	Empathic mirroring and resonance, empathic listening to and understanding of narcissistic challenges, working through perceived failures of empathy by the therapist	Exploring, confronting and interpreting narcissistic defences and transference – in particular the patient's aggression, envy, contempt and devaluation of the therapist
Psychotherapeutic stance in the encounter with the patient	Participating observer who is present as a subject; containing and empathically mirroring self-object	Predominantly neutral, confronting and interpreting therapist who does not have the same presence as the subject
Intended structural changes	Establishing internal structure (cf. defects in the organization of the self)	Developing internal integration and more mature defences; modifying and overcoming pathological grandiose self, identity diffusion and defences organized around splitting
Key therapeutic treatment factors	Corrective experiences in interactions with the therapist as an empathically mirroring and/or idealized self-object; transmuting internalization of the therapist and interactions with the therapist as a self-object – including elements of real relation	Gaining insight into internal conflicts, aggression and envy; working through negative transference; analytical interpretation is the paramount treatment factor
Risks of therapeutic strategy	That the patient becomes too passively dependent on and fails to achieve delimitation from the therapist as a containing and empathic (idealized) self-object (cf. individuation); illusion of treatment process without anxiety and pain; underestimating the patient's resources and agency, infantilizing the patient; overlooking the self-object's own legitimate needs	That the patient feels criticized, disparaged, shamed and/or abandoned by 'neutral', confronting, implicitly moralizing and interpreting therapist; overestimating the patient's agency and ability to contain and deal with painful mental states

patient's aggression, envy and any psychopathic traits pollute the therapeutic space and should therefore be met with clear boundary-setting and an insistence, from the outset, on examining the dynamic background of the patient's destructive behaviour in the therapeutic space (Kernberg). Specifically, this implies, for example that, according to Kohut, aggression in the patient's interaction with the therapist (transference) should generally be understood as an indication that the patient has experienced ruptures or deficiencies in the therapist's self-object functioning. Kernberg would understand this aggression in relation to the actualization of unconscious aggression in the patient and the resulting distorted perception of and urge to control or 'dismantle' the therapist as therapist (Kernberg, 1984, p. 188). Kernberg thus mainly attributes aggression in the patient's transference to the patient's internal dynamic processes, while Kohut attributes more significance to relational processes and to something playing out between patient and therapist in the here-and-now. Thus, the therapist also – in part due to failures in their responsiveness to the patient's self-object needs – has a shared responsibility if the patient reacts with aggression, withdrawal or self-directed aggression in the interaction with the therapist.

Generally, Kohut views the patient's transference as reflective of the effort to establish a self-object relation in the therapeutic space and a desperate attempt to have the therapist meet self-object needs that have not previously been met by others – needs of admiration, warmth, validation, empathic mirroring, intimacy, identification or merger with an idealized other. On this point, Kohut describes different forms of object hunger (cf. above) and transference (see Chapter 5). Although Kernberg acknowledges Kohut's purely descriptive accounts of these dynamic processes and constellations in the transference, he does not view them primarily as reflections of the patient's attempts to satisfy archaic and, essentially, understandable and legitimate narcissistic needs.

Kernberg is more interested in how transference in patients with NPD, in his opinion, will always be dominated by the patient's sometimes more or less covert – and sometimes unconscious – anger, envy and contempt directed at the therapist and, not least, by the patient's fear of becoming dependent and feeling lesser than, inferior to or shamefully inadequate in relation to the therapist (Gabbard & Crisp, 2018, p. 83). The specific manifestations of what Kohut views as actualization of archaic self-object needs in transference are viewed by Kernberg as indications of the patient's resistance to treatment – resistance to acknowledging and understanding aspects of their own self, including anger/rage and envy – that is actualized in the therapeutic space. Kernberg also argues that Kohut tends to overlook the patient's anger and negative transference, which block the patient's ability to 'hear' the content of the therapist's verbal interventions and use these as a basis for self-reflection and for developing a deeper understanding of themself (Ermann, 2020, p. 117).

Conversely, based on Kohut's understanding, we may argue that the patient will not be able to 'hear' what the therapist says until the therapist's verbal interventions are provided in a way and in a relational atmosphere that makes it possible for the patient to listen (Wolf, 1996, p. 134). In practice, this means that the patient should, at the very least, experience that their basic self-object needs are seen, mirrored and acknowledged by the therapist. Thus, it is not only – perhaps not even primarily – the therapist's ability to deliver certain verbal interventions with a particular content that determines the outcome of treatment. The therapist's more personal qualities, including the ability to establish contact and an emotional atmosphere in the therapeutic space that meets the patient's core self-object needs are at least as important (see Jørgensen, 2018/2019).

Based on Kohut's work, we can argue that aspects of the patient's emotional contact with the therapist as a self-object in itself contains key therapeutic treatment factors and, for example, that the therapist's empathic mirroring of the patient and ability to accept the patient's idealization contribute significantly to the development of internal structure and capacity to regulate own affects and impulses that is key in the treatment of pathological narcissism. Similarly, we can argue that therapist should to some extent and temporarily satisfy some of the emotional and relational needs that are actualized in the patient's transference, including satisfying self-object needs that were not seen and met sufficiently responsively by past self-objects. According to Kohut (1977, p. 30), essential transformations in psychotherapy do not take place 'in consequence of such supportive intellectual [cognitive] insights, but in consequence of the gradual internalizations' of the therapist way of acting as a self-object in interactions with the patient. '[T]he beneficial structural transformations occurring in a successful analysis do not take place as the result of insights' (p. 30) but are produced by the development of the internal structure that is lacking in the patient's personality, though transmuting internalization: a process driven by what unfolds at the different levels of contact between patient and therapist, including the therapist's ability to contain and offer responsive reactions – empathic but also as a subject that is clearly separate from the patient's self – to the patient's transference and acting in the therapeutic space in general.

On the other hand, referencing Kernberg, we could insist that what the patient really needs is to meet a therapist who, from an emotionally neutral, more observational and objective position can offer clarifications and interpretations of the patient's subjective experiences, thoughts, feelings and behaviour in the transference and the therapeutic space that help the patient to achieve greater self-insight and to integrate and modify their perceptions of self and others. There is reason to consider what it takes to help the patient overcome unrealistic narcissistic idealizations and expectations in relation to others, including the therapist. Should the therapist – primarily via specific interventions (technique); cf. Kernberg – clearly set boundaries for, reality-test and confront the patient with their unrealistic, infantile and grandiose expectations of the therapist? Or should the therapist – primarily via their contact with the patient; cf. Kohut – contain and, to varying degrees, satisfy some of the patient's needs for empathic mirroring and emotional contact with an idealized other (the therapist); a contact that gradually enables the patient to scale down their grandiose defence – in the form of grandiose self-perceptions and expectations of self-objects, developed in an attempt to deal with severe deficiencies in the early satisfaction of self-object needs – and take back/tone down their idealized perceptions of the therapist?

Pitfalls in the two models to be balanced in practice

It is debatable how much Kernberg's 'transference focused psychotherapy' (TFP) actually acknowledges the often significant role of nonverbal – not necessarily articulated and analytically interpreted – aspects of the interaction between patient and therapist as elements in healing pathological narcissism. For example, the activation of the patient's internalized object relations in a safe setting where they may be (cognitively!) contained and explored is considered a treatment factor in TFP (Diamond et al., 2022, p. 145). However, compared to Kohut's fairly overt therapeutic use of elements in the contact and the therapist's involvement in the interpersonal interaction with the patient, particularly in his later work, there are at the very least clear differences between Kohut's and Kernberg's relative focus and emphasis on the use of the therapeutic contact versus their focus on the patient's attainment of insight, including the systematic effort to uncover and articulate the conscious awareness of the patient's grandiose self in the therapeutic process.

Kernberg (1984, p. 184 ff.) is quite critical of what he perceives as Kohut's focus on the therapist's empathy at the expense of their objective neutrality, just as he believes that Kohut conflates different forms of idealization when he connects the therapist's acceptance of the patient's idealization with the therapist's position as the containing, accepting and empathic self-object, which in Kohut's understanding makes a considerable contribution to the patient's development process. According to Kernberg (1984, p. 85), this conflates idealization as a defence against aggression (cf. splitting, devaluation and idealization directed at the therapist), idealization as an attempt to deal with feelings of guilt (or, more likely, feelings of shame) and idealization associated with the patient's projection of their own grandiose perceptions onto the therapist.

In relation to all three forms of idealization – to which we might add idealization as a defence against envy of the therapist – Kernberg sees it as the therapist's task to uncover how the patient's idealization in the specific situation is connected with various other affects and defensive strategies. The task may be approached in a variety of ways, including with different degrees of empathy and confrontation. Furthermore, Kernberg (1984, p. 181) has pointed out that the severely narcissistic patient does not deny the separation or the existence of a boundary between the self and the therapist as the idealized self-object; cf. Kohut's idea that the self and the therapist sometimes merge in the patient's internal psyche – which, in a very concrete understanding would, in principle, indicate a psychotic level of functioning – but only denies (is unable to handle) the existence of any significant differences between self and therapist.

An overly concrete and rigid interpretation of Kernberg's treatment approach carries the risk that patients – particularly poorly organized patients with a fragile grandiose defence – are subjected to narcissistic injury and overwhelmed by narcissistic rage or, more likely, feel shamed and abandoned by a confrontational and emotionally withdrawn – at times perhaps silent – therapist, who sees the therapeutic space as an opportunity for the patient to come into contact with previously covert aspects of themself. A passive and almost silent therapist may intensify an already withdrawn and humiliated patient's destructive shame, painful emotional isolation and sense of being abandoned on their own in a situation characterized by overwhelming needs for nurturing contact (Livingston & Farber, 1996, p. 602). For a patient who is already tormented by destructive shame and perceives their own feelings and needs as unacceptable and wrong, therapeutic interventions that identify their needs as expressions of infantile greed or articulate their behaviour in interactions with the therapist as expressions of envy, masochism or vindictiveness may be perceived as not just another narcissistic injury but as shaming and devaluing (Wile, 1984).

The patient may come to perceive their subjective experiences and emotional yearnings as illegitimate and have their painful sense of having no right to exist confirmed, while their need for empathic mirroring and corrective emotional experiences – in which destructive interaction patterns are not repeated in the contact with the therapist – go entirely unmet. These are all dynamics of the therapeutic relationship that may have a negative effect on the therapeutic process and the narcissistically disordered patient's treatment outcome (Wile, 1984). Furthermore, although the therapist sees, acknowledges and validates the patient's emotional needs and need for new experiences in the interaction with the therapist as understandable in light of the patient's history, this does not necessarily imply that these needs should be satisfied. And it certainly does not imply that they cannot also be made the object of common exploration as an important part of the therapeutic process.

Kernberg's approach places much greater emphasis on enhancing the patient's self-reflection and cognitive self-perception than on the therapist's empathic understanding and emotional resonance in the contact with the patient (Fiscalini, 2004, p. 127). On the other hand, the Kohut-inspired therapist may be misled into 'pampering' or infantilizing the narcissistic patient, particularly in the case of vulnerable narcissism by acting too much as the good self-object that mainly aims to satisfy the patient's archaic self-object needs at the expense of the hard and often painful – but also necessary – effort to understand, with the patient, what is happening in the therapeutic relation and how this relates to and repeats key aspects of the patient's relational difficulties in other relationships outside the therapeutic space. Failing to also confront the patient with their destructive narcissism and its consequences, including how the patient's destructive narcissism is actualized in negative transference, may contribute to undermining the patient's agency and maturation process (Fiscalini, 1993b, p. 339 ff.).

Even though what plays out in the emotional and psychological contact will always have a crucial impact on the psychotherapeutic process and the treatment outcome, the therapist's satisfaction of the patient's self-object needs from the position of the good object will never in itself be sufficient to cure pathological narcissism. With Lacan – and, in practice, with Kernberg – we can say that it is always also the therapist's job to represent and defend the social order (Name-of-the-Father) and – like the symbolic father's role in the mother–child relationship – insist on the existence of and marking the distinction between self (the child) and other (mother), in this case, the boundary between the patient's and the therapist's selves that is a condition for psychological life and the development of independent subjectivity. With this, the therapist thus insists that the patient has not and never can merge with the therapist, corresponding to any fantasies about the ideal self-object or the paradisical self-object relation (Wilden, 1980, p. 281 ff.). At the risk of resorting to an overly categorical, black-and-white distinction, with Fiscalini (2004, p. 136), we may say that behind his patients' symptoms, Kohut tends to see the injured (good, innocent) child who needs to be contained, rescued and healed, while Kernberg tends to see the aggressive (bad, guilty) child who needs to be confronted with reality, (reality-)corrected and 'educated'.

This field of tension between Kernberg and Kohut is fruitful in many ways. Therapists need to strike a suitable balance between the two positions with a flexible understanding and therapeutic approach to their patients, as they continually attune their understanding and way of meeting the individual based on what they need right now, including to what extent the patient is currently dominated by grandiose versus vulnerable manifestations of pathological narcissism. As always, therapists need to be mindful of their own possible tendency to see and define their individual patients based on their own preconceived theoretical model, while also not following an arbitrary path without guidance from theory. In practice, this means that when working with a specific patient, the therapist cannot know, for example, what grandiose self-perceptions or masochistic traits may be based on, let alone how a patient's narcissistic subjective experiences and behaviour should be understood until they have been explored in a close dialogue with the individual patient as these perceptions, traits and acts play out. It will never be sufficient simply to refer to a diagnosis and a general theory about narcissism. The therapist will always need to develop a specific understanding with a focus on the individual's unique history, experiences and internal psychological dynamic (Fiscalini, 1993b, p. 319).

In addition, the individual patient will always need a combination of emotional response and responsiveness in the real relationship as well as more concrete interventions that stimulate the patient's curiosity, self-reflection and ability to have nuanced thoughts about their own and others' inner life and interpersonal interactions – a combination that must be continually attuned to match the individual patient's current state (level of functioning) and needs. Thus, the therapist should not seek to function as a mirror or an objective observer and interpreter of what the patient shows and tells in the therapeutic space. Instead, the therapist should try to be open to the unavoidable emotional effect of the interaction with the patient and reflect on and incorporate this into their understanding of the patient and what plays out in the therapeutic space. In doing so, the therapist should also consider how their own subjective experiences and needs influence their own being and acting in the therapeutic space and how the very act of containing and digesting/processing the patient's being, acting and projections in the therapeutic space – and offering a balanced reaction to it – can make a key contribution to the patient's change process. This may stem, for example, from the patient feeling seen, significant, contained and empathically understood perhaps for the first time in their life. These two levels of the therapeutic interaction will always influence each other, in the sense that the patient never just 'hears' the specific content of the therapist's verbal interventions. To varying degrees, the patient will also sense and react to the therapist's tone of voice and emotional reaction, the emotional atmosphere in the therapeutic space and what plays out in the nonverbal and emotional contact. In some cases, these latter aspects are more important to the patient than 'what the therapist says'. Similarly, the therapist should generally be attentive to the patient's tone of voice, emotional mood and nonverbal communication and not just the content of 'what the patient says' (Pick, 1985, p. 158).

Different variants of pathological narcissism?

For decades, there has been a form of consensus that the disagreements between Kohut and Kernberg in certain areas reflects the fact that they worked with different groups of narcissistically disturbed patients (Fiscalini, 1993a). Simply put, the claim is that the patients with pathological narcissism that Kernberg writes about and worked with in his psychotherapeutic practice were, on average, more severely disordered – with a lower level of BPO – and, not least, were more dominated by aggression and severe grandiose manifestations of pathological narcissism, while Kohut's practice and self-psychology theory were based more on patients with a personality organization at a somewhat higher level of BPO, with a much greater prevalence of vulnerable manifestations of narcissism (Kernberg, 2004a, p. 52).

It is difficult to determine to what extent the difference between the two theorists' understanding and proposed strategies for treating pathological narcissism can be explained by or reduced to the possibility that their work involves different subgroups of NPD. However, there is little doubt that Kohut's theory and treatment method are better suited for understanding and working with predominantly vulnerable manifestations of pathological narcissism, in which grandiose self components are often more split off or dissociated, and the self is flooded by destructive shame, depressive feelings and despair. Meanwhile, part of Kernberg's proposal for how we should treat patients with severe pathological narcissism is aimed more at patients with what he describes as malignant narcissism (see Chapter 3.1) and patients whose symptom image is clearly dominated by different forms of aggression and rigid grandiosity, while their access to shame and more depressive feelings may appear fairly limited (Jacoby, 2017, p. 120; Brauner et al., 2021, p. 319). Furthermore, we also always need to consider how the therapist's being and acting in the therapeutic space influences how the patient is and acts, how the patient's pathological narcissism specifically manifests itself in the therapeutic space. The patient's being and acting in the interaction with the therapist can never be understood solely with reference to the patient's inner life and dynamics alone.

3.6 John Steiner's contribution to the understanding of pathological narcissism

Withdrawal to a psychic retreat

The psychoanalyst John Steiner has described how emotionally vulnerable persons in particular may try to protect a fragile and exposed self by withdrawing from external reality and seeking refuge in a psychic retreat, like a shell, an internal bubble, a fortress or a bell jar that is fully or partially cut off from the outside world (Steiner, 1993); an island, a cave or a fortress where the self has full control over who and what is allowed in (Weiss, 2012, p. 312). We may view this as a strategy to protect a narcissistic vulnerable self or a defence of the self's narcissism. In some cases, this is more temporary, occurring when the self is under extraordinary emotional pressure. In other cases, it will have developed into a more permanent state or way of life. Steiner bases his work, in part, on Herbert Rosenfeld's (1971, 1990, p. 141 ff.) understanding of destructive narcissism and how the existence of such an internal hiding place may be a fruitful concept for understanding how patients with pathological narcissism attempt to survive psychologically. Rosenfeld (1971) associates the narcissistically disordered patient's withdrawal from the external world with Freud's concept of primary narcissism, in which the self lives mainly in their own inner world, without contact with external objects separate from the self (see Chapter 2.1). He tries to understand this particular autism-like state with reference to Freud's highly speculative death urge (drive). The latter is not tenable unless we interpret the death urge as a more metaphoric description of an internal (self-) destructive force within the self.

In relation to this point, the French psychoanalyst Andre Green (2004, p. 39) speaks of negative narcissism, in which the injured self that never really had their fundamental human need for contact with significant others met but was met with emptiness, indifference and disinterest (p. 248), has shut down emotional contact with the external world and seeks the emptiness, non-existence, indifference, gender neutrality, nothingness, anaesthesia and the dissolution of connections between the internal and the external world, between self and others, between the imaginary world and the real world (Green, 2004, p. 39).

Similarly, the psychoanalyst Neville Symington (1993, p. 39 ff.) has described how persons with pathological narcissism, as a result of early relational traumas or perceived psychological breakdowns, have abandoned, rejected or withdrawn from the good, life-giving object – that is a source of emotional life and vitality – and sought refuge in a magical imaginary world with no intimate contact with real others in the external reality. This is done in an attempt to escape their psychological reality and the psychological pain that may occur in contact with reality (Shoshani et al., 2006, p. 501 ff.). This sort of rejection or disruption of any intimate emotional contact with (potentially) life-giving objects may also cause the severely disordered patient to avoid or be unable to establish the emotional contact with the therapist that is crucial to the effect of the treatment – unless the therapist can gradually help the patient to learn to do so, mainly by insisting on establishing emotional and psychological contact with the patient at a pace that the patient is able to contain and deal with.

With Symington (1993, p. 3 ff.), we may see the patient's 'rejection' of contact with others (life-giving objects) as a result of not only severe deficiencies and traumatic experiences in early relationship but also of the patient's reactions to them in the form of various defences of the vulnerable self, including withdrawal to an inner universe people by imaginary objects. Naturally, psychotherapeutic work cannot erase early traumatic experiences from the patient's memory and history, but it can help change how the patient perceives, addresses and reacts on them in their current and future life.

We may observe this withdrawal to a self-constructed inner universe both in overtly narcissistic vulnerable patients and in patients who express grandiose self-reliance. Both try to protect their fragile self, self-image and self-esteem by avoiding or withdrawing from any form of intimate psychological and emotional contact with others out of fear that such contact may cause the fragile self to collapse or reveal a deep yearning for and dependence on others, which is perceived as unbearable and unacceptable to the self; cf. earlier traumatic experiences of being betrayed, abandoned or abused by supposedly good and life-giving attachment persons (objects).

Individuals with grandiose pathological narcissism may at times try to shut down or erase all loving and dependent parts of themselves and identify completely with their own destructive aspects; a strategy that may initially offer a sense of freedom, superiority and self-reliance (Rosenfeld, 1971, p. 174).

However, behind this facade and the mental withdrawal to a psychic retreat, they continue to be tormented by a deep longing for contact with others who can love, admire and nurture the self. The only possible exception is persons with severely malignant narcissism. They are not necessarily people who isolate in a concrete sense and avoid more formal exchanges with others. Instead their focus is often on avoiding intimate emotional contact and expressing their own affects and other mental states to others. In various ways, the self signals that it does not need others or needs communication or contact with others.

Modell (1980, p. 259) describes how these patients do not seem to relate to the therapist in the therapeutic space. They act as if the therapist is not even there, except, at best, as a sort of function, and they express a variant of non-communication with a non-person (the therapist). They may initially appear emotionally switched off or 'dead' and create an atmosphere of stagnation and mental death in the therapeutic space. This reflects their feeling of being dead and emotionally empty inside or a compulsion to shut down all emotions, as much as possible, out of fear that their emotions might otherwise get out of control and overwhelm the self and the external world. In some cases, this may be associated with the self's fear of – but also deep, denied yearning for – intimacy in the contact with the therapist (Modell, 1975, p. 275).

One of the key differences between pathological narcissism and more classic borderline disorders is that the yearning for contact (object hunger) is typically much more conscious and overt in persons with a borderline disorder, while it is much more denied and concealed by grandiose self-reliance in pathological narcissism (see Chapter 3.1). A patient who has sought refuge in a psychic retreat may have excellent formal contact with others. Thus, the phenomenon is in no way limited to persons with overt schizoid withdrawal and contactlessness. The core feature is the absence of intimate emotional and psychological contact with others and a pronounced tendency to shut down, become emotionally overwhelmed – by going into an emotional state of alert and becoming silent or aggressive – if others get too close and become too insistent in their invitation to deeper contact.

Denial of external reality

Steiner views the construction of such a psychic retreat as a pathological organization in which the personality is stuck in a state that involves what he calls a perverse pseudo-acceptance of reality (Steiner, 1993, p. 12). This is a narcissistic defence strategy that, on the one hand, allows the narcissistically vulnerable person to maintain exactly as much (or as little) real contact with external reality that the self appears normal. On the other hand, it also implies extensive denial of large parts of reality that, for various reasons, are too painful for the self to acknowledge. This may include, for example, past abuse and its catastrophic consequences for the ability of the self to be in intimate contact with itself and others or the fact that the self is slowly withering and dying or is not living but simply trying to survive, from day to day, in part as a result of having withdrawn from contact with others. According to Steiner (1993, p. 89 ff.), this represents a corruption of reality and the truth: based on a certain understanding of (parts of) reality, the self creates a version that, even though it has some connection to external reality, distorts and turns away from core aspects of 'truth' and reality.

Oedipus turns a blind eye to parts of reality

Steiner (1993, p. 116 ff.) uses Sophocles' classical play about King Oedipus to illustrate the human tendency to turn a blind eye to or deny parts of reality that for some reason are too unbearable and anxiety-producing to acknowledge. King Oedipus has unknowingly killed his father and subsequently married his own mother. As the story proceeds, it becomes increasingly obvious – in some sense also to him – that this is in fact the unbearable truth. However, he continues to lie to himself and try to convince himself that this cannot be true. By increasingly far-fetched means, he holds on to a version of reality that he is aware – if not necessarily in a fully conscious or detailed way – is not true. Steiner (1993, p. 116) argues that Oedipus both knows and does not know what he has done. He knows or has a, perhaps partially unconscious sense of, the truth but turns a blind eye to the truth about his actions and about who he really is: a son of the man he killed and the woman he is now married to.

Thus, King Oedipus is not just a story about uncovering the truth but just as much about how we can hide the truth from ourselves – and how unbearable it can be when the truth is uncovered. When the truth can finally no longer be denied, Oedipus's mother Jocasta kills herself, and Oedipus is so overwhelmed by shame that he blinds himself so that he can no longer look truth in the eye (Steiner, 1993, p. 122) or be confronted by others' gaze at the self and the unbearable shame it carries.

Related to the story about Oedipus, it could be argued that people with pathological narcissism who flee from external reality to seek refuge in a grandiose inner universe create their own internal reality and try to convince themselves that they can survive on their own and have no need for contact with others. However, as they are doing this, they maintain a sense that this is not (entirely) true. They turn a blind eye to truth, which is that they yearn for contact with others to love and admire the self. Their conscious perception of reality and the truth is not psychotic but distorted in ways that let them look away from and ignore unbearable parts of reality. More specifically, the self that has retreated into its own internal bubble may, to varying degrees, deny certain basic aspects of the human condition, for example that unless a person 'is themself' and reveals 'who they are' in interactions with others, they cannot be seen, met, recognized and perhaps admired for who they are. If we are not ready to see, listen to and give something to others, we will rarely be able to build and maintain relations in which we are seen, listened to and met in our own needs. If, for some reason, a person cannot be naked and emotionally present in intimate contact with others, their fantasies about close physical and emotional contact with the good object they dream about or yearn for in their psychic retreat cannot become concrete reality in actual external, physical reality.

Construction of an imaginary world

More specifically, withdrawing to a psychic retreat not only involves withdrawing from intimate contact with others and seeking social isolation. It also involves the construction of an internal imaginary reality or fantasy world where the person can experience a form of omnipotent control and imperviousness in relation to real others and external reality in general. Here, up to a point, the person can live inside an illusion of being emotionally self-reliant, with no need for anyone else (Modell, 1975, p. 276). However, to maintain this illusory universe, where key elements of reality are denied, it is crucial to avoid intimate contact with others, let alone aspects of the self, that are incompatible with the self's constructed fantasies of being emotionally self-reliant and entirely independent of others. Similarly, the self must avoid communicating affects that might signal its yearning or need for others, as this might cause the grandiose facade and the walls around the self's psychic retreat to crack (p. 276).

As Modell (1980, p. 261) has pointed out, these omnipotent fantasies of being emotionally self-reliant may originally have developed in reaction to – and as a way of dealing with (psychologically survive) – severe deficiencies in early parent–child (self-object) relations, in which the self found that the parents were unable to contain, protect and meet its basic emotional needs but instead perhaps violated the boundaries of the self or overwhelmed the self with their own affects. Thus, from an early age, the self learned that it has to rely on itself and protect its true self by avoiding intimate contact with others. Initially and superficially, this idealized internal world, detached from external reality, may feel safe, peaceful and associated with a form of calm, particularly in comparison to external reality, which may seem chaotic, incomprehensible and beyond the self's control in ways that appear to threaten the existence of the self.

However, this seemingly safe and peaceful state is always at risk of devolving into a death-like calm associated with stagnation, internal mental death, contactlessness, loneliness and a deep yearning for life, contact and living, rather than just surviving. Furthermore, the experience of the psychic retreat may at time be dominated by cruelty and threats to the self. Nevertheless, the prevailing experience, most of the time, is that life inside the internal bubble is less scary, more familiar, predictable and under the control of the self, and thus the self prefers this to contact with concrete other people and external reality (Steiner, 1993, p. 2). Once the self has withdrawn into their psychic retreat, time stops, no development is possible (Weiss, 2012), and the self has no intimate emotional contact with real others. Emotionally, the self is all alone and only has emotional contact with imaginary others in their private inner world, where the self is not, or only partially, delimited from others and has full control over fantasized others.

In this imaginary inner world, the self may be fully or partially merged with the good object and deny – avoid acknowledging – that real external objects are separate from and beyond the self's control (Steiner, 2014, p. 38). The self may to varying degrees feel sedated, 'put on hold' and emotionally shut down and may lose the ability to think. In a sense, the self may lose interest in the external world (Rosenfeld, 1971, p. 175) and, as in dissociative state, stare blankly into space, spending time on SoMe (social media) without being mentally present IRL (in real life), or take long baths that are subsequently perceived as 'black holes', where time stopped, and the self has no immediate recollection about what happened. To the outside world, the self may hide behind a wall of coldness, emotional indifference to others or grandiose self-reliance, which will normally keep others at a distance. In this way, the self signals to others to stay away and that the self has no interest in or desire for contact with others. While it can be quite painful to live much of one's life in this sort of inner world, cut off from intimate contact with others, the main problem when a patient withdraws into a self-constructed psychic retreat is that any deep psychological development will only be possible if the patient comes out of hiding and faces external reality (Steiner, 1993, p. 41), initially by gradually establishing emotional and psychological contact with a therapist (see Chapter 4.1).

References

Akhtar, S. (1992). *Broken structures: Severe personality disorders and their treatment.* Jason Aronson.

Akhtar, S. (2009). *The damaged core: Origins, dynamics, manifestations, and treatment.* Aronson.

Akhtar, S. (2021). Narzisstische Beziehungsgestaltung [Narcissistic relationship formation]. In S. Doering, H.-P. Hartmann, & O. F. Kernberg (Eds.), *Narzissmus: Grundlagen, Störungsbilder, Therapie* (2nd ed., pp. 454–465). Schattauer Verlag.

Altmeyer, M. (2000). *Narzissmus und Objekt: Ein intersubjektives Verständnis der Selbstbezogenheit* [Narcissism and object: An intersubjective understanding of self-sufficiency]. Vandenhoeck & Ruprecht.

Altmeyer, M. (2023). *Das entfesselte Selbst: Versuch einer Gegenwartsdiagnose* [The unleashed self: Attempt at a diagnosis of our time]. Psychosozial-Verlag.

American Psychiatric Association (APA) (1987). Diagnostic and statistical manual of mental disorders (third edition, revision; *DSM-III-R)*. American Psychiatric Publishing.

American Psychiatric Association (APA) (2013). *Diagnostic and statistical manual of mental disorders (fifth edition; DSM-5)*. American Psychiatric Publishing.

Ansell, E. B., Wright, A. G. C., Markowitz, J. C., Samislow, C. A., Hopwood, C. J., Zanarini, M. C., Yen, S., Pinto, A., McGlashan, T. H., & Grilo, C.M. (2015). Personality disorder risk factors for suicide attempts over 10 years follow-up. *Personality Disorders; Theory, Research, and Treatment*, 6, 161–167.

Bartholomew, K., Kwong, M. J., & Hart, S. D. (2001). Attachment. In W. J. Livesley (Ed.), *Handbook of personality disorders: Theory, research, and treatment* (1st ed., pp. 196–230). Guilford.

Biberdzic, M., Tan, J., & Day, N. J. S. (2023). It's not you, it's me: Identity disturbance as the main contributor to interpersonal problems in pathological narcissism. *Borderline Personality Disorder and Emotional Dysregulation*, 10, 1–12.

Binswanger, R. (2024). *Reden über Trieb, Sexualität und Gender: Grundlagen für die psychotherapeutische Praxis* [Talking about drives, sexuality and gender: Foundations for psychotherapeutic practice]. Psychosozial-Verlag.

Blasco-Fontecilla, H., Baca-Garcis, E., Dervic, K., Perez-Rodriguez, M. M., Lopez-Castroman, J., Saiz-Ruiz, J., & Oquendo, M.A. (2009). Specific features of suicidal behavior in patients with narcissistic personality disorder. *Journal of Clinical Psychiatry*, 70, 1583–1587.

Blasco-Fontecilla, H., Baca-Garcia, E., Duberstein, P., Perez-Rodriguez, M., Dervic, K., Saiz-Ruiz, J., Courtet, P., de Leon, J., & Oquendo, M. A. (2010). An exploratory study of the relationship between divers life events and specific personality disorders in a sample of suicide attempters. *Journal of Personality Disorders*, 24, 773–784.

Blasco-Belled, A., Tejeda-Gallardi, C., Alsinet, C., & Rogoza, R. (2024). The links of subjective and psychological well-being with the dark triad traits: A meta-analysis. *Journal of Personality*, 92 (2), 584–600.

Bogaerts, S., & Jankovic, M. (2024). Narcissism and relational capacity: The contribution of identity integration and social concordance. *Current Psychology*, 43, 3915–3927.

Bogaerts, S., Garofalo, C., Caluwe, E., & Jankovic, M. (2021). Grandiose and vulnerable narcissism, identity integration and self-control related to criminal behavior. *BMC Psychology, 9* (191), 1–11.

Bowlby, J. (2012). *A secure base: Clinical applications of attachment theory*. Taylor & Francis. (Original work published 1988)

Brauner, F., Müller, S., & Benecke, C. (2021). Scham, Neid und Wut – die zentralen Affekte des Narzissmus [Shame, envy and anger – the central affects of narcissism]. In S. Doering, H.-P. Hartmann, & O. F. Kernberg (Eds.), *Narzisssmus. Grundlagen, Störungsbilder, Therapie* (2nd ed., pp. 317–328). Schattauer Verlag.

Cain, N. M., Pincus, A. L., & Ansell, E. B. (2008). Narcissism at the crossroads: Phenotypic description of pathological narcissism across clinical theory, social/personality psychology, and psychiatric diagnosis. *Clinical Psychology Review*, 28, 638–656.

Caligor, E. (2013). Narcissism in psychodynamic diagnostic manual. In J. S. Ogrodniczuk (Ed.), *Understanding and treating Pathological Narcissism* (pp. 63–79). American Psychological Association.

Caligor, E., Levy, K. N., & Yeomans, F. E. (2015). Narcissistic personality disorders: Diagnostic and clinical challenges. *American Journal of Psychiatry*, 172, 415–422.

Caligor, E., & Stern, B. L. (2020). Diagnosis, classification, and assessment of narcissistic personality disorder within the framework of object relations theory. *Journal of Personality Disorders*, 34, 104–121.

Cohen, I. J., Tanis, T., Bhattacharjee, R., Nesci, C., Halmi, W., & Galynker, I. (2014). Are there differential relationships between different types of childhood maltreatment and different types of adult personality pathology? *Psychiatry Research*, 215, 192–201.

Cramer, P. (2011). Young adult narcissism: A 20 year longitudinal study of the contribution of parenting styles, preschool precursors of narcissism, and denial. *Journal of Research in Personality*, 45, 19–28.

Dakanalis, A., Clerici, M., & Carra, G. (2016). Narcissistic vulnerability and grandiosity as mediators between insecure attachment and future eating disordered behaviors: A prospective analysis of over 2.000 freshmen. *Journal of Clinical Psychology*, 72, 279–292.

Dashineau, S. C., Edershile, E. A., Simms, L. J., & Wright, A. G. C. (2019). Pathological narcissism and psychosocial functioning. *Personality Disorders; Theory, Research, and Treatment*, 10, 473–478.

Day, N. J. S., Bourke, M. E., Townsend, M. L., & Grenyer, B.F. S. (2020). Pathological narcissism: A study of burden on partners and family. *Journal of Personality Disorders*, 34, 799–813.

Day, N. J. S., Townsend, M. L., & Grenyer, B. F. S. (2022). Pathological narcissism: An analysis of interpersonal dysfunction within intimate relationships. *Personality and Mental Health*, 16, 204–216.

Dawood, S., Schroder, H. S., Donellan, M. B., & Pincus, A. L. (2018). Pathological narcissism and nonsuicidal self-injury. *Journal of Personality Disorders*, 32, 87–108.

Daws, L. (2024). *James Masterson. A contemporary introduction*. Routledge.

Dhawan, N., Kunik, M. E., Oldham, J., & Coverdale, J. (2010). Prevalence and treatment of narcissistic personality disorder in the community: A systematic review. *Comprehensive Psychiatry*, 51, 333–339.

Di Pierro, R., Di Sarno, M., Preti, E., Di Mattei, V., & Madeddu, F. (2018). The role of identity instability in the relationship between narcissism and emotional empathy. *Psychoanalytic Psychology*, 35, 237–243.

Diamond, D., & Hersh, R. G. (2020). Transference-focused psychotherapy for narcissistic personality disorder: An object relations approach. *Journal of Personality Disorders*, 34, 159–176.

Diamond, D., Levy, K.N., Clarkin, J.F., Fischer-Kern, Cain, N.M., Doering, S. Hörz, & Buchheim, A. (2014). Attachment and mentalization in female patients with comorbid narcissistic and borderline personality disorder. *Personality Disorders; Theory, Research, and Treatment*, 5, 428–433.

Diamond, D., Yeomans, F. E., Stern, B. L., & Kernberg, O. F. (2022). *Treating pathological narcissism with transference-focused psychotherapy*. Guilford.

Diamond, M.J. (2022). *Ruptures in the American Psyche: Containing destructive populism in perilous times*. Phoenix Publishing.

Dickenson, K.A., & Pincus, A.L. (2003). Interpersonal analysis of grandiose and vulnerable narcissism. *Journal of Personality Disorders*, 17, 188–207.

Doering, S, Hartmann, H.-P., & Kernberg O. F. (2021). *Narzissismus: Grundlagen, Störungsbilder, Therapie* [Narcissism: Basis, disorders, therapy] (2nd ed.). Schattauer Verlag.

Drozek, R. P., Unruh, B. T., & Bateman, A. (2023). *Mentalization-based treatment of pathological narcissism*. Oxford University Press.

Du, T. V., Miller, J. D., & Lynam, D. R. (2022b). The relation between narcissism and aggression: A meta-analysis. *Journal of Personality*, 90, 574–594.

Eaton, N. R., & Greene, A. L. (2018). Personality disorders: Community prevalence and socio-demographic correlates. *Current Opinion in Psychology*, 21, 28–32.

Egan, V., Chan, S., & Shorter, G. W. (2014). The dark triad, happiness and subjective well-being. *Personality and Individual Differences*, 67, 17–22.

Ehrenberg, A. (2004). *Das Erschöpfte Selbst: Depression und Gesellschaft in der Gegenwart* [The exhausted self: depression and society in the present]. Campus Verlag. (Original work published 1998)

Ehrenberg, A. (2011). *Das Unbehagen in der Gesellschaft* [The discomfort in society] (J. Schröder, Trans.). Suhrkamp Verlag. (Original work published 2010)

Ensink, K., Chretien, S., Normandin, L., Begin, M., Daigle, D., & Fonagy, P. (2017). Pathological narcissism in adolescents: Relationships with childhood maltreatment and internalizing and externalizing difficulties, *Adolescent Psychiatry*, 7, 300–314.

Ermann, M. (2020). *Narzissmus: Vom Mythos zur Psychoanalyse des Selbst* [Narcissism: From myth to psychoanalysis of the self]. Kohlhammer.

Fiscalini, J. (1993a). Interpersonal relations and the problem of narcissism. In J. Fiscalini & A. L. Grey (Eds.), *Narcissism and the interpersonal self* (pp. 53–87). Columbia University Press.

Fiscalini, J. (1993b). The psychoanalysis of narcissism. An interpersonal view. In J., Fiscalini & A. L. Grey (Eds.), *Narcissism and the Interpersonal Self* [pp. 318–348]. Columbia University Press.

Fiscalini, J. (2004). *Coparticipant psychoanalysis*. Columbia University Press.

Fjermestad-Noll, J., Ronningstam, E., Bach, B., Rosenbaum, B., & Simonsen, E. (2020a). Perfectionism, shame, and aggression in depressive patients with narcissistic personality disorder. *Journal of Personality Disorder*, 34, 25–41.

Fonagy, P. (2021). Persönlichkeitsstörungen und Gewalt: Ein psychoanalytisch-bindungstheoretischer Ansatz [Personality disorders and violence: A psychoanalytic-attachment theory approach]. In S. Doering, H.-P. Hartmann, & O. F. Kernberg (Eds.), *Narzisssmus: Grundlagen, Störungsbilder, Therapie* (2nd ed., pp. 83–128). Schattauer Verlag.

Fossati, A., Feeney, J., Pincus, A., Borroni, S., & Maffei, C. (2015). The structure of pathological narcissism and its relationship with adult attachment styles. *Psychoanalytic Psychology*, 32, 403–431.

Foster, J. D., & Brunelli, A. B. (2018). Narcissism and romantic relationships. In A. D. Hermann, A. B. Brunell, & J. D. Foster (Eds.), *Handbook of trait narcissism* (pp. 317–326). Springer Nature.

Gabbard, G. O., & Crisp, H. (2018). *Narcissism and its discontents: Diagnostic dilemmas and treatment strategies with narcissistic patients*. American Psychiatric Publishing.

Gao, S., Yu, D., Chan, K. L., Zhang, L., & Meng, X. (2024). The association between child maltreatment and pathological narcissism: A three-level meta-analytic review. *Trauma, Violence, and Abuse*, 25, 275–290.

Gazzillo, F., Lingiardi, V., Corno, F., Genova, F., Bornstein, R. F., Gordon, R. M., & McWilliams, N. (2015). Clinicians' emotional responses and psychodynamic diagnostic model adult personality disorders: A clinically relevant empirical investigation. *Psychotherapy*, 52, 238–246.

Giner, L., Blasco-Fontecilla, H., Perez-Rodriguez, M. M., Garcia-Nieto, R., Giner, J., Guija, J. A., Rico, A., Barrero, E., Luna, M. A., de Leon, J., Oquendo, M. A., & Baca-Garcia, E. (2013). Personality disorders and health problems distinguish suicide attempts from completers in a direct comparison. *Journal of Affective Disorders*, 151, 474–483.

Green, A. (2004). *Die tote Mutter: Psychoanalytische Studien zu Lebensnarzissmus und Todesnarzissmus* [The dead mother: Psychoanalytic studies on life narcissism and death narcissism] (E. Wolff & E. Kittler, Trans). Psychosozial Verlag.

Green, A., & Charles, K. (2019). Voicing the victims of narcissistic partners: A qualitative analysis of responses to narcissistic injury and self-esteem regulation. *Sage Open*, 9, 1–10.

Grijalva, E., Newman, D. A., Tay, L., Donellan, M. B., Harms, P.D., Robins, R.W., & Yan, T. (2015a). Gender differences in narcissism: A meta-analytic review. *Psychological Bulletin*, 141, 261–310.

Grover, K. E., Carpenter, L. L., Price, L. H., Gagne, G. G., Mello, A. F., & Tyrka, A. R. (2007). The relationship between childhood abuse and adult personality disorder symptoms. *Journal of Personality Disorders*, 21, 442–447.

Hare, R. (2003). *Hare's Psychopathy Checklist-Revised* (2nd ed.). MHS.

Hasin, D. S., & Grant, B. F. (2015). The national epidemiological survey on alcohol and related conditions (NESARC) waves 1 and 2: Review and summary of findings. *Social Psychiatry and Psychiatric Epidemiology*, 50, 1609–1640.

Hengartner, M. P., Ajdacic-Gross, V., Rodgers, S., Müller, M., & Rössler, W. (2013). Childhood adversity in association with personality disorder dimensions: New findings in an old debate. *European Psychiatry*, 28, 476–482.

Horney, K. (1939). *New ways in psychoanalysis*. Norton.

Horton, R. S. (2011a). Parenting as a cause of narcissism: Empirical support for psychodynamic and social learning theories. In W. K. Campbell & J. D. Miller (Eds.), *The handbook of narcissism and narcissistic personality disorder: Theoretical approaches, empirical findings, and treatments* (pp. 181–190). John Wiley.

Horton, R. S. (2011b). On the environmental sources of child narcissism: Are parents really to blame? In C. T. Barry, P. K. Kerig, K. K. Stellwagen & T. D. Barry (Eds.), *Narcissism and Machiavellianism in youth* (pp. 125–143). American Psychological Association.

Hörz-Sagstetter, S., & Kampe, L. (2021). Komorbidität [Comorbidity]. In S. Doering, H.-P. Hartmann, & O. F. Kernberg (Eds.), *Narzissmus: Grundlagen, Störungsbilder, Therapie* (pp. 216–224). Schattauer Verlag.

Huxley, E., & Bizumic, B. (2017). Parental invalidation and the development of narcissism. *The Journal of Psychology*, 151, 130–147.

Jacoby, M. (2017). *Individuation and Narcissism: The psychology of self in Jung and Kohut: Classic edition*. Routledge. (Original work published 1985)

Jaksic, N., Hanzek, M. S., Rebernjak, B., & Ogrodniczuk, J. S. (2017). Experience of shame mediates the relationship between pathological narcissism and suicidal ideation in psychiatric outpatients. *Journal of Clinical Psychology*, 73, 1670–1681.

Johnson, J. G., Cohen, P., Smailes, E. M., Skodol, A. E., Brown, J., & Oldham, J.M. (2001). Childhood verbal abuse and risk for personality disorders during adolescence and early adulthood. *Comprehensive Psychiatry*, 42, 16–23.

Johnson, J. G., Smailes, E. M., Cohen, P., Brown, J., & Bernstein, D. P. (2000). Associations between four types of childhood neglect and personality disorder symptoms during adolescence and early adulthood: Findings from a community-based longitudinal study. *Journal of Personality Disorders*, 14, 171–187.

Jørgensen, C. R. (2009). *Personlighedsforstyrrelser: Moderne relationel forståelse og behandling af borderlinelidelser* [Personality disorders: Modern relational understanding and treatment of borderline disorders] (2nd ed). Hans Reitzels Forlag.

Jørgensen, C. R. (2019). *The psychotherapeutic stance* (D. Silver, Trans.). Springer. (Original work published 2018).

Jørgensen, C. R. (2020). *Identitetskriser: Veje og vildveje for det fragmenterede moderne menneskes identitet* [Identity crises: Paths and detours for the identity of fragment modern people]. Hans Reitzels Forlag.

Jørgensen, C. R. (2024). *Understanding and working with shame: Psychotherapeutic, cultural and philosophical perspectives* (D. Silver, Trans.). Routledge. (Original work published 2023)

Jørgensen, C. R., & Bøye, R. (2022). How does it feel to have a disturbed identity? The phenomenology of identity diffusion in patients with borderline personality disorder: A qualitative study. *Journal of Personality Disorders*, 36, 40–69.

Jørgensen, C. R., Rasmussen, A.S., & Bøye, R. (2023). Level of identity in patients with borderline, narcissistic, avoidant and other specified personality disorder. *Nordic Psychology*, ahead of print: doi:10.1080/19012276.2023.2197561.

Jurist, E. (2021). Narzissmus und Sucht. In S. Doering, H.-P. Hartmann, & O. F. Kernberg (Eds.), *Narzissismus: Grundlagen, Störungsbilder, Therapie* (2nd ed., pp. 373–392). Schattauer Verlag.

Karterud, S. (1995). *Fra narcissisme til selvpsykologi: En innføring i Heinz Kohuts forfatterskap* [From narcissism to self psychology: An introduction to Heinz Kohut's writings]. Ad Notam Gyldendal.

Kaufman, S. B., Weiss, B., Miller, J. D., & Campbell, W. K. (2020). Clinical correlates of vulnerable and grandiose narcissism: A personality perspective. *Journal of Personality Disorders*, 34, 107–130.

Kealy, D., & Ogrodniczuk, J.S. (2011). Narcissistic interpersonal problems in clinical practice. *Harvard Review of Psychiatry*, 19, 290–311.

Kealy, D., Ogrodniczuk, J. S., Rice, S. M., & Oliffe, J. L. (2017a). Pathological narcissism and maladaptive self-regulatory behaviors in a nationally representative sample of Canadian men. *Psychiatry Research*, 256, 156–161.

Kealy, D., Laverdiere, O., Cox, D., & Hewitt, P.L. (2023). Childhood emotional neglect and depressive and anxiety symptoms among mental health outpatients: The mediating roles of narcissistic vulnerability and shame. *Journal of Mental Health*, 196, 24–32.

Keene, A. C., & Epps, J. (2016). Childhood physical abuse and aggression: Shame and narcissistic vulnerability. *Child Abuse & Neglect*, 51, 276–283.

Kernberg, O. F. (1975). *Borderline conditions and pathological narcissism*. Jason Aronson.

Kernberg, O. F. (1984). *Severe personality disorders*. Yale University Press.

Kernberg, O. F. (2004a). *Aggressivity, narcissism, and self-destructiveness in the psychotherapeutic relationship*. Yale University Press.

Kernberg, O. F. (2004b). *Contemporary controversies in psychoanalytic theory, techniques, and their applications*. Yale University Press.

Kernberg, O. F. (2014). An overview of the treatment for severe narcissistic pathology. *International Journal of Psychoanalysis*, 95, 865–888.

Kernberg, O. F. (2018). *Treatment of severe personality disorders: Resolution of aggression and recovery from eroticism*. American Psychiatric Association Publishing.

Kernberg, P. (2000). Developmental aspects of normal and pathological narcissism. In E. F. Ronningstam (Ed.), *Disorders of narcissism: Diagnostic, clinical, and empirical implications* (pp. 103–120).American Psychiatric Press.

Kjærvik, S. L., & Bushman, B. J. (2021). The link between narcissism and aggression: A meta-analytic review. *Psychological Bulletin*, 147, 477–503.

Klein, M. (1975). Some theoretical conclusions regarding the emotional life of the infant. In *Envy and gratitude and other works 1946–1963* (pp. 61–93). (Original work published 1952)

Kohut, H. (1971). *The analysis of the self*. The University of Chicago Press.

Kohut, H. (1977). *The restoration of the self*. The University of Chicago Press.

Kohut, H., & Wolf, E. (1978). The disorders of the self and their treatment: An outline. *International Journal of Psychoanalysis*, 59, 413–425.

Krizan, Z., & Johar, O. (2015). Narcissistic rage revisited. *Journal of Personality and Social Psychology*, 108, 784–801.

Lampe, S., Hamiliton-Giachritisis, C., Garner, E., & Walker, J. (2018). The role of narcissism in aggression and violence: A systematic review. *Trauma, Violence & Abuse*, 19, 209–230.

Levy, K. N., Clarkin, J. F., & Crow, T. M. (2021). Narzisstische Persönlichkeitsstörung: Prävalenz und Verlauf [Narcissistic personality disorder: Prevalence and course]. In S. Doering, H.-P. Hartmann, & O. F. Kernberg (Eds.), *Narzisssmus: Grundlagen, Störungsbilder, Therapie* (2nd ed., pp. 189–200). Schattauer Verlag.

Lihua, Z., & He, Z, (2021). Relationship between narcissism and aggression: A meta-analysis. *Acta Psychologica Sinica*, 53, 1228–1243.

Links, P. S. (2013). Pathological narcissism and risk of suicide. In J. S. Ogrodniczuk (Ed.), *Understanding and treating pathological narcissism* (pp. 167–181). American Psychological Association.

Littlebear, S., Lofties, E., & Mikolon, T. (2024). Counselor perceptions regarding narcissistic personality disorder, narcissistic traits, and domestic violence. *Contemporary Family Therapy*, 46, 231–240.

Lobbestael, J., Arntz, A., & Bernstein, D.P. (2010). Disentangling the relationship between different types of childhood maltreatment and personality disorders. *Journal of Personality Disorders*, 24, 285–295.

Marcinko, D., Jaksic, N., Izezic, E., Skocic, M., Suranyi, S., Loncar, M., Franic, T., & Jakovljevic, M. (2014). Pathological narcissism and depressive symptoms in psychiatric outpatients: Mediating role of dysfunctional attitudes. *Journal of Clinical Psychology*, 70, 341–352.

Maria, A. S., Reichert, F., & Renneberg, B. (2021). Zum Verhältnis von narzisstischer und selbstunsicherer Persönlichkeitsstörung [On the relationship between narcissistic and self-insecure personality disorder]. In S. Doering, H.-P. Hartmann, & O. F. Kernberg (Eds.), *Narzissmus: Grundlagen, Störungsbilder, Therapie* (pp. 62–69). Schattauer.

Mattia, J. I., & Zimmerman, M. (2001). Epidemiology. In W. J. Livesley (Ed.), *Handbook of personality disorders: Theory, research, and treatment* (pp. 107–123). Guilford.

Maxwell, K., & Huprich, S. (2014). Retrospective reports of attachment disruptions, parental abuse and neglect mediate the relationship between pathological narcissism and self-esteem. *Personality and Mental Health*, 8, 290–305.

McWilliams, N. (1994). *Psychoanalytic diagnosis*. Guilford.

Menard, K. S., & Pincus, A. L. (2012). Predicting overt and cyber stalking perpetration by male and female college students. *Journal of Interpersonal Violence*, 27, 2183–2207.

Meyer, B., & Pilkonis, P. A. (2011). Attachment theory and narcissistic personality disorder. In W. K. Campbell & J. D. Miller (Eds.), *The handbook of narcissism and narcissistic personality disorder: Theoretical approaches, empirical findings, and treatments* (pp. 434–444). John Wiley.

Miller, J. D., Crowe, M. L., & Sharpe, B. M. (2022). Narcissism and the DSM-5 alternative model of personality disorder. *Personality Disorders: Theory, Research and Treatment*, 13, 407–411.

Modell, A. H. (1975). A narcissistic defence against affects and the illusion of self-sufficiency. *International Journal of Psychoanalysis*, 56, 275–282.

Modell, A. H. (1980). Affects and their non-communication. *International Journal of Psychoanalysis*, 61, 259–

Møhl, B., Bech-Jessen, J., & Graugaard, C. (2019). Parafilier og parafile forstyrrelser [Paraphilias and paraphilic disorders]. In C. Graugaard, A. Giraldi & B. Møhl (Eds.). *Sexologi: Faglige perspektiver på seksualitet* (pp. 905–933). Munksgaard.

Mollon, P. (2020). *Pathologies of the self: Exploring narcissistic and borderline states of mind*. Confer Books.

Morgan, T.A., & Zimmerman, M. (2018). Epidemiology of personality disorders. In W. J. Livesley & R. Larstone (Eds.), *Handbook of personality disorders: Theory, research, and treatment* (2nd ed., pp. 173–196). Guilford.

Morrison, A. P. (1989). *Shame: The underside of narcissism*. Analytic Press.

Morrison, A. P. (2008). The analyst's shame. *Contemporary Psychoanalysis*, 44, 65–82.

Morrison, A. P., & Stolorow, R.D. (1997). Shame, narcissism, and intersubjectivity. In M. R. Lansky & A. P. Morrison (Eds.), *The widening scope of shame* (pp. 63–87). Psychology Press.

Neumann, E. (2017). Emotional abuse in childhood and attachment anxiety in adult romantic relationships as predictors of personality disorders. *Journal of Aggression, Maltreatment & Traumaz*, 26, 430–446.

Nguyen, K. T., & Shaw, L. (2020). The aetiology of non-clinical narcissism: Clarifying the role of adverse childhood experiences and parental overvaluation. *Personality and Individual Differences*, 154, doi:10.1016/.paid.2019.109615.

Nørgaard, N. L., & Simonsen, S. (2019). *Den ængstelige personlighed* (The anxious personality). Hans Reitzels Forlag.

Otway, L. J., & Vignoles, V. L. (2006). Narcissism and childhood recollections: A quantitative test of psychoanalytic predictions. *Personality and Social Psychology Bulletin*, 32, 104–116.

Paris, J. (2014). Modernity and narcissistic personality disorder. *Personality Disorders: Theory, Research and Treatment*, 5, 220–226.

Paulsen, J. A., Syed, M., Trzesniewski, K., & Donnellan, M. B. (2014). Generational perspectives on emerging adulthood: A focus on narcissism. In J. J. Arnett (Ed.), *The Oxford handbook of emerging adulthood* (pp. 26–44). Oxford University Press.

Pincus, A. L. (2023). Narcissistic personality disorder and pathological narcissism. In R. F. Krueger & P. H. Blaney (Eds.), *Oxford textbook of psychopathology* (4th ed., pp. 628–649). Oxford University Press.

Pulay, A. J., Goldstein, R. B., & Grant, B. F. (2011). Sociodemographic correlates of DSM-IV narcissistic personality disorder. In W. K. Campbell & J. D. Miller (Eds.), *The handbook of narcissism and narcissistic personality disorder: Theoretical approaches, empirical findings, and treatments* (pp. 167–180). John Wiley.

Rasmussen, K. (2016). Entitled vengeance: A meta-analysis relating narcissism to provoked aggression. *Aggressive Behavior*, 42, 363–379.

Riegel, K. D., Schlosserova, L., & Zbornok, T. S. (2022). Self-reported narcissistic traits in patients with addiction through the lens of the ICD-11 model for personality disorders. *Frontiers in Psychiatry*, 13, 1041480. doi:10.3389/fpsyt.2022.1041480.

Ritter, K., Roepke, S., Merkl, A., Heuser, I., Fydrich, T., & Lammers, C.-H. (2010). Komorbiditäten bei patienten mit einer narzisstichen Persönlichkeitsstörung im Vergleich zu Patienten mit einer Bordeline-Persönlichkeitsstörung [Comorbidities in patients with narcissistic personality disorder compared to patients with borderline personality disorder]. *Psychotherapie, Psychosomatik, Medizinischer Psychologie*, 60, 14–24.

Ritter, K., Vater, A., Rüsch, N., Schröder-Abé, M., Schütz, A., Fydrich, T., Lammers, C.-H., Roepke, S. (2014). Shame in patients with narcissistic personality disorder. *Psychiatry Research*, 215, 429–437.

Ronningstam, E. (2005). *Identifying and understanding the narcissistic personality*. Oxford University Press.

Ronningstam, E. (2011). Psychodynamic theories on narcissism and narcissistic personality. In W. K. Campbell & J. D. Miller (Eds.), *The handbook of narcissism and narcissistic personality disorder: Theoretical approaches, empirical findings, and treatments*, pp. 41–55. John Wiley.

Ronningstam, E. (2012). Alliance building and narcissistic personality disorder. *Journal of Clinical Psychology: In session*, 68, 943–953.

Ronningstam, E. (2021). *NPD Basic: A brief overview of identifying, diagnosing and treating narcissistic personality disorder* (4th Ed.). McLean Hospital, Harvard Medical School.

Ronningstam, E., & Gunderson, J. G. (1991). Differentiating borderline personality disorder from narcissistic personality disorder. *Journal of Personality Disorders*, 5, 225–232.

Ronningstam, E., & Maltsberger, J. T. (1998). Pathological narcissism and sudden suicide-related collapse. *Suicide and Life-threatening Behavior*, 28, 261–271.

Ronningstam, E., & Weinberg, I. (2023). Narcissistic personality disorder: Patterns, processes, and indicators of change in long-term psychotherapy. *Journal of Personality Disorders*, 37, 337–357.

Ronningstam, E., Weinberg, I., Goldblatt, M., Schechter, M., & Herbstman, B. (2018). Suicide and self-regulation in narcissistic personality disorder. *Psychodynamic Psychiatry*, 46, 491–510.

Rosenfeld, H. (1971). A clinical approach to the psychoanalytic theory of life and death instincts: An investigation into the aggressive aspects of narcissism. *International Journal of Psychoanalysis*, 52, 169–181.

Russ, E., Shedler, J., Bradley, R., & Westen, D. (2008). Refining the construct of narcissistic personality disorder: Diagnostic criteria and subtypes. *American Journal of Psychiatry*, 165, 1473–1481.

Russell, G. A. (1985). Narcissism and the narcissistic personality disorder: A comparison of the theories of Kernberg and Kohut. *British Journal of Medical Psychology*, 58, 137–148.

Schalkwijk, F., Luyten, P., Ingenhoven, T., & Dekker, J. (2021). Narcissistic personality disorder: Are psychodynamic theories and the alternative DSM-5 model for personality disorders finally going to meet? *Frontiers in Psychology*, 12, 676733.

Sedikides, C., Rudich, E. A., Gregg, A. P., Kumashiro, M., & Rusbult, C. (2004). Are normal narcissists psychologically healthy? Self-esteem matters. *Personality Process and Individual Differences*, 87, 400–416.

Set, Z. (2021). Mediating role of narcissism, vulnerable narcissism, and self-compassion in the relationship between attachment dimensions and psychopathology, *Alpha Psychiatry*, 22, 147–152.

Shoshani, B., Soshani, M., & Becker, M. (2006). From lifegiver to mutual nurturance: A relational perspective on Symington's monadic view of narcissism. *Psychoanalytic Dialogues*, 16, 499–517.

Simonsen, S., & Euler, S. (2019). Avoidant and narcissistic personality disorders. In A. Bateman & P. Fonagy (Eds.), *Handbook of mentalizing in mental health practice* (pp. 351–367). American Psychiatric Publishing.

Simonsen, S., & Simonsen, E. (2011). Comorbidities between narcissistic personality disorder and axis-I diagnoses. In W. K. Campbell & J. D. Miller (Eds.), *The handbook of narcissism and narcissistic personality disorder: Theoretical approaches, empirical findings, and treatments* (pp. 239–247). John Wiley.

South, S. C., Eaton, N. R., & Krueger, R. F. (2011). Narcissism in the official psychiatric classification systems: Toward DSM-5. In W. K. Campbell & J. D. Miller (Eds.), *The handbook of narcissism and narcissistic personality disorder: Theoretical approaches, empirical findings, and treatments* (pp. 22–30). John Wiley.

Steiner, J. (1993). *Psychic retreats: Pathological organizations in psychotic, neurotic and borderline patients*. Routledge.

Steiner, J. (2014). *Seelische Rückzugsorte verlassen. Therapeutische Schritte zur Aufgabe der Borderline-position* [Leaving psychic retreats: Therapeutic steps to abandon the borderline position]. Klett-Cotta.

Stinson, F. S., Dawson, D. A., Goldstein, R. B., Chou, P., Huang, B., Smith, S. M., Ruan, W. J., Pulay, A. T., Saha, T. D., Pickering, R. P., & Grant, B. F.. (2008). Prevalence, correlates, disability, and comorbidity of DSM-IV narcissistic personality disorder: Results from the wave 2 national epidemiologic survey on alcohol and related conditions. *Journal of Clinical Psychiatry*, 69, 1033–1045.

Symington, N. (1993). *Narcissism: A new theory*. Karnac.

Talmon, A., & Ginzburg, K. (2021). The differential role of narcissism in social-personality research. In W. K. Campbell & J. D. Miller (Eds.), *The Handbook of narcissism and narcissistic personality disorder: Theoretical approaches, empirical findings, and treatments*. (pp. 133–145). John Wiley.

Tolstoy, L. (2010). *Anna Karenina* (A. & Y. Maude, Trans.). Vintage Books. (Original work published 1878)

Torgersen, S., Czajkowski, N., Jacobson, K., Reichborn-Kjennerud, T., Røysamb, E., Neale, M. C., & Kendler, K. S. (2008). Dimensional representation of DSM-IV cluster B personality disorders in population-based sample of Norwegian twins: A multivariate study. *Psychological Medicine*, 38, 1617–1625.

Torgersen, S., Kringlen, E., & Cramer, V. (2001). The prevalence of personality disorders in a community sample. *Archives of General Psychiatry*, 58, 590–596.

Torgersen, S., Lygren, S., Øien, P. A., Skre, I., Oustad, S., Edvardsen, J., Tambs, K., & Kringlen, E. (2000). A twin study of personality disorders. *Comprehensive Psychiatry*, 41, 416–425.

Trull, T. J., Jahng, S., Tomko, R. L., Wood, P. K., & Sher, K.J. (2010). Revised NESARC personality disorder diagnoses: Gender, prevalence, and comorbidity with substance dependence disorders. *Journal of Personality Disorders*, 24, 412–426.

Urbonaviciute, G., & Hepper, E. G. (2020). When is narcissism associated with low empathy? A meta-analysis. *Journal of research in Personality*, 89, 1–19.

Van Schie, C. C., Jarman, H. L., Huxley, E., & Grenyer, B. F. S. (2020). Narcissistic traits in young people: Understanding the role of parenting and maltreatment. *Borderline Personality Disorder and Emotion Dysregulation*, 7, 10. doi:10.1186/s40479–020–00125–7.

Van Schie, C. C., Jarmen, H. L., Reis, S., & Grenyer, B. F. S. (2021). Narcissistic traits in young people and how experiencing shame relates to current attachment challenges. *BMC Psychiatry*, 21, 246. doi:10.1186/s12888–021–033249–4.

Vater, A., Ritter, K., Schröder-Abé, M., Schütz, A., Lammers, C.-H., Bosson, J. K., & Roepke, S. (2013a). When grandiosity and vulnerability collide: Implicit and explicit self-esteem in patients with narcissistic personality disorder. *Journal of Behavior Therapy & Experimental Psychiatry*, 44, 37–47.

Vater, A., Roepke, S., Ritter, K., & Lammers, C-H. (2013b). Narzisstische Persönlichkeitsstörung. Forschung, Diagnose und Psychotherapie [Narcissistic personality disorder: Research, diagnosis, and psychotherapy]. *Psychotherapeut*, 6, 599–615.

Velotti, P., Rogier, G., & Sarlo, A. (2020). Pathological narcissism and aggression: The mediating effect of difficulties in the regulation of negative emotions. *Personality and Individual Differences*, 155, 1–6.

Walter, M., & Bilke-Hentsch, O. (2020). *Narzissmus: Grundlagen, Formen, Interventionen* [Narcissism: Foundations, forms, interventions]. Kohlhammer.

Weidmann, R., Chopik, W.J., Ackerman, R.A., Allroggen, M., Bianchi, E. C., Brecheen, C., Campbell, W. K., Gerlach, T. M., Geukes, K., Grijalva, E., Grossmann, I., Hopwood, C. J., Hutteman, R., Konrath, S., Küfner, A. C. P., Leckelt, M., Miller, J. D., Penke, L., Pincus, A. L., Renner, K.-H., Richter, D., Roberts, B. W., ... Back, M. D. (2023). Age and gender differences in narcissism: A comprehensive study across eight measures and over 250.000 participants. *Journal of Personality and Social Psychology: Personality Processes and Individual Differences*, 124, 1277–1298.

Weiss, H. (2012). Utopien und Dystopien als Orte des seelischen Rückzugs [Utopias and dystopias as places of spiritual retreat]. *Psyche*, 66, 310–330.

Widiger, T. (2011). The comorbidity of narcissistic personality disorder with other DSM-IV personality disorders. In W. K. Campbell & J. D. Miller (Eds.), *The handbook of narcissism and narcissistic personality disorder: Theoretical approaches, empirical findings, and treatments* (pp. 248–260). John Wiley.

Widman, L., & McNulty, J. K. (2010). Sexual narcissism and the perpetration of sexual aggression. *Archives of Sexual Behavior*, 39, 926–939.

Widman, L. & McNulty, J.K. (2011). Narcissism and sexuality. In W. K. Campbell & J. D. Miller (Eds.). *The handbook of narcissism and narcissistic personality disorder: Theoretical approaches, empirical findings, and treatments* (pp. 248–260). John Wiley.

Wile, D. B. (1984). Kohut, Kernberg, and accusatory interpretations. *Psychotherapy*, 21, 353–364.

Winnicott, D. W. (1971). *Playing and reality*. Routledge.

Wilden, A. (1980). *System and structure: Essays in communication and exchange*. Tavistock Publications.

Wilson, S., Stroud, C. B., & Durbin, C. E. (2017). Interpersonal dysfunction in personality disorders: A meta-analytic review. *Psychological Bulletin*, 143, 679–734.

Wolf, E. S. (1996). *Theorie und Praxis der psychoanalytischen Selbstpsychologie* (Theory and practice of psychoanalytic self psychology). Suhrkamp Verlag.

World Health Organization (WHO) (1992). *The ICD-10 classification of mental and behavioural disorders: Clinical descriptions and diagnostic guidelines*.

World Health Organization (WHO) (2021). *ICD-11 diagnostic guidelines* (unpublished draft for research use).

Yakeley, J. (2018). Current understanding of narcissism and narcissistic personality disorder. *BJPsych Advances*, 24, 305–315.

Zabel, L. (2019). *Narzisstische Depression: Theorie und Konzepte in Psychiatrie und Psychoanalyse* [Narcissistic depression: Theory and concepts in psychiatry and psychoanalysis]. Psychosozial-Verlag.

Zeigler-Hill, V., & Jordan, C. H. (2011). Behind the mask: Narcissism and implicit self-esteem. In W. K. Campbell & J. D. Miller (Eds.), *The handbook of narcissism and narcissistic personality disorder: Theoretical approaches, empirical findings, and treatments* (pp. 101–115). John Wiley.

Zimmernan, M., Rothschild, L., & Chelminski, I. (2005). The prevalence of DSM-IV personality disorders in psychiatric outpatients. *American Journal of Psychiatry*, 162, 1911–1918.

4 Psychotherapeutic understanding and treatment of NPD

This is a fake heading: delete at typesetting stage

Several structured and partially manualized methods have been developed for psychotherapeutic treatment of more severe personality disorders, with subsequent presentations of modified versions directed specifically at treating NPD. This applies in particular to transference-focused psychotherapy (Yeo-Yeomans et al., 2015), which has been developed further to provide treatment for NPD (Diamond et al., 2022), and mentalization-based psychotherapy (MBT; Bateman & Fonagy, 2004, 2016), for which a group of authors have proposed a version that targets NPD (Drozek et al., 2023). Furthermore, it can be argued that Kohut's self psychology-based treatment method was developed from the outset to treat various degrees of pathological narcissism (Kohut, 1971, 1977; Wolf, 1996). To provide treatment to persons with pathological narcissism, therapists need to be trained and have received supervision in one of the widely recognized psychotherapeutic treatment methods aimed at personality pathology. They also need to possess a certain degree of curiosity about and be ready to examine their own reactions and presence in the therapeutic process and in the contact with patients. The latter is important because psychotherapeutic treatment of personality disorders will inevitably involve and challenge the therapist as a person, in the sense that the personality-disordered patient will always actualize and act out their psychological difficulties in the interpersonal and emotional interaction with the therapist in the therapeutic space, given that personality disorders must essentially be understood as relational disorders (Jørgensen, 2009).

Helping people with pathological narcissism is not a technical process, it is a human process that revolves around establishing and being in psychological and emotional contact with the patient. It requires well-honed responsivity – the ability to continue to sense what the patient needs and attune one's actions accordingly – and the ability to remain fully attentive in and of the moment in the meeting with the patient and their relational and inner psychological life. To provide real help to people with severe personality disorders and pathological narcissism, the therapist has to make themself and their responsiveness as a subject available to the patients in the

DOI: 10.4324/9781003744962-4

therapeutic space. This means being 'personally' and emotionally present and drawing on the full spectrum of one's emotions and emotional responsiveness in the effort to understand what particular challenges this individual is facing in relation to being in contact with themself and others. This in no way implies sharing personal details or difficulties with the patient – the therapist's personal life has no place in the therapeutic space – but it involves remaining as fully present as possible in the emotional and psychological contact with the patient.

This is a complex task which cannot be reduced to specific techniques that can be described in manuals or guidelines. That would reflect a mindset and strategies from the domains of administration, standardization and heightened efficiency that are incompatible with psychological thinking and in-depth psychotherapeutic work. Psychotherapy should not be handled by technicians, method-based service providers or civil servants but by individuals who are capable of being psychologically and emotionally present in the psychotherapeutic space and in contact with the patient and to engage in dynamic psychological thinking. None of these are skills that can be acquired primarily by reading quantitative empirical studies or treatment manuals, which are by definition based on and reflective of extensive simplifications of reality, including internal psychological processes and the complex processes in the psychotherapeutic space and in the interaction between patient and therapist. On the other hand, acquiring knowledge about pathological narcissism and the basic elements of psychotherapeutic work can be an important part of the foundation for being present, containing and thinking nuanced psychological thoughts about how the individual person's unique difficulties are expressed in the therapeutic space and in the interaction with the therapist.

NPD as a relational disorder – that is cured relationally

Personality disturbances have their origin in interpersonal relations and are also maintained and manifested through disturbances of interpersonal relations, including the relationship with a therapist (Jørgensen, 2009). Specifically, this means that the core of pathological narcissism will always play out in front of the therapist in the therapeutic space, where the patient, through their way of being and acting in the interaction and contact with the therapist (or the occasional absence of contact), demonstrates what is the core of their difficulties. Thus, it is also via the interactions with the patient that the therapist has the opportunity to reduce and, to varying degrees, cure the patient's pathological narcissism, including through 1) the shared exploration of what happens in the therapeutic relationship, 2) the gradual establishment of an ever deeper emotional and psychological contact with the patient, in which 3) the pathological patterns that have maintained the patient's pathological narcissism are not repeated to the same degree and the patient thus 4) can attain new, corrective emotional experiences in the relationship with the therapist.

The core of the difficulties of someone living with a personality disorder will thus always play out in the patient's way of relating to and interacting with the therapist in the therapeutic space. They will play out in the patient's transference, the therapist's countertransference and the various ways in which these interact with and influence each other in an ongoing intersubjective exchange. One implication of this is that the therapist's ability to establish and remain in emotional and psychological contact with the patient is crucial for the psychotherapeutic process, including in situations when the patient becomes anxious and withdraws from contact or attacks the therapist in order to protect their vulnerable self. For the therapist, this is not primarily about learning a set of specific techniques that they can turn to when a certain standard situation arises in the therapeutic space. Interpersonal contact and interactions are complex processes that cannot be standardized and thus cannot be established or handled by means of standardized interventions.

Developing the ability to provide psychotherapy has more to do with acquiring more general psychotherapeutic competencies and with continually honing one's ability to be present in, handle and use the emotional and psychological contact with the individual patient. This is done through a combination of theoretical studies, systematic training, experience and ongoing supervision. This perspective stands in some contrast to the common view in certain professional environments that considers it possible and meaningful to develop very specific and carefully described techniques for treating patients with each of the, by now, numerous psychiatric diagnoses. When the therapist has acquired the basic elements and technical skills in one, or perhaps more, of the widely recognized psychotherapeutic methods, they should instead focus on developing more personal qualities, including their ability to remain psychologically and emotionally present in the contact with the patient and to capture how the core of the individual patient's difficulties will always be manifested in the therapeutic space, not least in the here-and-now interactions with the therapist. The therapist thus relies on their ability to capture, articulate and use what plays out in the therapeutic relationship in the moment, treating it as key therapeutic material and crucial elements in the psychotherapeutic process, combined with their ability to listen to and understand the individual patient. Based on their human and professional judgement, the therapist then determines what is the best possible strategy and specific intervention in relation to the specific patient here and now.

The big, complex – and interesting – questions about what constitutes the core and the effective factors of the psychotherapeutic process, which we are touching on here, will not be explored further in the present context (see Jørgensen, 2019). The intention is not to present yet another new proposal for a coherent method or special technique for the treatment of NPD. From a dynamic relational perspective, such a project would be rather pointless, in the sense that the core of a person's unique psychological constitution and current psychological difficulties could never be narrowed down to a specific diagnosis to be treated with a similarly specific method that has been described in great detail. The ambition is, in a sense, much more modest, namely to point to some elements that it is important to be mindful of in therapeutic work with individuals who struggle with pathological narcissism. In this context, pathological narcissism should be understood more broadly than the specific diagnosis of NPD.

In the following outline of key challenges and themes in the psychotherapeutic treatment of pathological narcissism, the term 'pathological narcissism' thus refers to a range of pathological dynamic processes, including internal psychological and, not least, relational processes that are associated with and manifestations of pathological narcissistic issues and difficulties. These are challenges and themes that therapists can expect to encounter in a wide range of patients with varying degrees of personality disturbances. The reflections and recommendations concerning psychotherapeutic work with pathological narcissism are thus far from limited to the much too narrow and – as hopefully demonstrated over the previous chapters – in many regards problematic *DSM-5* diagnosis of NPD. They will instead, to varying degrees, be relevant and applicable to psychotherapeutic work with most severe and moderate forms of personality pathology that involve grandiose and, in particular, vulnerable manifestations of narcissistic pathology, including patients with borderline disorders (Jørgensen, 2009). The following discussion and recommendations for psychotherapeutic work with pathological narcissism are based on a fundamentally dynamic relational understanding of and approach to psychotherapy (Jørgensen, 2009, 2018, 2023). The focus is not on patients with malignant pathological narcissism, which Kernberg describes as a severely disturbed subcategory of pathological narcissism that is particularly difficult or perhaps impossible to treat psychotherapeutically, in part due to prominent dissocial/psychopathic, paranoid and sadistic traits that may be destructive to the therapeutic relationship and the possibility of establishing a viable treatment alliance, given the patients' often strong urge to control and intimidate the therapist (Caligor et al., 2015, p. 418).

Treatment prognosis and outcome

Historically, clinical psychology has shown remarkably little interest in the empirical study of the treatment of pathological narcissism. This may be due to a number of factors, including the above-mentioned problems related to the formalized diagnosis of NPD, which has caused the prevalence of NPD to appear fairly low in both general population studies and clinical populations. This has led to the impression that pathological narcissism is a relatively rare problem in psychotherapeutic clinics. Furthermore, many may find patients with grandiose pathological narcissism unlikable, difficult, bordering on offensive in their arrogant self-sufficiency, which may have led to diminished interest in understanding and helping these people. Moreover, individuals with predominantly grandiose narcissism in particular are unlikely to seek help, and when they do come into contact with the healthcare system, their treatment may appear as a very demanding task, and since they are typically also quick to break off treatment, empirical studies with this patient group can be particularly challenging. Generally, more severe symptoms, perception of subjective distress and some degree of acknowledgement of one's own share in perceived difficulties will increase the motivation for seeking and remaining in treatment. These conditions are often absent or poorly represented in persons dominated by grandiose narcissism.

There also seems to be a certain professional consensus that psychotherapeutic work with patients who have pathological narcissism can be relatively challenging, in part because the narcissistic patient can be both intensely dismissive, demanding and aggressive towards the therapist. In addition, it is also widely understood there is a considerable risk that patients with pathological narcissism will terminate the treatment prematurely. A few studies have found that NPD is associated with increased risk of treatment dropout (Hilsenroth et al., 1998; Ellison et al., 2013). A number of factors related to pathological narcissism may be associated with a significantly poorer treatment prognosis, particularly when many of them coincide. Among these factors are the following (Kernberg, 1975, p. 285 ff.; Vater et al., 2013b, p. 609; Weinberg & Ronningstam, 2020, p. 125):

- Highly self-destructive behaviour, for example in the form of attempted suicide, various forms of substance abuse and repeated relational ruptures
- Severe dissocial or psychopathic traits (cf. malignant narcissism), which may play out in relation to the therapist in the form of threats, lying and failure to disclose information that is essential to the treatment (not driven by anxiety)
- A high degree of arrogance and self-sufficiency that also plays out in relation to therapists
- Relationally toxic defence strategies manifested as intense criticism and disparagement of, contempt for, attacks on and strong attempts to control therapists
- Strong denial of any need for help from or dependence on others
- Persistent failures of attempts to complete education or hold a job, repeated perceived defeats, which lead to shameful – but denied – perceptions of the self as inferior and inadequate
- Chronic anger, aggression or narcissistic rage that plays out in ways that are toxic to the patient's relationships, including with therapists
- Massive envy of and urge to compete with therapists
- Apparent lack of interest in own inner life and psychological processes – has difficulty dealing with the possibility of multiple perspectives on reality
- Poor access to and ability to articulate or otherwise communicate feelings and other mental states that the person generally tries to shut down or act out

- Chronic sense of boredom, meaninglessness, inner death and emptiness – and a resulting urge to seek stimulation to 'feel alive' (cf. also various types of risk-seeking behaviour)
- Unable to take responsibility for own actions and acknowledging own share in perceived difficulties; highly externalizing defence
- Is in a social position or relational constellation that offers good opportunities for acting out toxic urge for dominance, power and self-staging without immediate negative consequences for the self.

While the absence of the negative prognostic factors listed above may give cause for some degree of optimism about the treatment, studies have also identified a number of positive prognostic factors in persons with pathological narcissism (Kernberg, 1975, p. 285 ff., 2018, p. 192; Walter & Bilke-Hentsch, 2020, p. 134):

- That the patient's history includes at least one stable and giving relationship with a parental figure (self-object) who acted as a credible source of love, nurture and positive attention for the self
- That the patient at some time had a love object who was not devalued and discarded
- Signs of a wish/yearning to be met with nurture and love that seems to enable a certain capacity for acknowledging the self's dependence on others
- Espousing, to some degree, more mature values that are not solely focused on the self's own victories and successes
- A certain capacity for emotionally appreciating and understanding the value of art, culture, literature and science, as it reflects an ability to look beyond oneself and one's own immediate needs
- A reasonable degree of impulse control
- A certain capacity for experiencing guilt (cf. relative absence of dissocial behaviour and a reasonable degree of superego integration)
- A reasonable degree of tolerance to anxiety
- Capacity for containing a certain measure of grief and depressive affects
- At least some capacity for seeing and recognizing therapists and others as autonomous subjects, separate from oneself.

Generally, patients with relatively more predominant vulnerable narcissism will be more accessible to psychotherapeutic treatment and have a better treatment prognosis, compared with patients with more predominant grandiose narcissism. This applies in particular in combination with dissocial, sadistic and perhaps paranoid traits. Some of the listed prognostic factors may also affect the therapist's countertransference, which may in itself add to both positive and negative (cf. positive versus negative prognostic factors) relational processes between patient and therapist (see Chapter 4.3) and thus also influence the treatment effect.

Due to the fairly limited amount of empirical research into pathological narcissism, there are no large-scale well-designed empirical studies of the effect of psychotherapeutic treatment of pathological narcissism. Thus, in that sense, there is no specific evidence-based method for the treatment of pathological narcissism (Caligor et al., 2015; Levy et al., 2021). However, there are a number of theoretically well-founded methods for the treatment of NPD (Weinberg & Ronningstam, 2020, p. 123) – particularly theoretical models based in psychoanalysis – and there seems to be a certain consensus on psychotherapy as the treatment of choice for NPD (Choi-Kain, 2020). A number of authors recommend using one of the approved (evidence-based) methods for the treatment of BPD modified and adapted to the particular needs and challenges of paticnts with NPD (Caligor et al., 2015, p. 420). In addition to TFP, MBT and psychotherapy based on Kohut's self psychology, as mentioned above, this might also include schema-focused therapy (SFT) (Young & Flanagan, 2000; Young et al., 2006). In any case, there is good reason to assume that NPD requires long-term psychotherapeutic treatment provided by specially trained and experienced psychotherapists. So far, there is no evidence that pharmaceutical treatment would have any effect on the core elements of pathological narcissism (Yakeley, 2018, p. 310; Ronningstam, 2022, p. 386), although medicine might in some cases offer temporary relief from certain accompanying symptoms, such as sleep problems, anxiety and affective dysregulation (depression).

4.1 General principles for working with pathological narcissism

Normally, it takes time to establish an actual treatment alliance in which the patient with pathological narcissism has a genuine interest in understanding themself and what is happening in the self's interactions with others. Generally, the typical patient with NPD will not show any real interest in or curiosity about others' reactions and what happens inside them – apart from insights they might use to satisfy their own immediate needs. This also applies to the therapist, who may initially be met with detached indifference, varying degrees of hostility or intense idealization. Patience, flexibility and a sense of subtle shifts in the patient's mental state in the therapeutic space are therefore important elements in treating this patient group. From the outset, the therapist should strive to create a containing and caring atmosphere in the therapeutic space, where the therapist acts, as much as possible, as the stable and reliable other who explicitly notices and offers empathic, validating and understanding response to the patient's subjective perceptions, emptions and other mental states (Modell, 1976, p. 291); cf. Winnicott's descriptions of a 'holding environment'.

The patient should feel that the therapist meets them with empathic resonance and tries to create an atmosphere in the therapeutic space that offers a suitable self-object matrix or a healthy self-object environment for the patient and thus acts as a counterweight to the patient's past negative self-object experiences and enhances the patient's self (Wolf, 1996, p. 139). The therapist should strive to be the reliable and emotionally accessible other who sees the patient and their 'true self' by taking an interest in, seeing and trying to make contact with the self behind the presented facade that the self puts up to hide from what is perceived as a threatening outside world. The therapist should meet the patient as a 'you', a subject, an equal who has significance and value regardless of how they may appear and act in the contact with the therapist.

No matter how the patient acts in the therapeutic space, including whether the patient seeks refuge behind an arrogant and devaluing facade or, conversely, is taciturn, unapproachable and seeks refuge in their psychic retreat, the therapist should strive to meet the patient with a curious, interested and accepting attitude and always avoid acting in ways that might appear critically disparaging or distancing or have the character of various types of defence against – or counterattacks in reaction to – the patient's attacks on the therapist. Particularly for patients with more severe pathological narcissism characterized by significant deficits in personality organization, the atmosphere in the therapeutic space may in itself have a curative effect, and at the very least it is always a crucial condition for the possibility of therapeutic change (Modell, 1975, p. 281, 1976, p. 304). Furthermore, the therapist should always seek to maintain that the perfect and flawless therapist who never makes 'mistakes' does not exist and thus strive to be the good-enough therapist, a human being who inevitably makes mistakes but consistently seeks to acknowledge, articulate and incorporate these missteps into the therapeutic work in ways that will hopefully help the patient.

The core of narcissism plays out in the therapeutic space

The key focus of psychotherapeutic work with pathological narcissism is how the patient's narcissistic grandiosity and vulnerability manifest themselves in the patient's ways of being, interacting and engaging in contact (or not) with the therapist. How the patient's self-image and self-esteem may fluctuate between, on the one hand, grandiose perceptions of the self's exceptional character and self-sufficiency and, on the other hand, convictions of the self's profound inadequacy, vulnerability and dependence on attention and admiration from others. The therapist should help the patient register and put these diverse manifestations of pathological narcissism into words. This should, ideally, happen at a pace that is not perceived as causing narcissistic injury and which lets the patient withdraw or counterattack the therapist, who is perceived as a threat to the patient's fragile internal balance. The therapist should be genuinely interested in understanding what the patient's experience is when their self-image and self-esteem suddenly shift in ways and at times that are completely or partially unpredictable to the patient.

Together, the patient and the therapist should attempt to arrive at an understanding of what is the basis and the driver of these shifts between the individual patient's grandiose self-perceptions, contempt for others and a need to withdraw from interpersonal contact versus painful vulnerability, fear of being exposed as shamefully inadequate and great need for attention, admiration and recognition from others. All things being equal, these shifts will also play out in the therapeutic space, where they may be associated both with recurring dynamic psychological processes inside the patient and with processes in the interaction with the therapist in the here-and-now. This may unfold, for example, in the form of rapid shifts between the patient feeling victimized by the therapist's perceived betrayal, injury or abuse – while perhaps still having a strong need for support and validation from the therapist – and the grandiose, arrogant and toxically aggressive patient who attacks and abuses the therapist (Kernberg, 2019, p. 963 ff.).

Furthermore, the patient will demonstrate in vivo in the therapeutic space what strategies they typically use in their attempts to cover up, deal with or compensate for sudden shifts in self-image and self-esteem. The core of the patient's pathological narcissism will thus be actualized and manifest itself in the interaction with the therapist. This contains great challenges as well as possibilities for the therapeutic work, as the therapist needs to notice and respond as aptly as possible to these actualizations of the patient's difficulties, which is in itself associated with significant therapeutic treatment factors (cf. 'corrective emotional experiences'). These actualizations also offer an opportunity for exploring the core of the patient's challenges – with the patient – as they play out in vivo in the therapeutic space.

The ongoing attention to and therapeutic use of the actualization of key dynamic psychological processes and recurring relational patterns in the patient's interactions with the therapist also include the therapist's reactions to the patient's ways of being and acting in the therapeutic space: the therapist's experience, how the therapist has an urge to react and what the therapist has an urge to say to the patient. The therapist's countertransference thus contains invaluable information about the patient's difficulties and about the sort of reactions that the patient typically encounters and contributes to sparking in others (see Chapter 4.3). Besides, the therapist's ability to pick up on the beginnings of problematic interaction patterns from the patient's life in the therapeutic space and react differently than the patient is used to is a key treatment factor in working with pathological narcissism. The patient's transference and the therapist's countertransference thus form crucial building blocks in the psychotherapeutic treatment of NPD.

The basic elements of treatment

The basic elements of the psychotherapeutic treatment of pathological narcissism are the same as in the treatment of other types of moderate and severe personality disorders. In that sense, therapists should follow the same basic approach as they do, for example, for borderline personality disorders. The psychotherapeutic stance and the ongoing work with what plays out in the treatment relationship are not fundamentally different from the psychotherapeutic treatment of other relatively severe personality disorders (see Jørgensen, 2009, 2018/2019). Still, it could be argued that psychotherapeutic work with pathological narcissism presents at least five mutually connected challenges that to some degree are specific to the work with this particular patient group:

1 The therapist needs to establish emotional contact and develop a treatment alliance with a patient who either signals a distinct disinclination to engage in this way (cf. predominantly grandiose narcissism) or is very shy and has difficulty engaging in intimate emotional contact (cf. predominantly vulnerable narcissism).
2 The therapist should be prepared to work with the patient's narcissistic defence in form of grandiose perceptions and arrogant rejection of the therapist and their offer of help or, conversely, the patient's tendency to dissociate, withdraw from emotional contact and/or seek refuge in their psychic retreat at sometimes just very minor steps towards making emotional contact with the therapist or painful parts of themself and their history.
3 The therapeutic work and the establishing of emotional contact will sometimes activate profound destructive shame in the patient, who feels exposed and humiliated when they come into contact with or reveal aspects of themself that are normally shut down or split off/dissociated.
4 The therapist will need to deal with the patient's sometimes extreme narcissistic vulnerability, which places high demands on the therapist's empathy, responsiveness, flexibility and ability to modify their strategy, interventions and way of being in contact with the patient to match what the patient needs and is able to contain in the given moment – something that may vary quite considerably over the course of a session. In this regard, too, the therapist will need to remain attentive to 'where the patient is at', meaning what the patient needs in the moment, and be agile in attuning their acting in the therapeutic space accordingly.
5 The therapist needs to be able to contain, recognize and, to some extent, satisfy, in particular, the severely disturbed and predominantly narcissistically vulnerable patient's self-object need for empathic mirroring and closeness to an idealized other (the therapist) – a need that was not met in the patient's earlier deficient self-object relations. In parallel with this, it is important to maintain and continually defend the framework of the therapy against expected challenges from the patient.

The dynamic relational treatment of pathological narcissism has two overarching goals:

1 Enhancing the patient's ability to contain, accept and thus also integrate different aspects of themself and their history, which will typically have been characterized by splitting/dissociation, internal polarization and

deficient integration. This happens primarily – but not exclusively – in the emotional and psychological contact and in the interaction with the therapist, as the patient over time internalizes the therapist's way of meeting and reacting to different aspects of the patient, including shameful and vulnerable self components (behaviour, needs, emotions and other mental states), that manifest themselves in the therapeutic space. This includes how the therapist contains and responds to the patient's emotional yearnings and needs (self-object needs) in the therapeutic space.

2 Enhancing the patient's capacity for self-reflection and thus the patient's ability to take charge over and create their own, more nuanced narrative about themself and their life; enhancing the patient's ability to take a step away from, have nuanced thoughts about and understand their own subjective experiences, emotional states and (impulsive) reactions, including any lack of reaction stemming from (vulnerable, loving, angry) parts of the patient's self having been and being shut down or dissociated. This happens primarily – but far from exclusively – via the common exploration of what is playing out in the patient, the therapist and, not least, their mutual interaction in the therapeutic space, including triangulation and reflection on transference and countertransference from different perspectives.

Encountering grandiose and vulnerable manifestations of narcissism

As discussed in the previous chapters, it is potentially problematic and not meaningful to apply a categorical distinction between grandiose and vulnerable narcissism. Both manifestations or aspects of pathological narcissism will almost always be present and in play in the individual patient, albeit in varying blends and combinations, with some exceptions among patients with severely malignant narcissism and heavy comorbidity of psychopathic/antisocial traits. Nevertheless, the following discussion will briefly make this distinction between the two 'variants' of manifestations of pathological narcissism. This is done in order to outline how patients whose immediate presentation is currently, or perhaps slightly more generally, dominated by either grandiose or vulnerable narcissism can in some regards be expected to appear and react differently and will thus also need a slightly different response from the therapist in some regards.

The common core of pathological narcissism, which is particularly relevant and always plays out, in varying ways, in the contact with the dynamic relational therapist, revolves around fundamental difficulties with establishing and being in equal relationships (see Chapter 2.3). Relationships are basically regarded as a struggle for dominance/submission, control, who is entitled to what and from whom, who is being humiliated versus humiliating the other, who is superior versus inferior – cf. one being idealized versus one idealizing the other – or who may risk being exposed as shamefully inadequate and inferior in relation to whom. The patient will often be convinced that dyadic relationships necessarily involve one person being 'one up' (superior, admired) and one who is 'one down' (inferior, envious); that relationships will always be defined by a competition for attention and about who is stronger, smarter and being admired for having most to offer or being the more 'valuable' person.

These perceptions of what constitutes the core and what is at stake in interpersonal relationships naturally make it challenging to develop the trust in a specific other, including a therapist, that is necessary for opening up to the other and allowing them to get close and have an impact on the self. The patient who perceives all relationships as being organized around competition and around who can humiliate whom may perceive the therapist's friendly and welcoming demeanour and empathy as shameful humiliation – a sign that the therapist perceives the patient as weak and as someone who is in need of kindness – and react with aggressive rejection (Schalkwijk et al., 2021, p. 4). Opening themself to contact and speaking about their difficulties, revealing distress and loneliness, will make the patient even more vulnerable to being emotionally affected, losing control and feeling embarrassed, shameful, humiliated or exploited – all states that are associated with unacceptable weakness. Thus, it takes great trust in the other, trust that the other is not going to exploit, humiliate or ridicule the self when the patient leaves themself open to intimate emotional contact and to contact with previously 'forbidden' or dissociated aspects of themself and their history, such as perceived abuse, an upbringing characterized by neglect, painful bullying and loneliness related to aspects of the self that could not be lived out. Establishing that kind of trust takes time and requires patience from both parties.

As mentioned above (see Chapter 3.1), patients with predominantly vulnerable manifestations of pathological narcissism may appear closely related to BPD. On the surface, however, their sense of identity typically appears more stable, and they contain a variety of grandiose perceptions, just as they may, to varying degrees, feel entitled to special treatment. In some cases, these perceptions do not become evident until after prolonged contact with the narcissistic patient, but they are not nearly as common among patients with BPD. When the therapist meets patients with predominantly grandiose manifestations of pathological narcissism, the differences in relation to BPD are far more apparent, solely because of the fairly apparent grandiose self-image in NPD, which are not normally seen – at least rarely to the same degree – in persons with BPD. Furthermore, from the outset, the therapist may experience a wall of non-contact from a patient with pathological narcissism. It may seem impossible to establish any intimate emotional and psychological contact with the patient, who may appear almost aggressively dismissive or remarkably evasive and unreceptive to the therapist's invitations to contact. By comparison, patients with BPD will often appear almost to hunger for contact or will at the very least be much easier to establish a certain level of emotional contact with. For patients with comorbid NPD and BPD, the situation is more complicated (see Chapter 3.1 and 3.2).

Reactions to perceived narcissistic injury

Both patients with predominantly vulnerable and patients with predominantly grandiose manifestations will typically be characterized by a marked tendency to experience narcissistic injury, but they often tend to react fairly differently when they feel injured or find that their self, social position, status or role is threatened. Precisely because the narcissistic patient has such a low threshold of perceived injury and expects criticism, threats, humiliation, shaming and ridicule around every corner, the patient will in practice inevitably feel threatened and injured by the therapist. Any intervention that is not perceived as perfect mirroring of the patient's self and current state and needs may potentially be experienced as a narcissistic injury. When that happens, it is essential for the therapist to notice and focus on this and use it as valuable therapeutic material. Generally, the patient's great sensitivity to perceived narcissistic injury makes the therapist's tact, flair and ability to time and communicate their interventions with sufficient empathic sense for what the patient needs and is able to contain in the moment extra important.

What we are discussing here should not be understood as clear-cut either–or categories. It is really a matter of degrees and various blends of or balances between vulnerable versus grandiose elements or manifestations of pathological narcissism in the individual patient which the therapist needs to notice and seek to consider in their ways of interacting and handling the contact with the patient. That pathological narcissism has two such seemingly incompatible manifestations – and that the individual may rapidly alternate between vulnerable and grandiose narcissism, which in a sense coexist in the patient's internal psychological dynamic – makes the work with this group of patients more challenging but also even more interesting.

A patient with predominantly grandiose narcissism will typically be more inclined to react to perceived narcissistic threats or injuries by the therapist with contempt, cold arrogance, attacks on the therapist or fairly transparent attempts to control or assume a dominant position in relation to the therapist, who may be perceived by the patient as inferior or incompetent (Crisp & Gabbard, 2020, p. 145). The patient tries to compensate for an underlying feeling of inferiority through what may appear as forced and feigned confidence (Brauner et al., 2021, p. 320). Similarly, the patient may try to deal with the activation of shame in the therapeutic space through devaluation of or attacks on the therapist, who is a witness to and perceived as being to blame for the activated feelings of shame. Perhaps, the patient will attempt to shed their own shame by acting in ways that cause shame in the therapist (cf. projective identification; Ogden, 1979; Jørgensen, 2018/2019, p. 249 ff.). The patient may react with resentment and outrage over the therapist's alleged professional incompetence or cynicism or the accusation that the therapist only has this job for the money or social status that it brings – notions that often contain projective elements in the sense that these accusations will often provide insight into the perceptions and psychological processes that dominate the patient's interior and relational universe.

As described by Rosenfeld (1987, p. 116), a patient with severe grandiose narcissism may perceive their own omnipotent defence as a 'good friend' and view anyone who tries to make the patient face reality and acknowledge their need for interpersonal contact as a serious threat to this 'friend' – the patient's grandiose self-image. Thus, the therapist should be prepared to be met with anger, contempt and devaluation (Rosenfeld, 1987, p. 131). When this happens, it is important to try to decode the patient's contempt as an expression of the patient's defence of a fragile self – a defence that might be activated precisely because the first small opening to contact with the therapist might be appearing.

By contrast, a patient who is dominated by more vulnerable manifestations of pathological narcissism will typically react to perceived narcissistic threats and injuries by being visibly hurt, disappointed, sad, dismayed and overwhelmed by intense destructive shame. The patient may also feel inferior and appear as the rejected and passive victim of a mean and insensitive therapist (Crisp & Gabbard, 2020, p. 145; Brauner et al., 2021, p. 319). Generally, the patient expresses how difficult and painful it is to be around others (including the therapist), to be in contact with themself and to be in therapy. Taken together, this may make the therapist find the work with this patient difficult and feel that they are either repeatedly injuring or becoming emotionally overinvolved in the patient – both of which are situations that are potentially shameful to a therapist (Britton, 1998, p. 47).

In some cases, the patient may withdraw from contact, seek refuge in their psychic retreat, perhaps drug themself with alcohol, drugs or sedatives. Or they may split the therapist's voice, tone and nonverbal communication off from the content of the therapist's verbal interventions in an attempt to protect themself against interventions that might threaten the patient's constructed image of and relationship to the therapist which they need to hold onto in order to be able to be in the therapeutic space. Some of the therapist's actions and interventions aimed at confronting the patient – or bringing them into contact – with reality may be perceived not just as narcissistic injuries but as attempts to drive the patient out of the Garden of Eden, the 'pure' and conflict-free relationship they need to have with the therapist (Weiss, 2012, p. 316).

Alternatively, the patient may turn to self-harm in an attempt to alleviate the unbearable psychological pain that was triggered because the patient once again felt injured, betrayed and hurt – for which the patient may blame themself, since the self appears to be so shamefully defective and inferior that it deserves to be betrayed and injured. These are all reactions that may give rise to feelings of guilt in the therapist's countertransference along with shameful doubts about the therapist's ability to understand and help the patient. In comparison with a patient dominated by grandiose narcissism, the clearly narcissistically vulnerable patient has much less agency and is much more likely to react with passive withdrawal in a victimized position than with more active and action-oriented strategies. However, both strategies should be viewed primarily as attempts to protect an exposed, vulnerable and uncomfortable self against perceived threats and injuries.

The patient's withdrawal to a psychic retreat in the therapeutic space

The patient's withdrawal to their psychic retreat (cf. Chapter 3.6) will not necessary manifest itself in very specific standardized ways. In principle, there are no limits to how this might play out in the interaction with the therapist, but it will often be in the form of tense silence, emptiness, boredom and meaninglessness or absence of perceived meaning in the therapeutic space, where it may feel as if time has stopped or slowed down to a glacial pace. The therapist may feel intensely cut off from emotional and intimate psychological contact with the patient and feel an urge to establish such a contact with the patient and to fill out the perceived emptiness with words or interventions in an attempt to escape the diffusely uncomfortable emptiness and silence in the therapeutic space. Here, the therapist's countertransference may thus play a crucial role, and it is therefore important to be mindful of and continually reflect on it (see Chapter 4.3). Furthermore, a sort of power struggle may arise in the therapeutic space, as the therapist tries to bring the patient out of their internal bubble, while the patient, on the other hand, reacts to the therapist's invitations to contact by enhancing the defences around their psychic retreat (Symington, 1993, p. 77). The patient may feel – and explicitly state – that life in the psychic retreat is better, more secure and more intense than the external reality. During much of the initial part of the treatment, the patient may also fear that if they share experiences from their psychic retreat with the therapist, it will lose its emotional power and thus its potential to serve as a safe retreat where they can be alone and feel in control. In regard to this, the therapist needs to be mindful of the possibility that the patient may have developed a form of dependence on the perceived security and satisfaction of certain needs that are associated with withdrawing to the psychic retreat. If and when the patient begins to take steps to come out of their retreat, they will inevitably be confronted with 'reality', which may involve painful losses, shameful aspects of the self, anxiety and contact with unbearable experiences. This painful content includes the consequences, for better or for worse, of establishing emotional contact with and being seen by others – the ability of others to see and react to aspects of the self and its history that the patient does not want others to see and has therefore tried to hide or split off. When the patient works up the courage to come out of hiding, it may further become difficult to maintain the grandiose self-perceptions that have helped keep a shameful and 'dangerous' narcissistic vulnerability in check. In the encounter with another, these grandiose perceptions of self and reality threaten to collapse, which can it itself be anxiety-provoking and activate painful feelings of shame.

The silent patient

When the patient's silence is driven by fear of contact with the therapist, it will often be unhelpful if the therapist also remains silent for long periods of time (Symington, 1993, p. 65). The silent therapist may contribute to the repetition of a painful pattern as the patient may have been met with silence and lack of responsiveness from significant others previously in their life (cf. the emotionally 'dead', absent or depressive parent). The patient has given up on trying to 'wake' the other up and has instead learned to withdraw into their psychic retreat and/or dissociate (Green, 2004, p. 255). Alternatively, the patient may have experienced significant others failing to see, contain and deal with important aspects of the self, including strong affects and yearnings. As a result, the patient may have learned to shut down and hide these aspects behind a wall of silence and apparent self-sufficiency in an attempt to protect themself, the other and their fragile contact. The point here is that it may be unhelpful if the therapist remains silent for just several minutes, although this depends to a high degree on what the mood is during this silence in the therapeutic space and, not least, how the patient perceives it. In some cases, it may be a good idea to ask the patient explicitly: 'It is my impression that the silence in the room right now is safe and pleasant. Do you feel the same way, or does it feel different to you?'; 'None of us has said anything for some time now. How do you experience the silence in the room, is it unpleasant, does it make you feel insecure, and do you need for someone to say something, or is it a safe and nice silence?' In relation to this point, it is important to note that a lot may be going on in the nonverbal contact, including in both the patient's and the therapist's inner universes, even if there is no verbal communication.

The very talkative patient

Other patients may flood the therapeutic space with chatter that has no emotional content or connection to the patient's inner life (Modell, 1980, p. 259). This may represent the patient's attempts to maintain control over the therapist and over what is happening in the therapeutic space. At the same time, it prevents the therapist from establishing intimate contact with the patient, given that the patient may perceive any initiation of emotional contact as a potential threat to the sentries guarding their psychic retreat. One example would be the patient who comes into every session having seemingly 'prepared' lots of material to share with the therapist. The patient may fill up the therapeutic space, from start to finish of each session, with stories without any affective charge, unless the therapist insists that the patient pause so that they can explore together what this is about. This is all done in a more or less unconscious attempt to avoid intimate contact with the self and the therapist. The therapist might say, 'I have noticed that you often have a lot of things that you want to tell me – which is good and important.

But sometimes, I get the feeling that you have so much you want to share that it's difficult for me to ask you any questions or dwell on any of it. What do you think of that – is that something you recognize from other situations?'; 'I wonder what this might be about – what do you think it would be like for you if you made more room for me to dwell a little more on what you say and ask some follow-up questions to the significant things you are telling me? Might that be nice for you? Or do you think it would make you feel a little insecure, afraid of losing control – perhaps you're not sure if I might choose to focus on things that you don't feel like coming into contact with and discuss with me?'

The patient with fragmented language

When a patient has withdrawn mentally to their psychic retreat, sometimes their verbal communication comes to be dominated by noticeable ruptures and disruptions that can make it more difficult for the therapist to decode and understand what the patient is in fact trying to communicate. In some cases, this will be driven by profound ambivalence in relation to the patient's yearning for contact with the therapist and a desire to share painful experiences with the therapist versus fear of contact with the therapist and aspects of the self that have been shut down but which may be on the cusp of breaking into the patient's consciousness as a result of what is happening in what is perhaps the tender, initial contact with the therapist and in the therapeutic process. Specifically, the patient may break of mid-sentence, as if the patient suddenly interrupts or stops themself from sharing something important with the therapist. Suddenly, the patient shuts down emotionally, perhaps explicitly saying to the therapist that they cannot or do not want to continue talking about an emotionally significant topic that is the focus of the therapeutic work in the moment, because it is becoming too emotionally overwhelming (or shameful) for the self (Modell, 1980, p. 259 ff.).

This may be seen as a sort of unconscious destruction of language and of the content of the verbal communication, as connections between thoughts and feelings, words and reality, internal and external reality, and different parts of reality are unconsciously attacked and destroyed. This is done out of fear of how establishing these connections might bring the patient into contact with unbearable aspects of their inner life and own history, such as how something that is playing out between patient and therapist in the moment and what is the current topic of focus in the therapeutic process may suddenly prove to have strong emotional links to – and contain recurring elements of – traumatic events in the patient's history; links that may be perceived as a dire threat to the self's fragile self-image, self-esteem and control over the boundaries of their psychic retreat.

As for the patient's levels of psychological functioning and personality organization, Steiner (1993, p. 28 ff.) situates a patient's withdrawal to a psychic retreat in the transitional area between Melanie Klein's (1946/1975) descriptions of the paranoid-schizoid and the depressive position. This will not be discussed further in the present context (see Jørgensen, 2009, p. 262 ff.), but in Steiner (1993, p. 34) this transitional area is associated, in part, with an overwhelming fear of losing the good object (the therapist or others) and related paranoid fantasies – and, not least, with a painful experience of having already lost it, which involves profound mourning and sadness. The latter is also associated with an experience of not just losing control over the good object but also fear of not being able to protect the good object against the self's own inherent destructiveness and greed. The patient's yearning for the good object, for contact with and possession of the object, is so overwhelming that the patient fears that this in itself may destroy the good object or send it fleeing.

Inviting the therapist into the psychic retreat

Some patients with pathological narcissism will try to deal with their painful fear of losing the good object – in this case the therapist – by 'inviting' the therapist into their psychic retreat. In this fantasy, the patient can be in close contact and have long 'conversations' with the therapist and have the experience of merging with and having some control over the therapist in their inner universe. This fantasy may also imply that what is playing out in the therapeutic space is regarded as less important. This is seen, for example, in the patient who brings the therapist into their psychic retreat where they can show and tell the therapist things that the patient was never able – or dared – to share in the therapeutic space. In the short term, this may pose a problem for the treatment, because the patient may have a sense that they have 'already' shared things that were in fact only 'brought up' in the psychic retreat. The patient may also have a sense – or convince themself – that it may not be very important to share these things with the 'real therapist' in the therapeutic space. In this form, the psychic retreat has a regressive function, because it replaces the concrete external reality and contact with the therapist that hold the potential for change.

In the long term, however, this may help the patient open up to the therapist in the therapeutic space. The patient's conversations with the therapist in the psychic retreat then serve as a form of rehearsal of and preparation for telling the 'real therapist', whose reactions are not under the patient's control the way they are in the fantasy of their encounter in the psychic retreat (Weiss, 2012, p. 311 ff.). All things being equal, however, the only real treatment effect comes from actual conversations with the real therapist in the therapeutic space, although we should not underestimate the significance of the patient's internalization of the therapist as the good object and their subsequent internal dialogues with the therapist. The crucial distinction is whether the internalization of and internal dialogues with the therapist serve as a defence against and a replacement for the real contact and dialogue with the actual therapist in the therapeutic space.

The client tries to turn the therapeutic space into a new retreat

Alternatively, the patient may try to turn the therapeutic space into a new retreat or an extension of their existing psychic retreat that is not part of the external reality and where the patient, in collusion with the therapist, can deny and avoid confronting parts of the external reality. Thus, the patient may – with the therapist – try to (re)discover a paradisical and peaceful state in the therapeutic space and in the relationship with the therapist (Steiner, 2020, p. 19). When this happens, the therapist and the therapy are incorporated into the patient's defence against frightening changes, and the therapist may be seduced into acting in ways in the therapeutic space that help to preserve the patient's pathological narcissistic organization (Steiner, 2014, p. 129). As long as the patient is successful in this, without being matched by the therapist's successful insistence on the existence of the external reality, the patient's psychological development will be paused or, at best, proceed at a much slower pace than necessary. On the other hand, this may also provide a significant opening for the therapeutic space and the relationship with the therapist to develop into a transitional area in between the internal and the external reality, where the patient and the therapist together can 'play with' different perspectives on reality, provided that the therapist is able to hold onto the external reality and the framework of the therapeutic space.

Reactions to perceived threats to the retreat

The patient's attempts to reshape the therapeutic space may be seen an indication that the patient's transference is dominated by illusory perceptions that the patient regards as crucial to the psychological survival of the self and which would be shaken and threatened by collapse if or when they inevitably are confronted with reality. This occurs, for example, when the therapist is separated from the patient and, in that sense, beyond the patient's omnipotent control and may react to the patient in ways that are perceived as a threat to the patient's self. Or it occurs when the therapist marks the boundaries of the therapeutic space and the therapeutic relationship – boundaries that are incompatible with the patient's fantasies of a form of merger with or ideal contact with the therapist.

In practice, the patient may, for example, get furious when the therapist marks the boundaries of the therapeutic relationship, or they may withdraw from contact with the therapist in an attempt to protect themself by seeking refuge in their psychic retreat. Alternatively, the patient may become sad when they feel that they have lost or been abandoned by the therapist. The patient's magical thinking may collapse: fantasies that simply being in contact with the ideal other – the idealized therapist – will somehow magically bring change, without any need for hard therapeutic work. These fantasies may be associated with the patient's difficulties with containing and dealing with the therapist's dual presence in the therapeutic space as a person – a human subject in an equal relationship – and as a therapist in a setting where the role of therapist always comes first. Thus, it will never be possible to realize any dreams or magical thinking the patient may have about the ideal relationship with the 'other' (the therapist) in the external reality, outside the therapeutic space. This is the case, even if the patient may yearn for and dream of being able to have the therapist as a sort of infinitely giving self-object, meaning that the patient, so to speak, wants to 'have' the therapist as a person rather than as a therapist (cf. Modell, 1975, p. 280).

The treatment of pathological narcissism aims to enable the patient to gradually acknowledge their need for others, for the good object that is separate from the self, an autonomous subject beyond the self's control. Furthermore, the self should be able to contain the reality that it may lose the good object but also that the self may be afraid of destroying the good object and their relationship with it if they fail to protect it from their own destructiveness, greed and what the self perceives as their persistent tendency to destroy good objects and their relationships with them (cf. perceptions of their own destructiveness and of having a toxic self).

For a patient who has sought refuge in a psychic retreat in order to protect their fragile true self against the threat of exposure (Modell, 1991), even small, cautious steps out of this internal bubble may be associated with intense anxiety and a feeling of being naked, transparent and unprotected and of having their shamefully inadequate self exposed (Steiner, 2006, p. 67). In this situation, any emotion may feel too intense and impossible for the self to contain (Bion, 1967, p. 108), and thus the self shuns emotions and tries to keep them under strict control. This may also be driven by worries about the catastrophic consequences that the patient fears – perhaps backed up by previous relational experiences – will be the result if the self actually comes out of hiding and comes into contact with and reveals their emotions in interactions with others.

Psychotherapy involves seeing and being seen – coming out of hiding

Psychotherapeutic work is associated with seeing and being seen, understanding and being understood (Steiner, 2006, p. 11). Thus, it is quite understandable that going into therapy can cause anxiety and ambivalence associated with moving in and out of one's internal bubble, where the fragile self is protected from harm – or with being in the transitional area between the internal and the external reality, between continuing to hide in one's own inner world and finding the courage to enter into contact with the therapist and facing the external reality. When the therapist helps bring the patient out of their internal bubble in the therapeutic space, and when the patient has repeatedly felt emotionally overwhelmed by this and, to varying degrees, had to withdraw from contact by being silent, staying away from subsequent sessions or attacking the therapist, the therapist may feel guilty over what may seem like a violation of the patient's boundaries. The therapist may feel that they have subjected a vulnerable patient to emotional harm by being too insistent in their invitations to contact and their focus on significant – but perhaps dissociated or denied – aspects of the patient's self and history. Provided that the therapist manages to dose these invitations to contact with aspects of the patient's self in the therapeutic relationship in ways that are attuned to what the individual patient is capable of containing, they should remember that establishing emotional contact and an encounter with reality – in suitable doses – is a necessary condition for the narcissistically disordered patient to move forward and develop the ability to leave their psychic retreat on a more permanent basis.

One patient with powerful and painful perceptions of being fundamentally wrong and unwanted is persistently preoccupied with the notion of being a heavy burden on the therapist: she is not 'entertaining' or 'interesting' enough and is convinced that it must be a huge strain for the therapist to be in contact with her (which it is not), particularly if (when) she briefly shows sides of herself that she normally puts a great deal of energy into keeping tucked away, hidden behind a 'cheerful' and, in a more concrete sense, well-functioning facade. She is convinced that if she is more 'herself' and shows these shameful and 'defective' sides of herself – self components associated with deep sadness and emotional strain but also with potential rage and sexually challenging behaviour – she will do irreparable damage to the therapist and to their mutual relationship. When she is struggling and comes into contact with these aspects of herself, she feels the urge to skip therapy sessions or to withdraw from the emotional contact with the therapist in the therapeutic space and hide in her psychic retreat. There, she can shut down her emotions – according to her, in order to protect both the therapist and herself against these 'dangerous' and 'repulsive' parts of the self.

In therapy, it becomes clear that these parts of the self and her attempts to keep them at bay are associated with experiences that her parents – for reasons that seem predominantly related to their own psychological difficulties – were unable to contain and care for her. This applies especially to parts of her self related to powerful affects (anxiety), need for nurture (greed), impulses (anger) and inadequately developed sense of 'appropriate boundaries' (invasive, intimidating insistence on contact). What she initially needs is for the therapist to 'take her by the hand' and go with her into the dark recesses of her inner world and history, where these defective and shameful experiences and self aspects are hidden. Importantly, the therapist needs to do so without any changes in the therapist's basic way of being present and in emotional contact with her. Over time, she will be able to perceive this as disproval of her past conviction that any contact with and opening into these parts of the self would destroy and scare others (the therapist) off and cause her to be left alone to deal with these unbearable aspects of herself and her history.

To the best of their ability, the therapist should support the patient who has been hiding inside their internal bubble but who may now be venturing out by helping them to contain and deal with their reactions to the established contact with the therapist and previously split-off or non-integrated self aspects. This may be done, for example, by helping the patient pace their departure from their psychic retreat to prevent them from establishing a contact with the therapist that is too intense and risks overwhelming the patient emotionally. In some cases, it may be helpful explicitly to register and recognize when the patient ventures out, and emotional contact is established in the therapeutic space (Steiner, 1993, p. 10). Next, the therapist and the patient can work together to explore what the patient fears if they move out of the bubble and into a closer contact with both the therapist and previously sealed-off self aspects, which are typically more vulnerable and, in the eyes of the patient, contemptible, inferior and shameful self aspects and experiences. In practice, this is an exploration of the psychological function of the psychic retreat, which may vary considerably from one patient to another. Initially, the shared attention should generally be directed at the surface and psychological function of the internal bubble – when and how it becomes apparent that the patient has moved into their psychic retreat and what this does for the patient. Next, the therapist may perhaps invite a closer exploration of the contents of the internal bubble and of the patient's thoughts, feelings and experiences when they are in the internal bubble (Volkan, 1979, p. 429).

In relation to this, the therapist should note that their interventions and (particularly, their emotional) presence as a person may be perceived as an attack on and a threat to the patient's psychic retreat that may make it necessary for the patient to resist or even attack the therapist and their work. This applies in particular to the effort to establish emotional and psychological contact with the patient here and now and with certain aspects of the patient and their history. Particularly when the patient feels extra vulnerable or emotionally thin-skinned – and perhaps feels that their delimitation of their own self and inner life from the therapist is challenged – the patient may need some form of very specific control over the therapist. This may involve, for example, that for shorter or longer periods of a session, the therapist is 'not allowed' to look at the patient, because this is perceived as intimidating and as a threat to the patient's fragile self-image, self-definition and self-control, as the therapist's gaze threatens to flood the patient's self with unbearable feelings, including destructive shame and fear of losing themself. Or the therapist's gaze may be perceived as a provocation, a challenge to the patient's grandiose self and a potential narcissistic injury that may lead to a strong urge for a counterattack on the therapist.

Generally, the therapist should strive to contain and accept this, while being mindful of how the establishment of this sort of relational constellation in the therapeutic space may contain elements that repeat destructive relational patterns from the patient's past relationships, which it may be necessary subsequently to address and explore with the patient. For example, how might the demand that the therapist not look at the patient contain elements that repeat relational patterns and strategies for protecting a vulnerable exposed self that are familiar to the patient from previous relationships and situations? Might it be related to emotions and methods for self-protection that the patient has experienced in or used in connection with past abuse or perceived betrayals? And might these old patterns and defence strategies have been activated in the therapeutic space because the patient in some sense felt intimidated, betrayed or threatened by the therapist's way of being and acting shortly before this occurred?

Finally, these dynamics may be associated with the patient coming into contact with parts of themself and their history that are so shameful and associated with so much self-contempt that it would be unbearable to have them exposed, met by the therapist's gaze and brought outside the inner space where they were previously hidden and repressed. In any case, the therapist should note that the patient's withdrawal to their psychic retreat and their avoidance of contact in the therapeutic space are also a way of avoiding contact with the external reality. They are a withdrawal to an inner space where the self does not have to encounter reality and where grandiose fantasies may be dominant, and everything seems possible and permitted (where the social order has been suspended), free from reality testing and correction (Steiner, 1993, p. 3). Even if it may seem understandable in the moment that the patient would need to retreat in order to protect a vulnerable self, the therapist should always be mindful of the destructive effect of this strategy, which is an obstacle to the patient's possibilities of development, including developing the ability to remain in emotional contact with non-destructive aspects of themself and with others.

In particular, interventions that focus explicitly on the patient and their inner life, history and emotional relationships may be perceived as intimidating and threatening by the narcissistically vulnerable patient. In some cases, it may be helpful to apply more therapist-focused interventions that appear to place the focus more on the therapist (Steiner, 1993, p. 133): 'When we approach the topic what happened to you during the early part of your life, are you then convinced that I find you disgusting and that I feel contempt for you?', 'I wonder if you worry that if you allow me and the therapy to become important to you, I am going to become intimidating and impossible for you to keep at arm's length?', 'I had the impression that you felt a little insecure a moment ago when I asked you what happened between you and your father?' Generally, patient-centred interventions have a more direct focus on having the patient speak about their inner life and understand themself, while the main intention of therapist-centred interventions is to enable the patient to feel seen, mirrored and understood by the therapist (Steiner, 2006, p. 12).

Development of a treatment alliance

Establishing emotional contact and developing a treatment alliance with the patient is much more important for the course of treatment and the treatment outcome than the specific choice of treatment method (Gabbard & Crisp, 2018, p. 72). The two tracks are interrelated, and establishing a treatment alliance requires a certain element of 1) mutual trust and agreement about the 2) goal and 3) method of the treatment – three elements that are all challenging to patients with pathological narcissism. Patients dominated by more grandiose aspects may be particularly disinclined to submit to the therapist's chosen treatment method and presented boundaries around the therapeutic space. More than a century ago, the psychoanalyst Karl Abraham (1919/1999, p. 256) described how sensitive narcissistic patients may be to reactions from the therapist that injure their ego feeling and how they may expect the therapist to simply satisfy their exacting needs. Furthermore, they do not accept the therapist in the role as a 'father' figure with the authority to control what is going to happen in the therapeutic space but mount a narcissistic defence against the therapist's person, work and method. Patients with predominantly grandiose narcissism may have a strong urge to dominate the therapist and the treatment relationship, like any other relationship, and they may be highly sensitive to perceived differences in power and status in the treatment relationship, including the perception that the therapist is somehow abusing their power or looking down upon the patient and disrespecting them as a person (Weinberg & Ronningstam, 2020, p. 130).

In some cases, the grandiose narcissistic patient may try to turn the therapy into an abstract discussion or debate between equals about the therapist's treatment theory and method or attempt to switch the roles in the therapeutic relationship by shifting the focus to the therapist and beginning to deliver therapeutic interventions of a sort – all in an attempt to avoid being put into a subordinate and less powerful position in relation to the therapist (Abraham, 1919/1999, p. 256 ff.). The therapist needs to be prepared for and able to handle this. It may be viewed as aspects of the patient's pathological narcissism, which may occasionally have a rather prominent place in the transference. This further underscores the importance of explicitly defining and explaining the patient's and the therapist's respective roles and tasks in the therapeutic space from the outset, even if the patient is not initially quite ready to accept the therapist's definition of the therapeutic space and the boundaries defined by the therapist. Clarifying the framework of the treatment also involves making it clear from the outset that psychotherapeutic treatment is not a pain-free quick fix but a process that takes time – months or, in many cases more realistically, years – and hard work from the patient as well as emotional and contact with painful feelings and aspects of themself and their history.

The narcissistic patient's sense of entitlement may also manifest itself in the patient acting out a strong urge to challenge or even violate the therapeutic framework and the therapist's professional and personal boundaries. When this happens, the therapist should bear in mind that the patient's violations of the therapeutic framework may be driven by many other motives and psychological processes besides reluctance to submit to the therapist's authority and agenda. It could spring, for example, from a yearning for close contact with the therapist as a self-object or a poor sense of interpersonal boundaries due to a lack of boundaries in the patient's childhood family or general relational history.

The patient's reluctant acknowledgement of their need for help

Reaching agreement about treatment goals requires that the patient, to some extent, acknowledges that they have a problem that is not just about how others disparage and fail to appreciate the self but that the self also has a share in what brought the patient into treatment, and that the patient is ready to share this with the therapist. However, it is far from given that the narcissistically disordered patient is ready to acknowledge that they actually have relatively serious problems, need help and therefore need to share their difficulties with the therapist. In some cases, the patient may initially present a few relative trivial problems that are not fully in accordance with the therapist's assessment and with any information the therapist has from other sources. The patient may tend to focus primarily on and talk about more grandiose elements and self-perceptions, while parts of the self that are associated with shame, psychological pain, inferiority and feelings of inadequacy are not revealed and are certainly not included in the patient's initially presented stories about themself (Choi-Kain et al., 2022, p. 41) or are only briefly mentioned and massively minimized.

This may reflect an attempt to avoid any loss of face and maintaining strict control with what the therapist needs to know. The patient may compartmentalize, dose which experiences and information are shared with the therapist and have their own agendas in and for the treatment, which are not necessarily shared with the therapist (Ronningstam & Weinberg, 2023, p. 341). In this way, the patient tries to maintain control and keep the upper hand in relation to the therapist and the therapeutic space and avoid the exposure of shameful aspects of the self and the revelation of self as defective, inferior and abnormal in the eyes of the therapist. To some extent, the patient also avoids coming into contact with and confronting their difficulties and painful aspects of themself and their history. In these situations, it may be helpful explicitly to articulate and validate the patient's need for control and, over time, to explore what this strong urge for control springs from and why it is so important for the patient to keep the therapist at a distance. In any case, it is important for the therapist to remain mindful of how a potential wall of grandiosity and arrogance – also in the meeting with the therapist – should be regarded as a mask that helps the patient defend against and cover up narcissistic vulnerability, shame, insecurity and susceptibility to injury (Walter & Bilke-Hentsch, 2020, p. 137).

For example, the patient may begin by briefly outlining some rather diffuse and abstract problems or problems that fairly quickly – in the patient's presentation of reality – are defined as 'somebody else's problems': problems caused by others for which the patient bears no responsibility. For example, the patient may be deeply lonely and yearn for contact with others but initially presents this as a problem based on others being self-centred and failing to acknowledge the self's many qualities, essentially because they are jealous. Or the patient may be a young man who withdraws from contact with others because he is worried that others might discover how boring, defective and inadequate he really is and then abandon him – but he describes the issue as having to do with others withdrawing from him and saying immature and ridiculous things about him behind his back. Thus, miraculously, the presentation becomes part of his attempt to convince himself that these people are in fact inferior, not worth bothering with and insignificant to him – even though he in fact yearns for contact with them and longs to be part of their group.

Focusing on the patient's perceived problems – and realistic goals

In defining the initial treatment goals, it is important to base the discussion on the problems presented by the patient, including using the words that the patient uses to describe their difficulties: 'You have told me that you are often "on autopilot" when you are with other people – I wonder if you have the same feeling right now?' 'Do you think there could be a connection between this feeling of being on autopilot when you're with other people and your feelings of loneliness?' It will also be helpful for the therapist to refer to what the patient said in order to build a 'we-feeling' and a common understanding of what 'we' are talking about and what 'we' are going to work on together (Levy, 2012, p. 896). Initially, the therapist should avoid challenging the patient's own descriptions of their difficulties and instead invite the patient to describe them in more detail and to explain more specifically when and where they appear. One example would the patient who describes that she struggles to be herself and to be fully present around others, which contributes to a vague feeling of emptiness, meaninglessness and loneliness (Caligor et al., 2015, p. 420). Or the patient who describes having difficulty controlling his temper, anger and resentment in recurring conflicts with others; perhaps he may have begun to wonder why he keeps ending up in conflicts, and he may have briefly entertained the notion that it could be related to something in himself, rather than everyone else being self-centred jerks, as he has been convinced for many years.

Another example would be the patient who describes how her self-esteem can vary wildly and occasionally drops so low that she is ready to do anything to escape a feeling of being wrong and defective. She finds it very difficult to share this feeling with anyone, for fear that they will look down on her and find her 'weird'. Generally, the therapist should not just listen to the patient's generalizing and non-specific descriptions of themself and their relational difficulties but should continue to ask for specific examples, events and experiences in which the phenomena that the patient describes in general terms manifest themselves more specifically. Gradually, this may be supplemented with efforts to explore these specific situations, together with the patient, in order to paint a more nuanced image of the patient's challenges: what did the patient and others say and do; specifically, how did the patient perceive that in the specific situation, and what thoughts and feelings is this likely to have caused in the patient and in the others involved in the situation (Dimaggio & Attina, 2012, p. 925)?

As a main rule, the therapist should always seek to formulate one or more explicit, realistic and specific treatment goals that are clearly and meaningfully related to what the patient wishes to change (Weinberg & Ronningstam, 2020, p. 125). This is important for the patient's treatment motivation and helps reduce (the often considerable) risk of dropout, and it should be addressed in connection with the diagnostic assessment or, at the latest, during the initial therapeutic sessions. An active involvement in articulating the specific treatment goals also helps strengthen the patient's experience of agency and control in the therapeutic space and keeps the fear of dependence, submission and humiliation at bay (Diamond et al., 2022, p. 151).

Gradual development of trust and establishment of contact

The final and most important element of the treatment alliance, establishing a relationship based on mutual trust, is closely associated with enabling the patient to dare to be open to emotional and psychological contact with the therapist – a big step for a narcissistically vulnerable patient that may be associated with considerable insecurity and fear of repeating past negative experiences from contact with others. Pathological narcissism is accompanied by often severe deficiencies in basic trust of other people and in the ability to feel secure in contact with others, typically rooted in severe deficiencies in the early self-object relations (Altmeyer, 2023, p. 78). The patient's reluctance to establish close emotional contact with the therapist stems from their need to protect the vulnerable self from renewed disappointment over self-objects' (in this case the therapist's) betrayal, inaccessibility and inability to contain the self and offer empathic mirroring (Kohut, 1977, p. 151). Thus, developing this aspect of the treatment alliance takes time and requires patience from the therapist. Over and over again, the patient will need to experience that their fear of being humiliated, ridiculed and misunderstood by the therapist – as they have been in previous relationships – is not going to be realized in the therapeutic space.

In a sense, during much of the initial stage of the treatment, patients can be said to test, over and over again, whether they can in fact trust the therapist by checking how the therapist reacts when they act in certain ways, describe certain events in their life or open up to emotional contact with the therapist: if I tell the therapist a little more about how my parents never really took an interest in me, how will you react? If I open the door ever so slightly to my sexual difficulties, are you going to humiliate me and ridicule my masculinity, or will you be able to understand how painful this is to me? If I tell you how hard it is for me to sense how others are doing, and how I use and exploit my husband without giving him anything in return, will you think that I'm a terrible person and walk out on me, or will you help me understand why I am – or feel that I am – like that? When I briefly hint at having been subjected to sexual abuse, are you going to notice, or will you ignore it, the way my mother did – and if you notice, will you see me as a damaged, filthy, repulsive non-human, as I see myself, and abandon me?

Initiating psychotherapeutic treatment can in itself activate the patient's urge to protect their threatened and vulnerable self by keeping the therapist at a distance, not allowing the therapist and the therapy to have any impact and hiding behind a facade of arrogance, feigned indifference and lack of engagement in the treatment. If the therapist and the therapy begin to make a real difference, the patient might become dependent on the therapist and thus on something outside the self's control. This will be a huge challenge to the narcissistic patient, who is convinced of the need to remain self-reliant and to avoid becoming dependent on anyone, because past experience tells them that they can trust no one but themself. Furthermore, grandiose self-perceptions and perfectionist ego ideals – as a defence against shameful feelings of inferiority and inadequacy – can complicate the development of a therapeutic alliance and the treatment in general, as they will typically make the patient reluctant to open up to the therapist (Fjermestad-Noll et al., 2020b, p. 24).

After some time, it may sometimes be helpful to articulate and focus joint attention on how the patient's attitude and behaviour in the treatment relationship seem to keep the therapist at a distance and prevent the therapist and the therapy from becoming important to them (Wein-Weinberg & Ronningstam, 2020, p. 131); cf. in particular the anxious avoidant and dismissive attachment style (see Chapter 3.2). The therapist should always do this with clearly conveyed respect and understanding for the patient's need to do this but may gradually engage in joint reflection on how the patient's need to keep the therapist at a distance might relate to their need to remain independent of others (cf. fear of dependence), maintaining control in contact with others (cf. fear of any loss of control and of exposing shameful aspects of the self) and defend their honour and dignity (cf. fear of coming into contact with disclosure of 'forbidden' feelings, such as sadness/crying, vulnerability, inferiority and feelings of inadequacy). To the best of their ability, the therapist should do so based on a fundamental understanding of how the patient's avoidant and dismissive behaviour in the therapeutic space reflects their survival strategy, which was developed for a (potentially understandable) reason, rather than manifesting some sort of (potentially narcissistically injurious) personal rejection of the therapist (Weinberg & Ronningstam, 2020, p. 131).

The therapist as a participating observer

The dynamic relational therapist's position in the psychotherapeutic space is perhaps best described as that of a participating observer. The therapist should strive to be fully present as a person and a subject in the contact with the patient and in the interpersonal – verbal and nonverbal – interaction in the therapeutic space. They should also persistently invite to and attempt to establish emotional and psychological contact with the patient that is attuned to what the patient is able to contain and handle without becoming emotionally overwhelmed. Thus, one key element in the meeting with the patient is to be present, be involved as a person – with the full spectrum of one's psychological and emotional resources – and to engage in the interaction with the patient in the therapeutic space. The patient is perceived as an equal in an intersubjective meeting, and while the patient's diagnosis, such as pathological narcissism, may suggest that certain ways of meeting and understanding the patient are better and more helpful than others, it only offers partial insight into who the patient is as a person, what this particular person is struggling with in their life and how this can be expected to influence and play out in the patient's meeting with the therapist. This stands in contrast to the neutral and emotionally distanced technician who – somewhat simplistically put – primarily meets the patient as a diagnosis to be cured through the application of a standardized method.

The other core aspect of the dynamic relational therapist's meeting with the patient is for the therapist to regularly take a step away from their interaction with the patient in the therapeutic space and, as much as possible, observe and reflect on it from an outside perspective. The therapist is emotionally alive, present and accessible in the interaction with the patient while simultaneously detaching themself from the interaction (Steiner, 2020, p. 14) and reflecting on it, with a fundamentally psychotherapeutic stance (Jørgensen, 2019). A task that is sometimes described as the therapist's role-responsiveness, meaning that the therapist accepts and leaves themself open to the role they are assigned by the patient – while preserving their ability to register and reflect on the interior experiences, reaction inclinations and emotional reactions that this leads to (Diamond et al., 2022, p. 153). To do this, the therapist needs to be sufficiently good – there is no such thing as the perfect therapist, and to some extent anyone will be able to do this – at simultaneously containing, registering and having nuanced dynamic psychological thoughts about what is happening right now in the patient, in the therapist and in the interaction with the patient. The psychotherapeutic stance and the psychotherapeutic gaze not only include the patient but also the therapist and their involvement in the interaction with the patient (Jørgensen, 2018/2019).

Listening with genuine interest, empathic mirroring and verbalizing

Patients with pathological narcissism will often tend to deny parts of reality that challenge, in particular, their grandiose self-perception and perceptions of the self as exceptional (Caligor & Stern, 2020, p. 107). Their primary wish is for the therapist to confirm their existing thoughts and perceptions (Kernberg, 2018, p. 166), and they may be provoked and feel threatened when the therapist, through their interventions, present and represent a different perspective on reality. The patient may feel abandoned, rejected, threatened or invaded by a sadistic object (Kernberg, 2014, p. 876). This group of patients often have limited and generally quite poor experiences with close interpersonal contact. Hence, establishment of contact in the therapeutic space should happen at a pace and in way that the patient is able to handle without needing to withdraw and seek refuge in their psychic retreat.

As a result, during much of the initial stage (months) of the treatment, the therapist may need to focus mainly on listening, asking about and empathically mirroring what the patient is telling and revealing during the therapy hour. Interventions that challenge the patient's established perceptions of reality and their defence strategies should mostly wait until a later stage. This depends to a high degree on the level of the patient's personality organization. Since patients with severe pathological narcissism typically have a relatively low level of borderline personality organization, they should initially be met primarily by an empathically mirroring and understanding therapeutic stance, although there may be a need to clearly mark the therapeutic boundaries. Better organized patients, on the other hand, will be able to handle more confrontational interventions at a much earlier stage of treatment. In any case, the therapist should continually verbalize selected elements of their observations and reactions to what the patient says and does in the therapeutic space – not as objective facts but as something that the patient can use as they like (cf. Hirsch, 1993, p. 315).

Particularly during the early stages of treatment, it may be helpful if the therapist focuses on conveying their genuine curiosity and interest in the patient's subjective experiences, perspective on reality and inner life through follow-up questions about what the patient has shared. Furthermore, the therapist may continually explicitly convey their attention to and interest in any recurring patterns in the patient's experiences, feelings and behaviour. The therapist should also continually validate the patient's experiences as meaningful and comprehensible (Weinberg & Ronningstam, 2020, p. 128; Choi-Kain et al., 2022, p. 39). In some cases, the patient's verbal communication will have a primarily performative function, in the sense that the patient primarily uses it to mark their grandiose self and their definition of reality to the therapist and to control and keep the therapist at a distance. Rather than challenging the validity and relevance of what the patient says, the therapist should initially show great interest in hearing more about what the patient is saying and showing. Both implicitly and explicitly, the therapist should let the patient know that their experiences are important and interesting – and more significant than the therapist's.

In the mentalization-based treatment tradition, this would be described as the therapist adopting a not-knowing stance, inviting the patient to engage in a curious exploration of their own self and their own subjective experiences and reactions, as the therapist continually validates the patient's subjective experiences as understandable and true to the patient (Bolm, 2021, p. 663). This approach helps to foster an equal relationship and minimize – but in no way eliminate – the risk that the patient might feel injured, threatened or humiliated by the therapist.

Relational constellations in the therapeutic space

The therapist should always consider what position the patient feels placed in – in the treatment relationship – and how this might bring up elements of repeating unbearable past experiences and relational constellations. For some people it may, for example, be unbearable to be put into a situation where they feel at risk, helpless, exposed and confronted with their great need for others, because they associate this with past experiences, when no one noticed or reacted to this. No one noticed the self's need for help and provided support, or perhaps the self's need for help was met with scorn, contempt or indifference. Over and over, they felt insignificant, abandoned and left in situations that they perceived as unbearable – and thus, they need someone else (the therapist) who is emotionally accessible and who sees and understands the self emotionally and psychologically (Steiner, 2014, p. 12), when inviting a joint examination of the patient's experiences and reactions is not in itself sufficient.

Showing oneself to be vulnerable and in need of help from the other can be associated with profound anxiety and insecurity. Being the one to receive something from another – something that one needs and may risk becoming dependent on – may produce a feeling of inferiority and of being in a humiliating situation, given the person's embarrassment and shame over their own needs and dependence. Some patients will attempt to escape this dreaded position by assuming a position of authority, agency and helping others, thus having the experience that others need the self.

Need for control and for being the one who can help others

One patient with severe narcissistic difficulties has a history of feeling abandoned and left in severely insecure and at times life-threatening situations, with no hope of anyone coming to her aid, and feeling severely exposed and helpless. The lesson she has taken from this is that she has to fend for herself. Being someone who helps others gives her a sense of security, control and perhaps superiority in relation to others. It lets her feel strong, powerful and that she is seen as 'someone who can get things done'. Simply being in contact with the therapist, which inevitably requires her to abandon her position as the one who helps others and accept help herself, is associated with intense anxiety and insecurity for her, given that the survival strategy she has developed is suspended, to some degree. Furthermore, it brings her into contact with unbearable helplessness, exposure and abandonment as well as the fear that no one will notice it and respond to her need for help. The situation is also associated with a certain ambivalence and urge to submit to – as well as daring to hope and trust in – the therapist. This all seems to spring from the experience of witnessing her father's recurring intense and at time life-threatening abuse of her mother, as part of the patient from a masochist position has identified with the mother as a victim to the father's severely dominant behaviour and injuries. Overall, the patient has significant challenges striking a suitable balance between dominance and submission, and in practice she is unable to engage in equal relationships.

Hiding vulnerability behind a grandiose facade

Another patient associates being in the therapeutic space with feeling very small, immature, weak, chaotic and confused and losing control. Whenever she finds herself in this position, it actualizes related experiences from earlier times, when she was in a vulnerable and exposed position and was overwhelmed by similarly unbearable feelings – and no one was present who could help her contain, understand and regulate these feelings. Her parents were typically physically and/or mentally absent (drunk). In her experience, no one is capable of containing and handling her when she is not hiding behind a grandiose facade and appearing strong and decisive. She does not dare to reveal these 'weak' aspects of herself in the therapeutic space, out of fear that the therapist will not be able to contain her and come to her rescue. When she was a little girl, her parents did not come to her aid but left her home alone or in various bars until late at night.

Appearance dominated by anger, outrage and resentment

During the initial stage of the treatment, some patients may have a strong urge and need to hold onto their existing grandiose self-image and perspective on reality. However, the therapist may also meet patients who are inclined to speak about and show their anger (narcissistic rage), outrage and resentment over others' behaviour and their perception of feeling poorly and justly treated by an evil and uncaring world and of not receiving the attention, respect and recognition they feel that they deserve. Initially, the therapist may – also explicitly – notice and accept this while explicitly asking whether the patient also experiences other feelings or mental states in connection with the events and interpersonal interactions that cause the expressed outrage and rage. Alternatively, the therapist may articulate what feelings and mental states the therapist comes into contact with when the patient describes their specific experiences: 'If I had been in your situation, I think I would have felt hurt and saddened to be treated like that' (Drozek & Unruh, 2020, p. 188). In some cases, this may serve as an opening to exploring subjective experiences, feelings and mental states that are notably absent from the patient's descriptions, including shame, sadness, insecurity and dependence. In addition, the therapist may – initially internally, without communicating this to the patient – consider what might be behind the patient's great need to fill the therapeutic space with resentment over others (Gabbard & Crisp, 2018, p. 68), why this appears to be necessary and what function it may serve in the patient's psyche.

Remarkable absence of anger and pride

Conversely, with predominantly vulnerable narcissism, it may be anger as well as pride in the patient's own actual qualities and accomplishments that seem strikingly absent from the patient's descriptions and which it may be helpful to direct the joint attention at. In some cases, the therapist may begin by noting the patient's qualities and perhaps describe how the therapist would have been angry if they had been treated as the patient describes it. In any case, this should continually be accompanied by a joint focus on why these feelings might be absent from the patient's subjective experiences and descriptions, given that the patient, for various reasons, may have difficulty containing and dealing with vulnerability and pride.

As described in particular in connection with mentalization-based therapy (Drozek & Unruh, 2020, p. 189; Drozek et al., 2023, p. 308 ff.), patients with a predominantly grandiose manifestations in particular may be very focused on themselves while showing limited interest in others. They may also be excessively focused on purely cognitive and very concrete external (behavioural) aspects of situations. Moreover, they seem to ignore or have much greater difficulty seeing and understanding more emotional and internal psychological aspects of interpersonal interactions. In extension of this, they may appear excessively convinced of the truth and significance of their own subjective experiences and their own perspective on reality – their authoritative version of reality and the truth – while others' experiences and perceptions of reality are ignored or disparaged as inferior or silly. This is all part of the patient's grandiose defence against doubt, vulnerability and fragile self-esteem, which the patient associates with unacceptable weakness and a grave risk of being injured, dominated and exploited by others. This may be viewed as a sign of imbalance and inflexibility in the patient's perception of reality. One way of addressing it may be what is known in the MBT tradition as 'contrary moves' (Drozek & Unruh, 2020, p. 189 ff.): an approach to the patient's material that develops their ability to perceive interpersonal interactions in a more nuanced manner, less shaped by rigid, narrowly focused and universal perceptions of other people and reality in general.

After the therapist has empathically validated and heard the patient's perspective on and subjective perception of interactions with others, which the patient will often describe in very general terms, the therapist invites the patient to briefly change focus and play with other possible aspects of a specific interpersonal interaction that the patient brought up. The therapist invites the patient to shift away from the very general, cognitive and behavioural focus to examining specific elements of the interpersonal interaction. In this exchange, the therapist also directs the dyad's joint attention at the specific situation, emotional aspects and possible internal psychological processes of the involved in individuals, initially primarily in the patient. In the long term, the therapist may supplement this with an invitation to reflect on how others might have perceived the specific situation and aspects of the specific interpersonal interaction, perhaps beginning by describing how the therapist might have perceived the situation if they had been one of the people involved in the described interaction.

Avoiding power struggles in the therapeutic relationship

As much as possible, the therapist should avoid getting involved and caught up in power struggles with the patient, including struggles about social status or dominance/submission in the therapeutic space, for example, by marking their control over the therapeutic space by being dominant and implicitly placing the patient in a subordinate position, which will typically be shameful and unbearable for the patient (Dimaggio, 2022, p. 415). The therapist should also strive to avoid adopting a normative and judgemental stance in relation to the patient (Caligor et al., 2015, p. 420). On the other hand, there are of course limits to the ways and extent to which the therapist will let the patient attack, disparage and injure them without explicitly commenting on and reacting to it. It will always be a matter of striking the best possible balance between, on the one hand, not being too touchy and maintaining one's ability to see the patient's fierce attacks as manifestations of their pathology and attempts to protect their vulnerable self and, on the other hand, responding to the patient's attacks with tact by clearly marking one's boundaries without counterattacking. Here, the therapist should bear in mind that simply ignoring or tacitly accepting intense injuries from the patient could be seen by the patient as confirmation that attacking and disparaging others is okay. This would send the implicit message that it is okay or, at least, acceptable that significant others perhaps injured or humiliated the patient in the past (Dimaggio, 2022, p. 415).

Triangulating interactions in the therapeutic space

One key therapeutic skill for handling the position of participating observer is the ability to triangulate. Simply put, this refers to the therapist's ability to take a step away from an interaction between two individuals, entities or factors – for example in a dyadic relationship, such as the interaction between patient and therapist – and observe, reflect on and understand it from an external, third perspective, based on psychotherapeutic theory and method (Grieser, 2015, p. 106). Similarly, the therapist may take a step away from and triangulate the interaction between the patient's verbally communicated material – what the patient says – and themself and their own immediate reactions to the material, again with support from their acquired theory, method and therapeutic experience.

In triangulating the dyadic interaction between the actions of patient and therapist in the therapeutic space here and now, the therapist uses this interaction as input for understanding the emotional and relational core of the patient's difficulties, as they are actualized and played out in the therapeutic space in the here and now. The narcissistically vulnerable patient who is trying to survive by forming a close attachment to an idealized other by keeping others at a distance, emotionally speaking, will display this behaviour in relation to the therapist. A patient dominated by grandiose narcissism who tries to protect their fragile self by hiding it behind a grandiose facade and keeping others at a distance by means of cold arrogance and clear contempt for others will do the same in the interaction with the therapist. On the one hand, this may of course complicate the establishment of a treatment alliance and the treatment relationship in general. On the other hand, it also offers an invaluable opportunity for the therapist to discover the patient's core difficulties and understand the dynamic psychological background of them in cooperation with the patient.

Triangulating what is playing out in the treatment relationship and in the therapeutic space in general can also help the therapist deal with emotionally challenging situations – again by taking a step away from what may feel emotionally overwhelming and perhaps stuck right now – and reflect on how this may be understood from an external perspective and in relation to the patient's pathology and their own personal limitations in their role as therapist. If the therapist finds a situation exceptionally difficult to handle and struggles to achieve enough emotional distance to have sufficiently clear and nuanced thoughts about it and understand what is going on, professional supervision may be helpful. For example, the therapist may feel shut out, isolated, lonely and professionally inadequate when working with a predominantly grandiose narcissistic patient who consistently meets the therapist with cold arrogance, indifference and intense devaluation as well as toxic verbal attacks on their person and professional competence. This may activate the therapist's own narcissism: narcissistic vulnerability and the need, for example, for a minimum of emotional contact and respect in the therapeutic space.

The therapist's ability to 'breathe' and reflect

To preserve the ability to breathe and have nuanced thoughts about what is going on in the patient's inner life and in the therapeutic relationship – which is the primary therapeutic task – it is important for the therapist, regularly throughout the process, to take a step away from this persistent and intense bombardment from the patient and reflect on how this may contain significant repetition of elements from the patient's relational life. This involves reflecting on how this illustrates what this particular individual does in their attempt to keep themself together, protect their fragile self and stabilize their self-esteem, which there is reason to think might collapse or prove severely dysregulated if the patient's current defence falls apart. The therapist tries to triangulate the destructive elements of the interaction with the patient and wonders: 'What is going on between us right now, and how does this repeat patterns from the patient's (and perhaps my own) life?'

Similarly, it may be important for the therapist to step away from and triangulate their interaction with a narcissistically very vulnerable patient with an obvious and very strong need for intimacy and continuous access to the therapist as the good self-object that the patient has been missing and yearning for all their life. It can be emotionally demanding, in many regards, as well as professionally challenging and interesting, to work with such a patient, who may initially signal that their main need – and preference – is to have the therapist in their life in other ways than as a therapist. The patient may signal that they need emotional intimacy and love more than they need invitations to examine and understand themself, based on what is happening in the relationship with the therapist and how it might contain significant information about what is the core of the patient's difficulties: the patient would rather be met and validated in their feelings for the therapist than examine these feelings.

The therapist may be deeply emotionally affected by this potentially very intense contact with a patient, which may in itself challenge the therapist's ability to have clear and nuanced thoughts. However, it is important to use what is playing out in this contact with the patient as a basis for understanding the patient and thus helping the patient better understand themself – and, not least, prevent destructive patterns from the patient's relational history from repeating themselves in the treatment relationship. What patterns from the patient's life are about to repeat themselves in the current therapeutic relationship? Or does this represent a new development, something that the patient has never previously experienced and therefore simply wants much more of? What sort of yearnings and needs does the patient come into contact with in the relationship with the therapist, and how does the patient try to handle these needs? Are they acted out, or does the patient attempt to shut them down – and if so, how should we understand that? Why does the patient try to shut them down? Is it because it is too shameful or 'forbidden' to have these yearnings and needs? And if so, how should we understand this experience in light of the patient's relational history?

The patient's ability to tolerate triangulation

The patient's ability to tolerate and deal with the therapist's articulation of the effort of triangulating what is playing out in the therapeutic space may contain information about the patient's level of personality organization. Triangulating the patient's relationship with the therapist, who has become the narcissistic self's perhaps most important self-object, may be perceived as an existential threat to the emotional resonance from the therapist that the patient so badly needs (Bolm, 2021, p. 662). Particularly in case of lower levels of organization, the patient will be more inclined to perceive the therapist's interventions as a deliberate challenge, provocation and threat to the patient's grandiose self-image or to feel betrayed, abandoned and left behind by the therapist when the therapist does not respond with sufficiently nurturing and loving empathic mirroring to the patient's self-object need in the real relationship. In this situation, anything coming from the therapist that is not in accordance with the patient's thoughts, convictions and perspective on reality – which implicitly also marks the therapist's separation from the self – may destabilize the patient's self (Kernberg, 2018, p. 166).

This also applies to interventions in which the therapist points to apparently contradictory elements of the patient's perceptions of self and others. This is an unavoidable part of the therapeutic work, but of course it may be described and communicated in different ways that seem more or less acceptable to the narcissistically vulnerable patient. For example, it will often be helpful to describe this as 'wondering' or to explain that there is something one 'needs some help understanding'. This directs the focus to the therapist, their inability to understand something and their need for the patient's help to understand, rather than directing the focus to the patient. For example, one patient may say that he does not care what various pathetic idiots might think about him while simultaneously seeming to react strongly to criticism, rejection and lack of explicit admiration from others. Another patient may seemingly avoid social events and intimate contact with others (in order to protect 'secret' perceptions of their own exceptional character and reduce their fear of shameful exposure and rejection) while simultaneously having a great need for others to see and confirm his accomplishments and what he stands for (Diamond et al., 2022, p. 152):

> I have been wondering about something that I don't quite understand – you're telling me that you don't really care what others think of you, but at the same time you're also saying that you find it exhausting to be around other people because it takes so much energy to figure out what others think about you. Maybe I'm just not really getting it, but perhaps you could explain how you see this?

Based on classic psychoanalytic theory, it could be argued that patients with severe pathological narcissism who struggle to deal with the therapist's triangulating interventions have relational challenges dating back to before the resolution of the oedipal conflict. This conflict revolves around the child's ability to deal with not being in an exclusive dyadic relationship, as dad, to put it in simplistic terms, intervenes in the mother–infant relationship and sets boundaries for this relationship. The child then has to deal with being on the outside, observing a dyadic relationship between two others that does not include the child, the relationship between mum and dad. A patient who cannot deal with the triangulation of relationships finds it difficult to be in a mature dyadic relationship, in which the self is separated from the other and is thus at risk leading a life without intimate contact with others, like Narcissus. Furthermore, pre-oedipal difficulties will often be rooted in unarticulated deficiencies in relationships (as opposed to conflicts that have been articulated), and they will therefore primarily play out in the nonverbal contact with the therapist – in unsymbolized, unarticulated aspects of transference and countertransference – which is also where it should primarily be addressed, particularly during the early stages of the treatment (Balint, 1968, p. 28 ff.).

Verbal language as a tool for evoking reactions in the therapist

In persons with pathological narcissism rooted in pre-oedipal deficits in personality organization, the verbal language may periodically take on a different function. The locutionary function of language – making an utterance with a particular meaning or reference via the concrete content of the verbal communication – is overlaid or superseded by a perlocutionary function, in which the primary intention of the verbal communication is to evoke a certain reaction in the interlocutor. In this case, verbal language mainly functions, or is used, in a performative manner. It is used as tool for affecting or evoking something in others – 'I am saying something in order to affect you or cause you to react in a certain way', 'I perceive what you're saying as an indication that you want to affect me or evoke a particular reaction in me' – rather than in a classic communicative sense, in which the verbal language is used to communicate explicitly stated content. Similarly, in some cases, the patient may appreciate the therapist's verbal communication more for its tone and the therapist's voice – which may calm the patient down and make them feel secure or, conversely, make the patient nervous and scared – more than for its semantic content (Britton, 1998, p. 50). For example, one patient explains how she sometimes listens to audio recordings of the therapist's voice when she feels nervous and scared and needs to calm herself down. What helps her in this situation is primarily the sound of the therapist's voice, not the specific content of what the therapist is actually saying in these recordings.

Specifically, this means that the therapist's triangulating interventions may be perceived as intentional rejection or threats to the self, not as attempts to understand what is actualized and going on in the therapeutic relationship. These challenges are associated with what Balint (1968, p. 87 ff.) calls the area of the basic fault, in which 'at any frustration these patients feel that it was intentionally inflicted' (p. 19), and the patient's nonverbal communication and nonverbal treatment factors of the therapist's work come into focus. Furthermore, both the patient and the therapist may feel that the therapeutic method – the process of working in the therapeutic space – is a threat to the fragile self and that the patient solely needs an infinitely empathic and passively understanding therapist, rather than a therapist who 'aggressively' insists on making meaning or imposing meaning on the patient (Britton, 1998, p. 49). This point will not be discussed further in the present context, but see the section on withdrawal to a psychic retreat above and Chapter 3.6 as well as Jørgensen (2019).

The therapist's failure to meet the patient's strong need for a self-object may weaken the self's internal coherence. This questions the classic notion of the neutral, emotionally reserved and periodically nearly silent therapist (Wolf, 1996, p. 109). Patients with a poor personality organization need a more visible and emotionally responsive therapist. Thus, when the patient's self-object needs are actualized in the transference, the therapist has to consider whether to respond by articulating and meeting these needs or whether to primarily invite the patient to engage in joint reflection – in part via triangulation – on what is happening right now in the therapeutic relationship and how it might shed light on the patient's relational difficulties and history. When working with better organized and predominantly grandiose patients, it may be more helpful to meet the patient's need for a self-object that is willing to be idealized while also, from a relatively early stage, drawing attention to the destructive consequences of the patient's grandiose self-perceptions and their behaviour in interpersonal relationships. This includes manifestations in the therapeutic space; cf. the earlier discussion of the relationship between Kohut's and Kernberg's approaches to pathological narcissism and how they are primarily helpful in relation to narcissistic patients with slightly different symptom pictures (see Chapter 3.5).

The therapist as a representative of 'reality'

On the other hand, if there is a collapse of the therapist's ability to take a step away, triangulate and reflect on what is playing out in the therapeutic space and how it relates to the patient's difficulties, the psychotherapeutic space itself will collapse. When this happens, the patient and the therapist will no longer be able to use what plays out between them to engage in a joint effort to understand the patient's difficulties and catalyse the psychological development in the patient that is the underlying rationale of psychotherapy. There will also be a risk that the therapeutic relationship stops being an intersubjective relationship and instead becomes either a 'non-relationship', with a poor separation between patient and therapist, or a relationship in which at least one party sees and uses the other as a soulless object for satisfying their own needs (Crisp & Gabbard, 2020, p. 152). The latter outcome is most apparent in the highly grandiose patient's use of the therapist as an audience for their own stories, while the therapist is not perceived, respected, acknowledged or treated as an independent subject. In this case, the therapeutic relationship is no longer characterized by emotional contact and mutual respect but is dominated by destructive complementarity, as one person affects the other, while this other has been reduced to an object that is being affected and has difficulty achieving enough distance to this situation to be able to have nuanced thoughts about and be less emotionally overwhelmed by what is happening in the relationship (p. 152).

The therapeutic relationship is always intersubjective. Thus, the therapist always already has a share in what is going out in the relationship and what perceptions the patient develops about the therapist and the therapy over time. For example, when a narcissistically vulnerable patient develops a strong need for the therapist to be available as a loving, admiring and empathically mirroring self-object, this also relates to how the therapist has been present and acted in the contact with the patient from the outset. Specifically, it points to how the therapist must always strive to strike the best possible balance between, on the one hand, being authentically emotionally present in the contact with the patient and meeting the patient with a loving gaze and, on the other hand, marking and defending the boundaries around the therapeutic relation and representing 'the law' (cf. Lacan): the separation of fantasy and reality in the therapeutic space. The therapist has to represent and defend the boundaries in and around the therapeutic space that, in addition to the purely ethical aspects, are an important part of the enabling the patient to triangulate: to observe and reflect on what plays out in the treatment relationship with an outside gaze. It also helps the patient to gradually let go of any fantasies that the contact with the therapist (the idealized self-object) is the only thing that could possibly fill out perceived internal defects, enable a form of permanent satisfaction of lifelong yearnings and thus cure the patient.

The therapist must be able to contain and, to varying degrees, meet the patient's self-object needs when these are actualized in the transference. However, it is also a part of the therapist's job to frustrate the patient's needs for and fantasies about the boundlessly satisfying self-object in a way that is as well attuned as possible to what the patient is able to handle at a given time; cf. Kohut's (1971, p. 50) concept of optimal frustration: bearable disappointments of self-object needs that promote the development of an internal personality structure. The specific implication of this can vary a great deal over time and, not least, across patients. The best achievable frustration of the patient is necessary for strengthening the patient's ability to distinguish between fantasy and reality – through the therapist's empathic but also firm and non-negotiable marking and defence of the boundaries around the treatment – and, over time, enable the patient to take care of themself and thus make the patient less dependent on continuous access to concrete others who can meet the patient's self-object needs (Karterud, 1995, p. 72 ff.). Conversely, the therapist who is excessively nurturing and who satisfies the patient's archaic self-object needs far beyond the parameters of the therapeutic setting – trying to be the perfect parent, 'partner' or friend and protector that the patient never had and may long for – may unconsciously strengthen the patient's unrealistic hope of being unconditionally and boundlessly loved and cared for by the therapist. This can make it even harder for the patient to deal with the inevitable frustrations associated with therapeutic work (Luchner, 2013, p. 229).

This also underscores that the patient's contact with the therapist as the good self-object is not in itself sufficient in the treatment of pathological narcissism, even though it will always be an important part of the treatment, especially with patients who have a poor personality organization. Establishing, maintaining – and conducting therapeutic work in – an emotional and psychological contact that is as authentic as possible is a crucial element of dynamic relational psychotherapy. Nevertheless, the therapist must always remain so clearly separate from the patient that they can function as 'the other', representing an external – empathic, understanding but also at times confrontational and reality-correcting – gaze on the patient's self that can promote the development of the patient's ability to observe themself from a balanced external perspective (Altmeyer, 2003, p. 224).

Vulnerable patients can be exceptionally sensitive to feeling betrayed and abandoned by the therapist and be constantly mindful of even the smallest signs of this. For example, the patient may feel painfully abandoned and left behind if the therapist is a little too clear in marking the boundaries around the therapeutic relationship and the therapeutic space or the separation between their own self and the patient's self (cf. the patient's possible need to feel like or very close to the therapist). Hence, the necessary marking of these boundaries – a marking that is necessary, particularly in the long term, for developing the patient's ability to mark and contain boundaries between fantasy and reality and between self and others – should always happen gently and in ways that are as well attuned as possible to what the patient is able to contain at a given time.

When the patient clearly finds that the therapist fails as a self-object – which will inevitably happen over and over again and in no way only when the therapist marks the boundaries around the treatment relationship and the therapeutic space – it may be important to address this explicitly. For one reason, it may be a condition for restoring the patient's trust in the therapist and in the patient's own self-object transference (see Chapter 4.2), particularly in case of severe perceived self-object failures. For another, it has an important therapeutic effect when the patient experiences that perceived relational ruptures can be healed and, not least, that the patient's experience of being let down and hurt is noticed and taken seriously. When the therapist explicit recognizes and regrets that their empathy and ability to serve as a self-object for the patient failed, that in itself contains important elements of validation of the patient's subjective experiences and emotional reactions. With this act, the therapist confirms that the patient in fact was let down and 'wronged' and that this was in no way the therapist's intention (McWilliams, 1994, p. 182 ff.). This is a reaction that the patient has typically not been used to from former self-objects when they failed the patient over and over again and proved unable to meet their developmentally appropriate self-object needs.

Furthermore, the therapist demonstrates live, in the here and now, how it is possible to acknowledge mistakes and inadequacies without being overwhelmed by shame or a collapsing self-esteem – and that, in the long term, it can be narcissistically satisfying and enhance one's personal integrity to dare to face the truth about oneself and one's own mistakes (Bueckler, 2010, p. 122). This can contain important elements of corrective emotional experiences for the patient, in the sense that the patient has the experience of being seen and treated as a person who can evoke empathic reactions (empathic responsiveness) from others and as a subject – a human being – who is of significance to others. The accumulation of countless such experiences in the therapeutic space will strengthen the vulnerable self and gradually help make the grandiose defence superfluous (Wolf, 1996, p. 150).

Illustration from psychotherapeutic treatment

This will briefly be illustrated with elements from a long-term psychotherapeutic process. The patient is a young man who grew up with severe neglect and repeated abuse. He is characterized by great narcissistic vulnerability behind a facade that in many regards is very well-functioning; he is almost insistently independent and reluctant to rely on anyone else. No one has ever looked after him, so from a young age, he has had to learn how to protect himself. His life so far has been dominated by profound emotional loneliness, as he has been emotionally compelled to focus on surviving but has had no room to live. For example, at the beginning of treatment, he has never been in an intimate and trusting relationship with another person. Gradually, however, he develops greater trust in the therapist, and for the first time in his life, he has the experience of being in close emotional contact with another human being without necessarily being overwhelmed by anxiety and shame and feeling compelled to flee, either by skipping the following sessions or by withdrawing to his psychic retreat. In this retreat, he is on his own, a situation he knows only too well from his external life, but he also feels of sense of security or, at least, a form of standstill and emptiness. These feelings may be painful, but they are also familiar and, to some extent, controllable, particularly in comparison with the external reality, where he must be constantly on guard and keep others at a distance.

The therapist has apparently become his most important self-object and is becoming increasingly important to him. He has also begun to appreciate the – at times quite intense – emotional contact with the therapist. This is also a source of concern for him, because he is beginning to experience signs that he has grown dependent on this contact and, thus, on the therapist. He perceives this dependence as 'life-threatening', because it makes him particularly vulnerable to the therapist's potential failures and to eventual 'abandonment' when the therapy is terminated. As the therapist has taken on growing emotional importance, the patient has also grown increasingly sensitive and vulnerable to even minor signs that the therapist feels contempt for him, is not interested in him or might be about to leave him. Furthermore, there is a part of the patient who wishes to have a different kind of relationship with the therapist; one in which the therapist is not his therapist but is closer and accessible well beyond the therapeutic sessions. At the same time, another part of the patient fears this possibility and would be completely unable to handle it were anything close to that ever to happen in the 'real world' and not just in his inner universe and retreat. At times, the patient thus feels trapped in a painful conflict between closeness and distance in relation to the therapist, which also manifests itself in dramatic shifts in the patient's behaviour in the interaction with the therapist. He alternately seeks closer contact and withdraws from the therapist; at times he is worried that the therapist might 'disappear', followed by periods when he considers terminating the treatment in an attempt to shut down sometimes overwhelming longing for more contact and a need for or dependence on the therapist that he perceives as a threat to the self and its autonomy.

For some time, this has been a persistent underlying theme in the therapy. During the first part of a session, the therapist relatively briefly summarizes the framework of the therapeutic space and why this framework is important for the therapeutic work. The therapist also seeks to associate the therapeutic framework as an indisputable reality with the patient's yearning for a different sort of relationship with the therapist. Presumably, he has only dared to come into contact with this feeling and, to some degree, share it with the therapist, because the therapeutic framework, so to speak, protects him from making his – as he perceives it still very dangerous – yearning for closer contact with others a concrete reality. Finally, the therapist briefly outlines how the therapeutic framework can produce feelings of great ambivalence in the patient: on the one hand, it protects him from what he fears but, on the other hand, it also prevents him from attaining what he simultaneously longs for. As this is being addressed, a tear rolls down the patient's cheek, and he grows silent. He withdraws emotionally from the contact with the therapist, and eventually the verbal communication threatens to break down as well, in the sense that the patient stops responding to the therapist's invitations to contact and to share what is happening inside him, or he offers very short replies. In many ways, the patient is signalling that right now it is too hard for him to be in the therapeutic space, and most of all he wants to leave. Ultimately, he leaves a few minutes before the session is over. When he leaves the therapeutic space, he simply says, 'I'm sorry.' The patient cancels the next session and, in every way, it is clear that something happened in this session that was overwhelming and very difficult for the patient to handle. It is also clear that the therapist did not manage to grasp and address it during the session.

At the beginning of the next session, the patient is again – or still – silent and emotionally shut down in a way that is remarkably similar to how he appeared at the beginning of the therapy course, before he had developed sufficient trust in the therapist to dare to allow emotional contact with both dissociated parts of himself and his history and with the therapist. From the outset, the therapist addresses the concrete events during the previous session, including saying that he is sorry that he apparently marked the boundaries of the treatment relationship in a way that made it difficult for the patient to remain in contact with the therapist. The therapist also shares his thoughts about how the patient may have experienced this and his intentions for – perhaps unnecessarily – providing a reminder of the boundaries of the therapeutic space.

Gradually, the patient opens up to describing his experience, and it becomes clear that he felt deeply let down and abandoned by the therapist as a self-object. It becomes clear that just prior to the previous session, the patient had decided to try something new in order to engage in closer contact with the therapist. In his perception, by so explicitly marking the therapeutic boundaries, the therapist leaves him or pushes him away. He feels that the therapist is abandoning him and that the therapist implicitly signalled for him to keep his distance. For good reason, these experiences were a narcissistic injury to the patient and contain repetitions of painful patterns from the patient's relational history. These are patterns that revolve around him being too much, too demanding, and being pushed away by significant others who, for various reasons – which had much more to do with them and their personal problems than with the patient – had difficulty containing him. The patient perceived that the therapist was pushing him away, just when he had decided to opening up to closer contact. This caused him to be overwhelmed by a severely shameful feeling of, once again, being revealed as wrong, as repulsive, as someone that no one wants to have anything to do with; someone that no one could love and who has no right to love anyone else, because he is so defective and inadequate, a dirty non-human – behind his, in many ways, well-functioning but also discreet facade and impressive ability to survive neglect and abuse.

Together, patient and therapist articulate the patient's experience in the previous session and his subsequent reaction of withdrawing to a psychic retreat and feeling the urge to sedate himself. Those are both strategies for protecting the patient's vulnerable self that the patient had otherwise, to a high degree, been able to leave behind. Together, they explore how what happened in the previous session contains a repetition of patterns from the patient's life. As they do this, they re-establish their emotional contact, and the patient is again able to be emotionally present in the therapeutic space. Part of the effective therapeutic action in this brief sequence from the therapeutic process is that the patient relives a familiar interaction pattern in which he is narcissistically injured and emotionally abandoned by his self-object, while the outcome is quite different from what he has been used to. In contrast to his earlier experiences, the therapist takes his subjective perceptions and emotional reactions – including his emotional pain over feeling let down and abandoned by the therapist as a self-object – seriously.

The patient has the experience that he and his emotional reactions are in fact significant to the therapist and affect the therapist. They impact and trigger emotional reactions in the therapist – and the therapist reacts responsively and with empathy to the patient's emotional reactions and needs. Not just in his role as a therapist but also in the real relationship and in his authentic emotional reactions to what happened during the session and how the patient subsequently felt, the therapist reacts in a way that is very different from what the patient has experienced in previous relationships, where he at best felt insignificant and more often as someone who was only a burden to others, who was too demanding and who ought to focus on satisfying other people's needs. By jointly working through a situation in which the therapist acted in a way that made the patient feel let down and abandoned by the therapist – and in an atmosphere in the therapeutic space where the patient feels seen as an equal human being – they restore their emotional contact, and the patient has a corrective emotional experience: he is important, he is met with empathic mirroring and responsiveness, and his feelings and needs are taken seriously.

The therapeutic work to repair these ruptures in the self-object relationship may cause the patient to gradually give up the notion of the boundlessly empathically mirroring and ideal self-object that picks up on and meets all the self's needs – a perception that is illusory in the real world. This allows the patient to gradually develop a more realistic but also more nuanced and grounded image of the therapist that includes flaws and deficits like everyone else: a process that involves elements of mourning work in the sense that the patient gives up a fantasized object, deeply coloured by the patient's own self-object needs and projective perceptions that it was necessary for the patient to construct and hold onto in order to maintain their fragile internal narcissistic balance (Steiner, 2020, p. 10; Boyer, 2022, p. 571) but which has gradually become, if not superfluous, then much less necessary in everyday life, provided that the patient is not subjected to new severe abuse and betrayals that might cause significant but typically temporary decline in functioning capacity in anybody.

Finally, the therapist's good-enough handling of this sort of situation in the therapeutic process also involves reflecting on why they felt the urge to mark the boundaries of the therapeutic space at this particular time and in this particular way. This includes whether it might be associated with the therapist's own countertransference and reactions that are not solely related to the patient's transference and behaviour in the therapeutic space. The psychotherapeutic stance not only applies to the therapist's relationship with the patient and the interpersonal interaction in the therapeutic space but also to the therapist and their own experiences and behaviour in the therapeutic space. Was the therapist's urge to mark the boundaries of the therapy, in this particular way and at this time, driven by an internal conflict in the therapist and an urge to control parts of the therapist's self that were activated in the interaction with the patient – or was the therapist's intervention a purely professionally informed reaction to the patient's behaviour in the therapeutic space?

Might the therapist also have come into contact with their own narcissism, a desire to engage in closer contact with the patient or convert the therapeutic relationship to a different form of relationship that is in no way possible in the therapeutic space and which the therapist thus tried to keep in check, not only in the patient but also in themself by reiterating the framework of the therapeutic relationship, even if this 'clarification' of the framework of treatment could be said to be therapeutically justified? In any case, the therapist has to be ready to recognize how the material playing out in the countertransference might be located in the transitional zone between subjective and objective countertransference. On the one hand, it may contain invaluable information about the patient's inner life and conflicts – here, for example, the patient's simultaneous yearning for and fear of closer contact with another person who is significant to the self – but, on the other hand, it may also be coloured by the therapist's own needs, yearnings and defence strategies (cf. Rohde-Dachser, 2024, p. 23).

In parallel with this work in and with the countertransference, the therapist has to bear in mind that if a patient seeks some form of contact in the real relationship with the therapist that seems to be replacing or compensating for the patient's lack of contact with others outside the therapeutic space, it is the therapist's responsibility to remind the patient – in an empathic and caring but firm way – that the point of the treatment is not for the patient to live and have their needs for emotional contact met (solely) in the therapy. Instead, the goal is to enable the patient to live and establish close emotional contact with others outside the therapy (Diamond et al., 2022, p. 384). As long as the patient is dominated by intense yearning for contact with the therapist in a real relationship, this may be perceived as painful rejection. It may thus be hard for the patient to realize that this is instead a sign of respect for the patient and their desire to get to a place where he can engage in equal relationships and deep emotional contact with others in 'the real world' outside the therapeutic space – and that the therapist's actions are dictated by the therapeutic framework and their joint therapeutic task that he is responsible for.

Detoxifying the patient's destructive shame

For most people, seeking treatment, asking for help and sharing one's psychological difficulties can be associated with shame. However, this reaction may be particularly pronounced in patients with pathological narcissism who have been trying protect a vulnerable self through grandiose self-perceptions and perfectionism – survival strategies that are hard to reconcile with having to tell a therapist about psychological and relational challenges and adopt a position where the patient may perceive themself as inferior and as a fragile victim. By sharing their difficulties with a therapist, patients will inevitably come into contact with vulnerable and shameful aspects of themselves. They may be at risk of being overwhelmed by shame and feeling an urge to trivialize their difficulties, avoid opening up completely and talking about the core of their difficulties, withdraw from contact and maybe even break off the treatment after just a few sessions. Thus, right from the initial contact, it is important for the therapist to be mindful of any feelings of shame in the patient and to explore, in an empathic and non-confrontational way, how the patient feels about seeking help and talking about their difficulties.

In many ways, destructive shame is an anti-therapeutic affect. It is associated with feeling unveiled and exposed as an inadequate and bad person and may thus be a powerful opponent in the therapeutic space, where we seek to examine and explore aspects of the patient that the patient perceives as inferior, socially unacceptable and repulsive (Wurmser, 1987, p. 64; Jørgensen, 2023/2024, p. 336 ff.). Shame is associated with a powerful urge to withdraw from contact and may thus stand in the way of the emotional contact that is a crucial element in dynamic relational psychotherapy. For that reason too, it is essential for the therapist to notice and deal with the patient's destructive shame, as well as possible, when it is actualized in the therapeutic space.

The therapist contains the patient's shame

As suggested earlier, working with pathological narcissism requires the therapist to be able to contain and respect patients who contain and sometimes fairly explicitly express feelings that are 'normally' considered socially unacceptable and which may lead to profound rejection or even social expulsion of anyone who expresses them; examples include envy, contempt, narcissistic rage, grandiosity and destructive shame (Choi-Kain et al., 2022, p. 40). Initially, the therapist's primary task is to show open and curious interest in these emotions and the relational context that they arise in as well as the purpose they serve for the patient. As much as possible, the therapist should be able to contain the patient's sharing acts and aspects of themself that may seem repugnant, asocial, socially unacceptable and shameful. Examples include the man who describes how he exploits and betrays his wife or the young woman who describes how she seduces the husbands of her female friends or how she lets her girlfriend pamper her while part of her feels contempt for the girlfriend and does not want to give her anything in return and thus try to create a more equal relationship. Or the patient who expresses envy of what she perceives as the therapist's highly privileged life and having it easy; a feeling that is understandable, given the patient's life, but which may challenge the therapist's ability to contain the patient.

When hearing these types of stories, the therapist's goal is to bear in mind that behaviour which may initially seem repugnant is related to the patient's narcissistic pathology. The therapist should always avoid becoming outraged, moralizing, judgemental or normative in relation to the patient and their material. Over time, it may be necessary for the therapist to confront the patient with the negative consequences of their actions to both themself and others. Unless the patient has clear dissocial and psychopathic traits, sharing this type of behaviour will be associated with intense underlying shame in the patient. To varying degrees, the patient will have been able to keep this feeling at bay through grandiose defence strategies, including perceptions of their own special qualities and status, which are perceived to make the patient impervious to normal social standards. The patient may despise and devalue the victims of their abusive acts and insist on being entitled to pursue their own needs – perhaps with reference to the abuse they suffered earlier in life.

As mentioned earlier, shame is perhaps the most significant emotion and affective driver of pathological narcissism (see Chapter 2.4). Shame is always a core underlying theme and a feeling that is inevitably activated in the therapeutic space whenever the patient's vulnerable self and narcissism are exposed. Thus, as part of the treatment process, the therapist needs to help the patient contain and gradually detoxify their destructive shame (Crisp & Gabbard, 2020, p. 145). In patients with predominantly grandiose narcissism, destructive shame may initially be disguised as – or veiled by – narcissistic rage and attacks on or contempt for the therapist, just as grandiosity and stories about the self's admirable qualities and successes may help provide distance to shameful parts of the self. As the patient gradually realizes that their grandiose self-perceptions are unrealistic and out of step with reality – which typically happens months, sometimes closer to a year, into the treatment process – the patient may show much more prominent and overt feelings of shame (Kernberg, 2018, p. 194).

Defence against shame

The literature describes a wide variety of defences against and strategies for dealing with destructive shame: attacking others, attacking the self (self-harm), withdrawing from contact, dissociation and other ways of shutting down the patient's own emotions, compulsive perfectionism (attempts to compensate for the self's inadequacy through concrete acts and accomplishments), and grandiose and excessive self-assertion as well as cold arrogance, contempt, disparagement and ridicule of others (Nathanson, 1994; Wurmser, 1987, p. 86; Jørgensen, 2023/2024, p. 149 ff.). All these defence strategies are closely associated with the many different manifestations of pathological narcissism, which underscores the need for the therapist to remain mindful of how the patient's way of being and acting can be closely related to and driven by underlying destructive shame.

The therapist's reactions to shame in the patient

The practical psychotherapeutic work with destructive shame will not be addressed in detail in the present context (see DeYoung, 2022; Jørgensen, 2023/2024, p. 323 ff.). Essentially, the key factor in psychotherapeutic work with destructive shame is how the patient perceives the therapist's reactions when the patient talks about and reveals shameful aspects of themself and their history. Destructive shame is a very painful intersubjective affect with roots in dysfunctional relations and disturbed contact that may be reduced and detoxified through new, positive experiences in the contact with the therapist. This way of detoxifying shame is particularly effective as the patient begins to perceive the therapist as a significant person (self-object) in their current life with a high degree of emotional and epistemic trust (Jørgensen, 2023/2024, p. 350). The core issue in detoxifying and healing the patient's destructive shame is the patient's internalization of the therapist's containing, empathically understanding and caring reactions when the patient exposes – talks about and displays – shameful aspects of their self and history. By modelling certain ways of being and acting in the therapeutic space, the therapist can help the patient develop their ability to observe, contain and reflect on themself without condemning, despising, disparaging or shaming themself (Wurmser, 1987).

One example would be the patient who is fundamentally convinced that she only has a right to exist if she is always ready when others need her help. Based on this assumption, she is quite shameful that the previous day, for the first time ever, she turned down a request for help from a close friend in a difficult situation. The patient's perception of always having to be ready to help others has clear grandiose elements, in the sense that she is also convinced that she is better at problem-solving than most people – a grandiose self-perception that has helped keep her painful perceptions of inferiority and insignificance in check. The therapist explicitly remarks how shameful it is for the patient to have turned down her friend and to share this story with the therapist – thus disclosing and coming into contact with this part of herself. At the same time, the therapist also seeks to introduce a more nurturing understanding – for very understandable reasons, the patient felt so drained the day before that she had to deviate from her pattern of always being there for others. She had to look out for herself to avoid having to spend the next several days in bed – which she knew from experience would have been the consequence – and skipping today's session.

In parallel with this intervention, the therapist directs their joint attention to how much she has been willing to sacrifice to help others – which in many ways is both laudable and impressive – but gradually also focuses on how this inclination towards masochistic self-sacrifice contains elements of repeating painful patterns from the patient's life and is associated with grandiose self-perceptions that protect her from self-hatred and thoughts about not having any right to exist. Simply reacting with caring understanding and empathic mirroring of the patient when she exposes these shameful aspects of herself, the therapist can help detoxify her destructive shame. In addition, working with contextualizing and understanding situations that cause her to become overwhelmed by shame can help reduce her shame.

Acceptance and validation as an antidote

When the therapist is perceived to accept, validate and recognize the patient as an equal and significant subject, despite their – universally human – flaws and deficits, this will serve as an antidote to shame. Similarly, the therapist's kind and caring gaze and empathic mirroring of the patient's inner life can enhance the patient's ability to reveal shameful self-aspects in the therapeutic space (Morrison, 1986, p. 369). Over time, the therapist's predominantly implicitly (nonverbally) conveyed understanding of human vulnerability and ability to validate and recognize shameful parts of the patient and their history help the patient get better at containing and accepting these parts of the self (Lecours et al., 2013, p. 140). To the extent that the insufficient integration of grandiose and vulnerable elements of the patient's pathological narcissism – and of the patient's self and identity – is driven by destructive shame, the therapeutic work of detoxifying and enhancing the patient's capacity for containing and regulating feelings of shame will also contribute to greater integration and a more stable organization of the patient's personality (Broucek, 1982, p. 373 ff.). This may also be understood as a gradual desensitization of the patient's sensitivity to shame and enhancement of the patient's affect tolerance as they come into contact with destructive shame in the therapeutic space again and again and discover that they can survive this feeling (Lecours et al., 2013, p. 138; Ritter et al., 2014).

It is not meaningful to prescribe certain interventions for the therapist to apply when the patient is struggling with destructive shame in the therapeutic space. How to be, act and react in the contact with the patient in these situations is much more important than the use of any specific verbal interventions. Similarly, what plays out in the not necessarily verbal contact and in the nonverbal interaction between patient and therapist is generally much more important for healing the patient's destructive shame than the specific content of the verbal communication. This does not imply that the topic of their conversation in the therapy space makes no difference – naturally, it should focus on issues that are emotionally significant to the patient and related to their psychological difficulties, including shameful parts of the patient's self and history. However, the way in which the patient and the therapist talk about the topic and developments in their emotional and psychological contact as they talk are much more important than any specific topic or specific verbal interventions. Establishing and maintaining a fundamentally positive, close and intimate emotional and psychological contact with the therapist that is continually adjusted – in terms of the degree of closeness and intensity – to the patient's current states and needs is an essential part of enabling the patient to feel safe enough to gradually dare to come into contact with and show the therapist the most shameful aspects of themself and their history – aspects that may potentially threaten the patient's fragile narcissistic balances when they surface.

Regulating the focus on shame

When the patient feels shameful over displaying or talking about certain aspects of themself and their past life – a life that may well have been dominated by early neglect, abuse, cynicism, contempt for and exploitation of others – it may be relevant to make this shame and its origin in the patient's history and resulting perceptions of self and others (cf. internal object relations) the focus of the therapeutic work. This includes a common interest in how the patient's experience of shame in the here and now may relate to the patient's self-perception. It also includes how the patient might imagine or perceive that the therapist is looking down upon or feeling contempt for the patient because the patient showed themself as vulnerable, insecure, small, immature and unable to articulate what they experience when their self-esteem collapses. Similarly, the patient may suddenly feel that the emotional contact with the therapist is so intense, intimidating and overwhelming – and brings them into contact with yearnings, emotions and self-aspects they may not have known that they had or thought they had managed to shut down – that they feel shameful and feel a strong urge to withdraw from contact, leave the therapeutic space or 'talk about something else'. In relation to this, it may sometimes – but not necessarily always – be helpful for the therapist to direct the joint attention to what is happening inside the patient right now and how it might be understood.

Finally, the therapist should help the patient regulate how much and how fast the patient comes into contact with shameful self-aspects in order to minimize the risk for the patient to be overwhelmed by destructive shame in the therapeutic space. Once patient and therapist have moved deep into a dark space characterized by intense destructive shame – for example by working with traumatic experiences when the patient was subjected to injuries or injured others – it can be difficult to get back out. This may hamper the therapeutic work and make it more difficult to maintain or re-establish the emotional contact with the patient, who had to withdraw from contact with the therapist and shut down their emotions (by dissociating, seeking refuge in their psychic retreat) in an attempt to reduce overwhelming shame.

It should be noted here that the experience of being so overwhelmed by destructive shame that it becomes impossible to articulate and work with this feeling in therapy – perhaps needing to break off a session and skip subsequent scheduled sessions – may in itself be associated with intense destructive shame and shameful perceptions of oneself as an 'inadequate patient who does not deserve to receive help', 'who wastes their own and the therapist's time' and so forth. Becoming overwhelmed by out-of-control shame in the therapeutic space may thus in itself lead to a narcissistic crisis by destabilizing the patient's self-esteem and the internal cohesion of the self (cf. internal splitting between vulnerable and grandiose self-aspects). For that reason too it is important for the therapist to try to regulate how much and how quickly the patient comes into contact with destructive shame and parts of themself and their history that will supposedly be associated with shame. The patient's level of personality organization affects their ability to contain and handle contact with destructive shame without dissociating, withdrawing from contact or fleeing into their psychic retreat.

Narcissistic injuries of the therapist

As mentioned earlier, in the effort to establish contact during the initial treatment phase, it may be helpful for the therapist to verbalize and validate the patient's perceived difficulties with trusting and working with a therapist whom the patient does not know and thus has no basis for knowing whether they are professionally competent and equipped to give the patient what the patient believes they need and deserve (Weinberg & Ronningstam, 2020, p. 130). Perhaps the patient thinks that the therapist is too young or too old, the wrong sex or the wrong sexuality – 'only a man can possibly understand what it's like to be a man', 'men can't be nurturing or understand how hard it is for me', 'a heterosexual/binary person couldn't possibly understand what it's like to be homosexual/non-binary' – or simply is not intelligent, experienced or skilled enough to understand and deal with the patient's particular difficulties. Whatever the therapist might think of these rather rigid perceptions of the world and of the therapist, it may be helpful to address them explicitly and, over the longer term, to examine the roots of these categorical perceptions together with the patient.

In doing so, the therapist should be mindful that they might perceive these de facto attacks on their personal and professional integrity as narcissistic injuries – for reasons that have to do with their own personal and professional experiences and history. Such perceived injury may increase the risk of unconscious reactions that are defensive, vindictive or otherwise unhelpful for the therapeutic process. The therapist may drop out of their professional role, feel personally offended, react personally wronged or struggle to maintain their fundamental psychotherapeutic stance in relation to the patient's and their own behaviour in the therapeutic space and what plays out between patient and therapist (Jørgensen, 2019), given that the ability to triangulate and act as a participatory observer may be compromised by emotional arousal.

The therapist's own narcissism and narcissistic needs may come into play in ways that are not helpful and which are harmful to the therapeutic work. If that happens, it may be necessary for the therapist to examine their countertransference, if necessary with help from a supervisor (see Chapter 4.3). In addition, there will naturally be a limit to the degree of injuries to one's professional and personal integrity and boundaries the therapist should contain, accept and address exclusively from a psychotherapeutic perspective without taking actual steps to look out for oneself – including demonstrating, in vivo, the significance of doing so – and to defend and preserve one's ability to think in the therapeutic space. No one will be able to think if they are persistently subjected to extreme narcissistic injuries, feel unsafe or fear for the patient's reactions to their interventions. This presents a somewhat different issue, which will not be further addressed in the present context.

4.2 Transference in pathological narcissism

According to Kernberg (1984, p. 197), the most important aspect of the psychoanalytic treatment of NPD is the systematic registration and analysis of the patient's pathological grandiose self, as it pervasively manifests itself in the patient's transference. Transference is an entrance – and often a shortcut – to the patient's internal psychological reality and how it plays out in concrete interactions with others (Diamond et al., 2022, p. 143). Thus, the core of pathological narcissism will always be evident in the patient's transference and its related processes in the therapist's countertransference; two key elements of the psychotherapeutic work that, as mentioned earlier, contains information of invaluable significance to the therapist's ability to understand and help the patient. Kohut (1968, p. 96 ff.) has described how the patient's self-object needs play out in different forms of transference in the interaction with the therapist. Thus, transference makes it possible for the therapist to gain insight into the core of the patient's difficulties even if the patient is not necessarily aware of them, let alone capable of articulating what they are. The patient does not describe the dynamic psychological core of their difficulties but shows them in their way of relating to and interacting with the therapist.

Simply put, the psychoanalytic concept of transference describes the phenomenon that the patient's perception of and reactions to the therapist are, more or less unconsciously, profoundly affected by the patient's experiences from past relationships with significant others. In concrete terms, this means that the patient is repeating patterns from their past experiences of and interactions with significant others in their current interaction with the therapist. The patient perceives the therapist in the same way that they have previously perceived significant others, just as their reactions to the therapist also tend to follow established patterns. These repetitions or re-enactments of interpersonal processes typically play out without the patient noticing that they are repeating old relational patterns. The patient is unaware or only partially conscious of and able to address these recurring interpersonal relational patterns, which are the core of their psychological difficulties but displays them live, here and now, in the way they relate to the therapist.

The patient who repeatedly felt that significant others viewed her as unwanted, too demanding and a nuisance if she showed signs of sadness or vulnerability while she received positive attention if she showed (feigned) strength, agency and high (grandiose) self-esteem – perhaps also if she appeared sexually attractive and flirtatious – will 'naturally' (unconsciously or, at least, without reflecting on it) expect the same to apply in the relationship with the therapist. The patient expects that the therapist, too, will perceive her as difficult and demanding and will judge her if she shows vulnerability. And on the other hand, she imagines that therapist might like her if she displays her usual slightly brazen and domineering grandiosity or if she is, discreetly or more explicitly, sexualizing in her contact with the therapist. She does not describe these features as key aspects of or specific manifestations of her relational difficulties – she is incapable of doing so, since she has only limited awareness of them. However, she demonstrates them in the way that she interacts with the therapist. She shows it by transferring core aspects of her past object relations to her present relationship with the therapist and living out what must be regarded as a false self, which was developed in an attempt to survive emotionally in a dysfunctional relational environment.

How the patient relates to and engages in the contact with the therapist – or tries to avoid contact in order to protect their vulnerable self from dreaded disappointment and injury – is a crucial element of the relational psychotherapeutic work with pathological narcissism. This involves both the real relationship and interaction between the patient's transference and the therapist's countertransference (see Chapter 4.3). The transference of patients with predominantly vulnerable narcissism will be shaped more by fear of being humiliated and overwhelmed by shame in the interaction with the therapist, while the urge to be seen and admired by the therapist is more prominent in patients with predominantly grandiose narcissism (Gabbard & Crisp, 2018, p. 85). Periodically, transference may also have the character of self-self-transference: in this case, the therapist may feel that they are not being seen and treated as an independent subject, delimited from the patient's own self, and that the patient primarily appears to relate to themself or to split-off/evacuated or unintegrated aspects of the self, which are transferred to the therapist (Kernberg, 2014, p. 867). In classic psychoanalysis and object relations theory, the main initial focus is on how elements of the patient's earlier relational constellations – or object relations – including core perceptions of self, others and interpersonal relationships, with their related affects, are repeated in the interaction with the therapist. In Kohut's work, the primary focus is rather on how fundamental emotional (self-object) needs – particularly narcissistic needs that have not been seen, mirrored and met in earlier self-object relations – dominate the patient's interactions with the therapist, as the patient's interactions with the therapist revolve around hopes and expectations that the therapist will satisfy previously frustrated self-object needs.

Different transference patterns

Based on Kernberg's object relations theory, Diamond et al. (2022, p. 175 ff.) outlined different transference categories or patterns that may be seen in patients with pathological narcissism. The actual manifestations depend on the individual patient's degree of personality organization. In particular, transference characterized by slightly more mature dependence and depressive feelings reflects a higher level of personality integration and organization. Below, some of Diamond et al.'s (2022, p. 176 ff.) transference categories have been combined into one:

1 Narcissistic transference characterized by emotional distancing and the absence of contact, as the therapist is seemingly too insignificant for the patient to show any real interest in them, or the therapist is devalued to prevent them from becoming significant to the patient. This transference may be driven by the patient's fear of rejection or of their own deep yearning for contact. In some cases, the narcissistic transference also plays out between the grandiose self and an (in the eyes of the patient) idealized omnipotent therapist.
2 An antisocial/psychopathic transference (cf. Kernberg's description of malignant narcissism associated with aspects of psychopathy), in which the patient's interaction with the therapist is driven by a conviction that all relationships are based on mutual exploitation, egocentric satisfaction of own needs, control and manipulation, while any notions of real concern and love are viewed as completely illusory or unattainable. The more prominent the psychopathic elements are, the more the transference will be characterized by callousness, cynicism and attempts to control and exploit the therapist.
3 A paranoid-narcissistic transference characterized by fear that the therapist may harm, punish or destroy the patient or, alternatively, by masochistic or sadomasochistic dynamic, as the patient feels that the therapist wants the patient to suffer, perhaps combined with a desire on the part of the patient to make the therapist suffer. This transference is most common in patients with severe malignant narcissism (Diamond et al., 2022, p. 366 f.).
4 Various levels of eroticized transference, in which the patient may be explicitly seductive and sexualizing from the outset in an attempt to cover up their own aggressions or achieve control over the therapist. Alternatively, the patient may gradually – over a longer period – become increasingly explicit in their yearning for and expression of loving and erotic feelings for the therapist, possibly combined with a preoccupation with – and jealousy of – the therapist's other patients and personal life and relationships. Gradual eroticization of the transference accompanied by loving feelings for the therapist will typically be a sign of relatively well-integrated object relations and a certain ability to love. Conversely, pronounced eroticization of the therapeutic relationship from the beginning of the treatment will typically be a sign that sexuality and sexual feelings are part of the patient's urge to manipulate, control and live out hostile feelings towards the therapist. The therapist's perception of sexual tension in the therapeutic space may be related to the therapist's own countertransference, but it may also be a sign that the patient seeks to shift the balance of power in the therapeutic space by eroticizing the

contact with the therapist (Weinberg & Ronningstam, 2020, p. 135). To do this, the patient tries, more or less unconsciously, to re-enact earlier perceived situations of seduction or abuse but now in the therapeutic space, where the patient is no longer in a passive position but in an active position and, to varying degrees, potentially as the abuser. Alternatively, the patient may, for various reasons, long for another and much closer form of contact with the therapist.

5 A dependent, possibly depressive transference, in which patient's narcissistic vulnerable self is dependent on the idealized therapist who protects and satisfies the patient's needs. The patient's self-perception may be characterized by feelings of guilt – or shame – and gratitude towards the therapist, who in some cases is perceived in a more realistic light, with flaws, shortcomings and vulnerabilities. Despite these flaws, the patient is very appreciative of the therapist. This transference may challenge the patient's perceptions of self-sufficiency and confront the self with a 'dangerous' dependence on the therapist. Thus, it may cause – and co-occur with – paranoid transference.

Arguably, these descriptions of transference patterns focus fairly exclusively on the patient, while the therapist's possible contribution to the development of various forms of transference are largely ignored. Furthermore, the transference in the individual patient is often too complex to fit neatly into any of the outlined categories. Nevertheless, these descriptions of various types of transference may be helpful for developing a nuanced understanding of the complex relational constellations and transference that will be at play in work with patients characterized by narcissistic pathology.

Transference in Kohut

Kohut describes two basic forms of transference: 1) idealizing transference influenced by the actualization of the patient's idealized parent imagos and 2) mirror transference dominated by the activation of the patient's grandiose self. Even though, to the untrained eye, the content of the transference – the perceptions, feelings and impulses that are actualized and played out in them – may seem highly immature, primitive and pathological, according to Kohut (1971, p. 213) they should be regarded as 'healthy and necessary maturational steps'. Transference regressions pointing back to these archaic needs that have not been met with resonance and understanding in the early self-object relations are thus 'neither ill nor ill' (p. 213). At various times in his authorship, Kohut describes transference types as narcissistic versus self-object transference (Kernberg, 1984, p. 185), based on the central and recurring point that the patient's transference is driven by and shows the patient's most important narcissistic needs. Thus, the therapist can gain insight into these needs in the patient by focusing on and trying to understand the patient's transference.

With Kohut we can say that the patient only truly becomes aware of and acknowledges their narcissistic needs when they encounter them in the transference. Here, they play out in vivo, and the patient comes into emotional contact with them in the interaction with the therapist. Only once the patient has acknowledged these needs as healthy, normal and necessary for their personal development can they 'undertake the task of gradually transforming them and of building them into the higher organization of the adult personality' (Kohut, 1971, p. 213). Unlike more classic psychoanalytic interpretations of transference (Freud, 1912/1957c), according to Kohut we should not primarily view transference as a distortion of the present driven by the past but rather as an expression of the patient's real emotional (self-object) needs in the present (Liebermann, 2013, p. 260). Thus, the therapist's ability to contain and mirror these needs is more important than complex interpretations of how the patient's transference may be associated with their history. Furthermore, Kohut (1971, p. 23) argues that a key criterion in diagnosing pathological narcissism is 'the nature of the spontaneously developing transference' in the patient's interactions with the therapist. As mentioned above, Kohut distinguishes between two forms of transference: mirroring transference and idealizing transference.

Mirror transference

In mirror transference, the patient's archaic grandiose self is activated, and the patient views the therapist as a self-object that is expected to mirror and confirm the patient's grandiose self and make the patient feel admired and special. These are experiences that the patient has not had in their early object relations and which they have therefore longed for much of their life. Mirror transference is dominated by needs for the therapist's acceptance, confirmation and admiration (Kohut & Wolf, 1978, p. 413), accompanied by a more or less pronounced urge for unlimited access to and a form of control over the therapist as the empathically mirroring self-object (Kohut, 1971, p. 120). Paradoxically, the patient may also feel that everything that is perfect and complete is concentrated in their own grandiose self (p. 106). This may be understood in relation to the patient's defence against dependence and their overwhelming need for 'the other', although this other will never be completely controlled by the self. The mirror transference allows for previously hidden parts of the patient's grandiose self to emerge and become the object of joint attention and exploration in therapy (p. 106).

Kohut (1968, p. 96) has described three subcategories of mirror transference, all of which are characteristic of patients with pathological narcissism:

1 An archaic form, in which the therapist is perceived as an extension of the patient's grandiose self and, in the patient's inner universe, is more or less merged with the patient's self.

2 A less archaic alter-ego or twinship transference, in which the therapist may be perceived as a separate individual but as more or less identical to or a mirror image of the patient's grandiose self.
3 Finally, the least archaic mirror transference in a narrow sense, in which the therapist is clearly distinct from the patient's grandiose self but is in fact only noticed and viewed as significant to the extent that the therapist satisfies the needs of the grandiose self.(Kohut, 1971, p. 114)

Particularly in the two former, more intense variants of mirror transference, the therapist is not, or only partially, perceived and recognized as a clearly delimited autonomous subject. According to Kohut (1971, p. 271), this may mean that the therapist is deprived of even a 'minimum of narcissistic gratification' in the therapeutic space. Intense mirror transference, in which the therapist may feel reduced to a function, a non-person, may thus challenge the therapist's own narcissism – particularly if the therapist loses sight of how the patient's transference is related to, and in vivo demonstrates, the core of the patient's narcissistic disorder.

Idealizing transference

Due to deficiencies in early object relations, the patient is driven by intense yearning for ideal objects. By being close to – or merging with – these objects, the patient hopes to be able to compensate for deficits in the internal structures of the self. This yearning is the emotional driver of the idealizing transference, which places the therapist into the position as the idealized object that the patient has been missing. The patient's need for intimacy to and varying degrees of merger with the idealized self-object is transferred to the therapist. The patient longs to be seen and loved as a unique and significant person by the idealized other (the therapist), and the patient's need to feel as the most important person in the world to the ideal other is transferred to the therapist (cf. Morrison & Stolorow, 1997, p. 63).

Kohut (1971, p. 8) describes the idealizing transference as the transference of an 'omnipotent and omniscient, admired and idealized, emotionally sustaining parent imago' to the therapist. Thus, the patient stabilizes their self and self-esteem by viewing – leaning on and seeking to be close to – the therapist as the ideal self-object (p. 105). The patient feels part of or closely connected to the therapist as the strong and powerful self-object. This provides a sense of strength that the self has been missing and which is absent if or when the patient is not connected to the therapist or feels that the connectedness is threatened. Intense idealizing transference makes the patient seek permanent closeness to the therapist. Thus, the patient may feel empty, powerless and highly vulnerable when they are separated from the therapist, particularly for prolonged periods in connection with holidays or long breaks during the treatment (Kohut, 1968, p. 88).

In the idealizing transference, the patient's perception of the therapist may be narcissistic in the sense that the therapist is not regarded as an autonomous subject that is distinct from the self but rather as a self-object in the transitional space between the internal and the external reality that is controlled by the self. The patient creates or constructs 'their therapist' based on their own fantasies and needs for a particular form of self-object, which may facilitate the development of a treatment alliance. Over time, however, it may also get in the way of the patient's ability to see and relate to the therapist as a separate subject in the real relationship. Thus, it may be necessary to explicitly address and focus on this in the therapeutic work. 'In the undisturbed [idealizing] transference the narcissistic patient feels whole, safe, powerful, good, attractive, active so long as his [the patient's] self experience includes the idealized analyst [therapist] whom he [the patient] feels he controls and possesses with a self-evident certainty that is akin to the adult's experience of his control over his own body and mind' (Kohut, 1971, p. 90). With Kohut, we can say that the patient's archaic need for an idealized self-object is reactivated in the relationship with the therapist. Over time, this may lead to the patient becoming dependent on the therapist, the therapeutic space and the therapeutic contact and dialogue as an adequate response to the patient's self-object needs. This includes elements of re-establishing an archaic self-object relation, only in a version that is far more benign for the patient, in the sense that the patient not only allows themself to come into contact with early self-object needs but also feels met with a very different degree of kindness and recognition than in earlier self-object relations (p. 46).

This also implies that the patient may react with deep despair, grief and rage when it becomes clear that they do not control the therapist and will not necessarily be able to have contact with and receive emotional nourishment from the therapist exactly when they need it. One example is a patient who – for a very legitimate reason – feels a strong need to be in contact with and talk to the therapist during a brief period while the therapist is away on a trip. When this proves impossible, he becomes so furious with the therapist that he burns an important text that he had previously written for the therapist; a text containing emotionally significant material about the patient's relationship with the therapist. Thus, the patient acted out his understandable narcissistic rage over the therapist's perceived failure as a self-object in a form of revenge involving burning a concrete object that was closely associated with his relationship with the therapist.

The narcissistically vulnerable patient may also be very sensitive to any signs of emotional withdrawal in the therapist. After a short break in the treatment, a patient expresses that she missed the therapist. She asks if the therapist also missed her – seemingly asking: Am I so significant to you that you might miss me, as I miss you? Whether the therapist missed the patient – or otherwise thought about her during this brief pause in the treatment – this is not a question he can readily answer, since the focus of the therapeutic work is not on his yearnings and needs but on the patient's. On the other hand, if he ignores and fails to answer the patient's question, she may take from it that her feelings for the therapist as a self-object are of no relevance to him and are not taken seriously. She may feel confirmed in her feeling of being insignificant, also to the therapist. The right answer for the therapist in this sort of situation will always depend on the concrete circumstances. Over time, the patient will gradually be confronted with the inherent asymmetry of the therapeutic relationship. To some patients, this may feel unbearable and may at times make it difficult for them to accept 'the good things' coming from the therapist, because this also confronts the patient with their own perceived shortcomings and perceived unbearable inferiority in relation to the idealized therapist.

Similarly, emotional closeness to the therapist may feel intimidating and as a threat to the exposed self and its fragile boundaries. When the patient feels that their boundless and constant access to the therapist, as the idealized self-object, is threatened, the patient's self-esteem may be destabilized, and the self may feel threatened by fragmentation or collapse. The patient may feel that life makes no sense and is not worth living if the therapist is not there for the self in the manner and to the degree that the self imagined and expected. This may happen, for example, if the therapist adopts a neutral and emotionally disengaged position – which the patient may perceive as cold and as an indication that the therapist does not care about the patient, that the patient is of no importance or value to the therapist – while suggesting how the patient's current conflict with their mother might be understood, when the patient's primary need is just for the therapist to mirror and understand how difficult it is for the patient to be in recurring conflicts with their mother and to side with the patient in these conflicts.

Dealing with the patient's transference

It is a core element of Kohut's psychotherapeutic method that the therapist should strive to meet the patient in a containing and empathetic way when the patient seeks to have the therapist see and meet emotional needs that have not been seen and satisfied in their early and typically deeply deficient self-object relations. Thus, the patient actualizes and acts out their self-object needs in the transference. During much of the initial stage of the treatment, some patients with pathological narcissism who have experienced severe failure from early self-objects will – simply put – primarily need the therapist's empathic mirroring, containing and understanding. These responses are a condition for the patient to establish the trust and internal structure necessary for 'hearing' and benefiting from interventions that are aimed more at enhancing the patient's conscious understanding of themself and their relationships (Kohut, 1977, p. 88).

Kernberg's TFP model for the treatment of NPD also recommends that during the initial stage of the treatment the therapist should primarily contain and address the patient's transference – projected parts of the self, dominant object relations, central affects and any remarkably absent affects, for example vulnerability or sadness – without challenging or throwing it back to the patient. This includes avoiding offering complex interpretations which the patient may perceive as a sign of the therapist's inability or unwillingness to contain the patient's projected and transferred affects and perceptions (Bromberg, 1998, p. 92; Diamond et al., 2022, p. 252 ff.). The therapist's primary task in this regard is to make the patient feel understood and to give the patient a sense that the therapist is interested in or understands what it is like to be the patient, understands their inner universe, feelings, yearnings, conflicted action urges and needs (Diamond et al., 2022, p. 255). Later in the treatment, the therapist may gradually introduce the notion that the patient's perception of and reactions to the therapist might be associated with parts of the patient's self and relational history. With this, the therapist can offer an in vivo demonstration of how reality can be viewed from different perspectives and thus enhance the patient's tolerance for ambiguity and the complexities of the real world (p. 280).

Validating and understanding the patient's (self-object) needs does not necessarily imply that the therapist should satisfy these needs, which are typically centred on needs for basic nurture, love and emotional contact with an ideal other. At the very least, however, the therapist should try, together with the patient, to contain, explore and understand the basis of these needs (Gabbard & Crisp, 2018, p. 98). When put into the position of the patient's perhaps primary self-object, the therapist should not enter into this role by 'being' or trying to act out the assigned position, including giving the patient the primary love that they may never have experienced. However, to the best of their ability, the therapist should be available as the object – the significant other – that the patient can direct their love and other powerful mental states and thoughts at. As Michael Balint (1968, p. 179) puts it, 'This difference between "giving primary love" and "offering oneself to be cathected by primary love" may be of fundamental importance for our technique.' This key distinction affects how we meet the patient and the more specific ways in which we should contain and intervene in relation to the patient's self-object transference. The therapist should not – and is not, in any meaningful way, able to – compensate for the profound deprivation of love and nurture that the patient has experienced so far in their life. However, the therapist should persistently – to the best of their ability – recognize and understand the patient's needs as they play out in the transference and communicate this understanding to the patient. At the same time, the therapist should also, to some extent, satisfy some of the patient's emotional and relational needs in the therapeutic space and within the conditions it implies (Balint, 1968, p. 180). This includes the need to be met by an empathic, responsive and loving gaze – to be seen and met as an equal and significant subject.

To the extent that the therapist is able to deal with the patient's sometimes intense yearning for empathic mirroring and to accept the patient's at times intense idealization and thus act as a self-object to the patient, this will – through transmuting internalization – help to repair the deficits in the patient's internal personality structure that are a result of severe deficiencies in earlier self-object relations and which, according to Kohut, form the core of pathological narcissism. The successful psychotherapeutic handling of the idealizing transference enables the patient to internalize the therapist as the idealized object – cf. internalization of the therapist as the good internal object that enhances the organization of the personality – while successfully working through the mirror transference transforms (matures) the grandiose self and supports the development of more stable and realistic self-esteem (Kohut, 1968, p. 101). Both processes are closely related to the concrete interaction between patient and therapist and thus in no way hinge solely on the specific content of the therapist's verbal interventions.

According to Kernberg – and to some extent in contrast to Kohut's recommendations – the therapist should always avoid satisfying the patient's needs in the transference and instead persistently insist on examining these needs. With Kernberg, we may argue that satisfying the patient's needs would inhibit the full expression of the patient's transference and contribute to the continuation of the patient's unconscious fear of their own envy and anger/hatred (Kernberg, 1975, p. 284 ff.). From the patient's perspective, by meeting their emotional needs, the therapist may be seen as trying to avoid being hit by the patient's envy and hatred; this could be perceived as a sort of confirmation of how toxic and dangerous these feelings supposedly are. In extension of this point, some authors have criticized Kohut for satisfying the patient's regressive needs rather than improving the patient's self-perception (Pulver, 1986, p. 137 ff.), which is widely regarded as an important element in curing pathological narcissism.

Another key therapeutic task in Kernberg's transference focused psychotherapy (Diamond et al., 2022, p. 143) is to identify and change the patient's dysfunctional, distorted and polarized perceptions of self and others, with their related affects, when these are activated and play out in the patient's transference and interactions with the therapist; a process that enhances the integration of the patient's identity. The transference and the patient's way of being and acting in the interaction with the therapist are thus viewed as an entrance to the patient's internal psychological reality and object relations, including the patient's grandiose self, hatred, envy and vindictiveness – but also their urge to dominate, devalue and control others, including the therapist. Explicitly addressing the patient's subjective perceptions of and behaviour in interactions with the therapist – and exploring possible connections between this and the patient's inner life and relational history – may transform the patient's dominant (distorted) perceptions of self and others.

Unlike Kernberg and others, Kohut does not view the idealized transference as reflective of a primitive defence (against envy, aggression directed at the therapist and so forth) that needs reality testing and correction. Rather, he views it as an expression of the patient's legitimate and – in light of the patient's relational history – understandable self-object needs, which manifest themselves in the transference and should be recognized, validated and gradually transformed into less archaic, more mature forms but which should not be dismissed, eliminated or regarded as inappropriate (Karterud, 1985, p. 60). Similarly, the therapist should signal that the patient's needs and expectations, as they are manifested in the mirror transference, are fully legitimate and understandable, which will counteract the patient's inclination to split off and deny parts of the self (Kohut, 1971, p. 175 ff.); cf. the vertical split of the self that isolates the grandiose self from the rest of the self and/or denies and possibly projects vulnerable parts of the self onto others, including the therapist. The yearnings and needs that the patient lives out in the mirror transference should be met with empathic mirroring, understanding and recognition, which will enable corrective emotional experiences and serve as a counterweight to earlier experiences from self-object relations characterized by severe (traumatic) deficiencies (Kohut, 1971, p. 191).

When the patient's archaic self-object needs are activated in the transference, the therapist cannot satisfy them at their original archaic level. For example, this may pertain to needs for basic bodily-physical contact, deep and close to infinite parental love or acceptance of limitless idealization. Instead, the therapist may, to varying degrees and within the non-negotiable boundaries of the therapy, meet derived needs for close emotional and psychological contact and admiration of the therapist – needs that the therapist should at least accept and acknowledge as legitimate and understandable, given the patient's history. Similarly, genuine feelings of love may arise between patient and therapist, which should not be denied or treated as taboo but which can also not be expressed in concrete acts. The patient's potential admiration of and feelings of love for the therapist should be given room to be addressed and explored in an atmosphere in which the therapist does not dismiss or otherwise disparage, trivialize or minimize the significance of these feelings, as this might be perceived by the patient as invalidating or delegitimizing significant parts of the patients self or emotions or treating them as taboo. Naturally, this may be a challenging balancing act for the therapist, who is responsible for upholding the framework of the therapy and should also avoid acting in ways that might support parts of the patient that might wish for a different form of relationship with the therapist and for the therapist to give up their therapeutic position.

Studies of transference in NPD

There are few empirical studies of the transference in patients with pathological narcissism (Alnæs & Høglend, 1985). Quite remarkably, these few studies do not involve the patients' own descriptions of their experiences and behaviour in the treatment relationship, only their therapists' accounts. The most interesting of these studies (Bradley et al., 2005) is based on psychologists' and psychiatrists' descriptions of their patients' (n=181) transference based on a questionnaire for documenting the therapeutic relationship. They also assess whether their patients meet each of the diagnostic criteria for personality disorders in the *DSM-IV*. The vast majority of the patients included in this study have a symptom disorder, primarily depression or anxiety. A small group (n=13) meet the diagnostic criteria for NPD; a predominantly grandiose narcissistic pathology. Based on factor analyses of the therapists' replies, the study identifies five specific factors or dimensions of the patients' transference. Two of them have a strong positive correlation with how many diagnostic criteria for cluster B personality disorders (including NPD) the patients meet: namely, one, that the transference is characterized by anger and entitlement and, two, sexualization (Bradley et al., 2005, p. 346). The latter may be related, in part, to the patient's attempt to establish some form of sexual contact with the therapist; a factor that is not very strongly associated with NPD but which must be assumed to be more closely related to borderline and histrionic PD.

The study also presents an overview of which descriptions of possible forms of transference, according to the therapists, are most and least characteristic of patients with NPD. Among the most characteristic, we find the patient's exaggerated need for admiration from the therapist, entitlement, alternating between idealizing and devaluing the therapist, being annoying/repulsive, demanding excessive contact/love from the therapist, wanting to have the therapist as a parent, being boring and playing the therapist off against others – all characteristics that, to varying degrees, are aligned with prevailing descriptions and perceptions of patients with predominantly grandiose pathological narcissism. At least as revealing is the therapists' assessment of which descriptions were least characteristic of the transference of their patients with NPD: being empathic to the therapist, triggering warm feelings in the therapist, being able to speak openly about their difficulties, being attentive to both verbal and nonverbal aspects of the therapist's communication, being good at reading social codes and working hard in the therapy.

Overall, this paints a picture of the transference in a group of patients who can be overtly challenging and produce a wide range of negative emotions in the therapist, particularly in therapists who are not familiar with how characteristic these transference constellations are of the key difficulties, particularly among patients with grandiose pathological narcissism. On the other hand, if the therapist is prepared for – and equipped to deal with – the transference in the engagement with the narcissistic patient, there is a better chance that the therapist will be able to contain and deal with the patient's transference in a qualified manner and will not be gripped by negative countertransference.

4.3 Narcissism and countertransference

The concept of countertransference is defined and understood slightly differently by different authors. In this book, it is used as a term for the therapist's subjective experiences and reactions in the interaction with the patient. The countertransference includes all the feelings, yearnings, needs, impulses, urges and other mental states that the therapist comes into contact with in the interaction with a given patient in the therapeutic space – and, in principle, also outside it, to the extent these can meaningfully be associated with the therapist's interactions with a specific patient. Originally, countertransference – for example in Freud's (1910/1957d, p. 78) work – was viewed solely as an obstacle to the therapy, as it was seen as an expression of the therapist's own internal hang-ups and 'resistance', thus hampering the therapist's optimal position as a neutral observer and the task of understanding and interpreting the patient's internal conflicts and transference (Sandler et al., 1979, p. 62 ff.).

Later, we have realized how much the countertransference can also enrich the treatment if the therapist is mindful of and able to decode their countertransference and thus use it to understand the patient, rather than acting it out in inappropriate ways in the interaction with the patient. The therapist's persistent attention to and reflections on their countertransference reflects a special way of listening to the patient that also involves nonverbal communication channels in the therapeutic space (Green, 2004, p. 79). In addition, it should be noted that the therapist's professional theoretical foundation, understanding of human nature and more specific understanding of pathological narcissism will inevitably affect the therapist's countertransference and psychotherapeutic stance – how the therapist meets and relates to people with pathological narcissism.

Countertransference as a nonverbal channel of communication

Just as the patient's transference in vivo – through their way of relating to and interacting with the therapist – displays the typically recurring patterns in the patient's interpersonal interactions, with their related thoughts, emotions, yearnings, defence strategies and needs, key elements of the therapist's subjective experiences, thoughts and emotions in the interaction with the patient will offer valuable insight into the sorts of reactions and interaction patterns the patient typically activates and encounters in their interpersonal relations. This all happens outside the verbal communication and possibly outside the involved parties' conscious awareness. The predominantly grandiose narcissistic patient who meets others with contempt and cold arrogance and makes others feel ill at ease and thus withdraw will generally act in the same way in their encounter with the therapist. Similarly, the therapist may experience a vague sense of discomfort and feel the urge to distance themself from the patient, perhaps concluding that the patient is not suited for psychotherapeutic treatment or refer them to a colleague.

This will play out in the patient's interactions with the therapist, without the patient necessarily being aware of it or perceiving it as a problematic, let alone being able to see how their behaviour in interpersonal interactions may generally be closely associated with – and a contributing cause of – the patient's painful loneliness and vague sense of alienation in interactions with others. Similarly, therapists with insufficient insight into their own countertransference and experience with decoding it as a source of important information about the core of the patient's difficulties and how they play out in the relationship with therapists may 'assess' that the patient is not suited for the treatment that the therapist offers. Perhaps, the therapist will then 'assess' that the patient is better off talking to another therapist – without realizing the extent to which this 'professional' assessment is driven by common forms of countertransference in the encounter with patients with grandiose narcissism.

As mentioned earlier (see Chapter 3.4), based on recurring patterns in their earlier relations, the patient will have developed internal mental representations of self, others and interpersonal relationships. These internal object relations subsequently serve as the basis of the patient's way of interacting with others (external object relations), including how the patient meets and relates to the therapist. The therapist's countertransference may thus provide the therapist with insight into the patient's internal, external and, to some extent, past object relations. If the therapist finds themself losing interest in the patient's longwinded stories about themself and struggles to pay attention when the patient is talking, this will often illustrate how the patient's behaviour in interpersonal interactions makes others lose interest in the patient and ignore what they are saying. Similarly, if the therapist finds that the patient's condescending comments and controlling behaviour is offensive and makes the therapist want to break free from and distance themself from the patient – or makes them feel unsafe and feel an urge to break off contact with them – this provides insight into how the patient generally acts and what reactions this way of acting typically activates in others. These reactions may be part of the basis of the patient's perceived loneliness and great unmet need for others to stay with and submit to the patient's agenda.

In addition, the patient may have developed different types of interpersonal defence strategies, in which parts of the patient's self, emotions and other mental states that, for various reasons, have been dissociated or split off – have not been integrated into the patient's personality – are evacuated and projected onto external objects, including the therapist. Thus, the therapist's countertransference may also contain important information about emotions and parts of the patient's self that the patient, for various reasons, is unable to contain; instead the patient tries to handle them by projecting or placing them outside themself. This phenomenon is also called projective identification (see Jørgensen, 2018/2019, p. 249 ff.). For example, the predominantly grandiose patient who perceives any sign of vulnerability or doubt as an expression of dangerous and pathetic (shameful) weakness may try to construct a grandiose facade that exudes an image of strength, authority and control. Behind this facade, the patient contains great vulnerability and doubt. However, the patient perceives these feelings as being so dangerous and unacceptable that they must be ejected by being projected onto the therapist. Next, the patient then meets any indication of vulnerability or doubt – or emotional sensitivity – in the therapist with mockery and contempt. The patient thus expresses contempt for what they consider the therapist's 'ridiculous' sensitivity, fragility and incompetence while these qualities in fact mirror parts of the patients own self that the patient struggles to contain and accept and thus feels compelled to split off and project onto the therapist. In concrete terms, the patient may evoke feelings of insecurity and uncertainty in the therapist by, for example, making condescending comments to and devaluing the therapist, threatening to complain about the therapist's alleged callousness and incompetence or acting in intimidating and transgressive ways in interactions with the therapist.

Thus, by listening to the countertransference, therapists can gain insight into key recurring patterns in the patient's object relations, dissociated feelings and parts of the patient that are not integrated into the larger self. However, in order to notice and incorporate these important elements of the patient's difficulties into the treatment, the therapist has to be open. This involves making oneself and one's psychological and emotional sensory capacity available in order to discover what position the patient is unconsciously trying to place the therapist in, through their actions in the therapeutic space. Is the patient trying to position the therapist as the idealized self-object, the inferior and despised object or the empathically mirroring self-object that is to protect and maintain the patient's vulnerable self or admire the patient's grandiose self? What emotions, yearnings and needs is the patient thus bringing into the therapeutic relationship? Does the patient have a strong need to be the dominant, controlling and superior subject in relation to an inferior object that submits to the patient's control and admires the patient's self and accomplishments? If so, how should we understand the patient's choice of seeking to establish this particular object relation constellation in the therapeutic space – what does this give the patient and protect them from? Will it satisfy the patient's need to feel independent and strong – and help them keep their vulnerability and fear of dependence and loss at bay?

Countertransference in different manifestations of narcissism

In the following, as we briefly zoom in on elements of the therapist's countertransference that are commonly seen in work with patients with pathological narcissism, it is important to bear in mind that the bulk of the existing theory and, in particular, empirical evidence in the field is mainly focused on the therapist's countertransference in the encounter with patients with predominantly grandiose manifestations of pathological narcissism. Consequently, this will also be the primary focus, in particular in the following section on empirical studies. Thus, the therapist's countertransference may be different, to varying degrees, when working with patients whose vulnerable manifestations of pathological narcissism are more prominent, although these patients will also have elements of grandiosity. In addition, there is reason to consider how it may impact on the therapist's perception of the patient's transference and their own countertransference if the therapist is trained in – and mainly embraces – either the self psychology tradition, with roots in Kohut's work (see Chapter 3.3), or the tradition of Kernberg's object relations theory (see Chapter 3.4).

Kohut thus encourages the therapist to focus mainly on the patient's internal (personality structure) deficiencies, yearnings, vulnerability and unmet self-object needs as they impact on the patient's transference, the treatment relationship and the therapist's countertransference, while Kernberg focuses much more on the impact of internal conflicts, aggression, envy and split-off parts of the patient's internal object relations on the transference and thus the treatment relationship and the therapist's countertransference. Simply put, therapists who base their work on Kohut's understanding of pathological narcissism will be much more tuned into vulnerable manifestations of pathological narcissism and tend to interpret symptoms of pathological narcissism as expressions of narcissistic vulnerability, while therapists based on Kernberg's interpretation of pathological narcissism will tend to see manifestations of grandiose narcissism and view specific symptoms through that lens. All things being equal, these variations in the understanding of the human psyche and fundamental understanding of what is the basis of the patient's way of acting in the therapeutic space will influence the therapist's countertransference, including the therapist's ability to contain the patient, how much it takes before the therapist feels injured by the patient's devaluation and contempt and so forth.

We should also be cautious about speaking in general terms about countertransference that is assumed to occur in the interaction with all narcissistically disordered patients. Both because there is a big difference in individual patients' transference and thus in the kind of countertransference they will typically activate in the therapist. And also, not least, because there may be considerable individual differences in individual therapists' perceptions of and reactions to a given patient's transference and way of acting in the therapeutic space. As mentioned earlier, the therapist is not just a neutral observer who only has 'objective' reactions and constructs 'objective' interpretations of the patient's way of acting in the therapeutic space. The therapist is inevitably a participant – and an involved subject with their own personal resonance – in the interaction with the patient, and thus the individual therapist's partially subjective inclinations to react in certain ways to the patient's way of being and acting will come into play. For example, there may be a big difference in the therapist's reactions to being intensely idealized versus being met with cold indifference and arrogance by a patient and treated like a soulless object that is solely expected to admire the patient and perform certain particular instrumental functions in the patient's universe.

What will typically be the common core of most therapists' countertransference when they encounter the patients' predominantly grandiose versus vulnerable narcissism is a – perhaps vague and not yet fully understood – feeling of not being seen and treated 'as themselves', let alone as a clearly distinct, equal and autonomous subject. This may be quite provoking and difficult to handle for some therapists, while others have an easier time containing and seeing how these experiences in the countertransference provides insight into the patient's pathology and how it plays out in the patient's interactions with others.

In any case, it is important for the therapist to have a certain insight into themself, their own relational patterns, yearnings, impulses and needs and their tendency to react in certain ways in different situations. This is an important part of the basis for the therapist to engage in qualified reflections on their countertransference and, not least, have nuanced thoughts about which aspects of their countertransference primarily say something about the reactions a given patient typically triggers and encounters in others (objective countertransference) and which aspects have more to do with the therapist themself and are thus less helpful for understanding the patient (subjective countertransference) (Jørgensen, 2018/2019, p. 241ff.). There can never be a categorical distinction between the two types of countertransference, since human interactions are, by definition, shaped by what happens between two subjects. That is not essential. What is essential is for the therapist to remain conscious of this distinction between two kinds of countertransference and continually include it in their reflections on how to understand the individual patient and how the patient's difficulties are embedded in interpersonal patterns – patterns that also play out in the therapeutic space and influence the therapist's own subjective experiences and reactions in the interaction with the patient.

The therapist's reaction to feeling reduced to an object

As underscored by Diamond et al. (2022, p. 28 ff.), among others, some of the traits that set NPD apart from the other PDs – particularly pronounced grandiosity, envy and arrogance – are characterized by not (just) being a problem for the patient but in many cases also for other people around the patient. They also give rise to negative countertransference which the therapist has to make efforts to contain, understand and deal with in order to minimize the risk of it compromising their treatment work. In the contact with a patient with a narcissistic disorder, the therapist may sometimes feel like a faceless spectator to the patient's stories and curated presentation of a self-sufficient self that does not need other people. In this situation, the therapist may struggle with boredom or sleepiness or the urge to withdraw from the patient (Modell, 1986, p. 294).

The therapist may feel reduced to a service function for the patient, with their only role being to listen to, confirm and admire the patient. The therapist does not feel seen and recognized as a real person or an equal subject and may have a sense of contactlessness, as if they are an isolated, barren planet orbiting around the sun (the patient). With Kohut (1971, p. 272), we have reason to consider whether the therapist's own narcissistic needs may make it difficult 'to tolerate a situation in which he is reduced to the seemingly passive role of being the mirror' to the patient's narcissism. It is part of the therapeutic task periodically to contain and accept being reduced to performing certain simple functions for the patient (Kohut, 1971, p. 273). Similarly, at other times, the therapist has to contain and accept the patient's admiration and idealizing transference (Kohut, 1968, p. 106; 1971, p. 264). In these situations, it is hardly just the therapist's technical skills and 'level of professional experience' but also their personality and 'current state of mind' that determines how the therapist responds to the patient's transference in their countertransference (Kohut, 1971, p. 270).

Some therapists may find it difficult to like the predominantly grandiose patient, who primarily meets the therapist with cold arrogance, devaluing and a remarkably self-centred approach to the world (Vater et al., 2013b, p. 609). A patient who for a variety of reasons – including, perhaps, fear of renewed betrayal and abandonment – tries to prevent the therapist from becoming significant to them, may make the therapist feel insignificant and irrelevant to the patient. Similarly, a patient who tries to resist their yearning for and/or fear of becoming dependent on the therapist may make the therapist feel alone, decoupled and without contact with the patient in the therapeutic space (Kernberg, 2018, p. 182). And when a patient meets the therapist with contempt, condescension and intense rejection – repeated rejections of the therapist's invitations to emotional and psychological contact – the therapist may feel an urge to withdraw from the patient (Tanzellini et al., 2017, p. 190). In some cases, this dynamic in the transference may be viewed as an expression of the patient's attack on the good object that, in earlier stages of the patient's life, was found to be unreliable and betrayed or abused the self (Lee & Levy, 2023, p. 186). Furthermore, the therapist's empathy, ability to be present and readiness to listen to what the patient tries to express via various communication channels may be compromised (Colli et al., 2014, p. 106). Most patients will have been victimized in various ways in earlier relationships and will often maintain this role of victimhood in the therapeutic space. Thus, that will be the relational constellation that most therapists are most familiar with in interactions with their patients. This too may make it challenging for many therapists to work with patients with predominantly grandiose narcissism, as their arrogance, contempt and aggressively controlling behaviour makes them appear and act much more as abusers in their interactions with the therapist, not as victims (Luchner, 2013, p. 224).

In extension of previous discussion of the therapist's way of dealing with negative countertransference, there may be reason to reflect specifically on at least two key questions in the encounter with the grandiose patient: what is it that the patient's expressed contempt and arrogance towards the therapist is intended to protect the patient from: what psychological purpose might this way of meeting the world serve for the patient? And is it conceivable that the patient has experience from their own life of being met and treated with contempt and indifference, corresponding to how the patient now meets and treats the therapist? If so, what was that like for the patient, how did the patient react to it? Again, the intention is to triangulate what is playing out in the treatment relationship and to explore possible connections between the patient's current transference (way of acting in interactions with the therapist), key elements of the therapist's countertransference and the patient's relational history.

The therapist's reaction to idealization

The patient's intense idealization may activate the therapist's own narcissism and grandiosity. Some therapists may find this flattering but also slightly uncomfortable (Gabbard & Crisp, 2018, p. 90). Others will feel a more or less unconscious urge to defend against this activation of their own grandiosity by rejecting the patient's idealization in various ways. The therapist may, for example, take on a more 'objective' ('neutral', emotionally withdrawn) and confrontational demeanour and find it difficult to maintain a fundamentally warm, accommodating and personal atmosphere in the therapeutic space (p. 77); 'The rejection may express itself through no more than a slight overobjectivity of the analyst's attitude or a coolness in the analyst's voice; or it may reveal itself in the tendency to be jocular with the admiring patient or to disparage the narcissistic idealization in a humorous and kindly way' (Kohut, 1971, p. 263). Basically, it will be problematic both if the therapist accepts the patient's idealization uncritically – because it produces a positive subjective countertransference and satisfies the therapist's own narcissistic needs – and if the therapist dismisses the patient's idealization without reflecting on it, perhaps because they find it difficult to contain the opposing and, presumably, predominantly negative feelings that it produces in the therapist's countertransference. In either case, the therapist will be at dire risk of losing their ability to maintain their fundamentally psychotherapeutic approach to what is currently playing out in the treatment relationship and of acting out elements of their countertransference in ways that are unhelpful or even harmful to the therapeutic work.

Therapists may differ in their professional opinion about the degree to which it is advisable to contain and accept the patient's idealization and, to varying degrees, satisfy elements of the patient's self-object need for the therapist to be the idealized other (parent imago), or whether the therapist should immediately interpret the patient's idealization as an expression, for example, of the patient's envy or aggression directed at the therapist's function as a therapist – cf. Kernberg's interpretation of the patient's idealization (see Chapter 3.4). In accordance with Kernberg's understanding of pathological narcissism, Diamond et al. (2022, p. 180) argue that, in particular, therapists with their own unresolved narcissistic conflicts (cf. the activation of the therapist's own grandiose narcissism) may be seduced by the narcissistic satisfaction of the patient's idealization and entertain illusory fantasies about the treatment, for example that contact with the therapist in itself can cure pathological narcissism (see Chapter 3.5). Furthermore, when meeting patients who, due to a history of severe neglect and injuries, appear as hurt, helpless victims, the therapist should be mindful of any tendency to meet them with exaggerated care and an urge to protect the patient. If this urge is acted out, it may contain elements of masochistic self-sacrifice and lead to feelings of guilt in the patient who will perceive themself as greedy, demanding and in infinite debt to the therapist (McWilliams, 2011, p. 282).

However, Diamond et al. (2020, p. 180) argue that it is also important for the therapist to perceive what it is the patient, so to speak, attempts to turn them into in their transference – which will also be manifested in the countertransference: what position the therapist is assigned in the patient's currently activated object relation and inner universe in general. Whichever way the therapist chooses to deal with the patient's idealization and the related countertransference, it is crucial to allow it to unfold and to reflect on how this idealization relates to elements of the patient's inner universe and narcissistic pathology as well as how the therapist is affected by and reacts to it. This includes how these reactions may relate to elements of the therapist's own psychology and narcissistic needs.

Studies of typical countertransference when working with NPD

In a number of empirical studies, therapists have been asked to describe their countertransference in interactions with their patients. Typically, the data was collected through self-report questionnaires covering a wide variety of possible forms of countertransference and including an assessment of the degree to which the patient has certain narcissistic traits or meets the formal diagnostic criteria for a personality disorder, including NPD. Most of these studies are only partially based on patients with a formal diagnosis of pathological narcissism and mainly examine possible correlations between the degree of pathological narcissism in the patient and the degree to which the therapist experiences various, primarily problematic forms of countertransference in the work with the patient (Betan et al., 2005; Rosberg et al., 2008; Colli et al., 2014). One study is solely based on therapists' work with patients with NPD (Tanzelli et al., 2017); however, the validity of the NPD diagnoses is difficult to assess. The patients in the other studies have a wide range of diagnoses. Most of the participating therapists are relatively experienced and work with various forms of psychotherapy.

Countertransference characterized by negative affects

Generally, the existing studies show that higher scores on measures of pathological (predominantly grandiose) narcissism are closely associated with the likelihood of therapists reporting a wide range of negative emotions and dynamics in the countertransference. In one study, based on patients with PD, therapists' reported negative countertransference is associated with poorer treatment outcomes (Rossberg et al., 2007). A related study, also based on patients with PD, also found a strong link between therapists experiencing positive emotions in their countertransference – particularly feeling that they are important to the patient – and good treatment outcomes. This latter study also found a strong correlation between negative emotions in the countertransference – particularly feeling inadequate and feeling a need to remain vigilant in the contact with the patient – and poorer treatment outcomes (Rossberg et al., 2008, p. 705). These findings underscores the importance of the therapist noticing which feelings dominate their countertransference and dealing with any negative countertransference.

The most interesting study in this field also sought to identify the most common countertransference emotions in the work with patients with narcissistic pathology. In this study, a small group of therapists reported countertransference emotions in their work with patients with NPD (Betan et al., 2005, p. 895). The most frequently reported countertransference emotions include feeling annoyed with the patient in therapy sessions, feeling used or manipulated and generally mistreated or abused by the patient, losing one's temper in interactions with the patient, feeling dismissed or devalued by the patient, feeling unappreciated by the patient, and worrying about saying the wrong thing that will make the patient explode, fall apart or walk out. The therapists also report that when they check their phone messages, they feel anxiety or dread that there will be a message from the narcissistic patient. At times, they report disliking the patient. They also report at times feeling an urge to say or do something aggressive and critical to the patient and having to make an effort to stop themselves from acting on it. Finally, the study lists the least likely feelings to occur in the countertransference in the treatment of narcissistic patients, based on the therapists' replies. This includes liking the patient very much and feeling compassion for them, looking forward to the sessions with the patient and feeling hopeful about the treatment outcome (p. 895).

Severe pathology related to more difficult countertransference

More generally, the existing studies find a strong correlation between the degree of pathological narcissism in the patient and therapists' likelihood to report countertransference related to feeling criticized and devalued, feeling helpless and inadequate and having angry and hostile feelings towards the patient (Tanzilli et al., 2017, p. 188). Furthermore, pathological narcissism is closely associated with a higher likelihood of feeling disengaged, a lower likelihood of having positive feelings for the patient and a lower likelihood of perceiving the therapeutic work with the patient as satisfying (p. 188). These correlations are stronger when the patient with NPD has comorbid traits from the other three cluster B personality disorders (p. 188), which typically indicates that the patient has a more severe disorder. This finding indirectly supports the clinical experience that more primitive, intense and chaotic transference in more poorly organized patients typically cause much more intense, more fluctuating and more chaotic countertransference, which it can be challenging for the therapist to contain and regulate (Kernberg, 2018, p. 59). In the work with more poorly organized patients, the countertransference may thus take on an intensely real character and be characterized by strong non-symbolized (non-mentalized) affects (beta-elements) and relational patterns or unintegrated elements of archaic object relations (stored in the procedural, not the verbal memory), which makes it harder for the therapist to take a step away from and reflect on the countertransference (Ermann, 2020, p. 124 ff.). This could be, for example, an experience of profound and unbearable loneliness that requires immediate action to escape or a feeling of being naked and defenceless in face of the patient's intense contempt and rage.

In extension of this topic, a study among experienced therapists (n=148), in which a subgroup of patients had narcissistic personality pathology (n=30), found that the more severely disordered the patient is – based on their level of personality organization – the greater is the likelihood that the therapist's countertransference is characterized by helplessness and feelings such as being overwhelmed and struggling to establish a good treatment alliance (Gazzillo et al., 2015, p. 242). The diagnostic assessment used in this study relied on the psychodynamic PDM system, rather than the *DSM* system, and most of the participating patients with narcissistic pathology have predominantly vulnerable manifestations of pathological narcissism. On the other hand, there is reason to assume that in most of the other existing studies, which used the *DSM* system's for the diagnostic assessment of the participating patients, the narcissistic pathology will be characterized by predominantly grandiose manifestations. Thus, it is interesting to note that this study finds that the patient's narcissistic pathology is associated with countertransference that is not only associated with anger and feeling criticized but also with an urge to protect and nurture the patient (p. 242). There is reason to assume that the latter pertains to the more vulnerable manifestations of narcissism in the patients in this study. However, we need more and larger studies before we can reach substantive and empirically founded conclusions about particular forms of countertransference in the work with patients characterized by vulnerable narcissism.

One study based on a broad group of patients in treatment, including patients with PD but only very few with NPD found, unsurprisingly, that a higher level of functioning in the patient is associated with more positive and fewer negative emotions in the countertransference (Colli et al., 2014, p. 104). Conversely, therapists feel more helpless, inadequate and disorganized in the work with lower-functioning patients (p. 105), which presumably includes patients with severe pathological narcissism. Generally, the lower the patient's level of functioning, the greater the risk of the therapist experiencing a wide range of negative emotions in the countertransference. Based on the participating therapists' descriptions of their countertransference in relation to patients with traits of various personality disorders, the authors describe what they view as typical traits of therapists' countertransference when working with patients with NPD. In addition to the above-mentioned tendency to become frustrated and annoyed, this also includes the tendency to feel bored and disengaged – reactions that appear to mirror feelings that are also often seen in patients with NPD – and to feel interchangeable, invisible and deskilled and that they could really be anyone to the patient, both as a person and as a therapist (p. 106).

Finally, therapists were found to associate working with NPD with being frustrated and losing focus during the sessions, so that their mind wanders to things other than what the patient is talking about; being dragged into processes that they are not aware of until after the session, and feeling compelled to set very firm limits with the patient (Tanzilli et al., 2017, p. 191). These are all experiences that suggest a predominantly negative and both personally and professionally demanding countertransference. The same applies, to some extent, to the therapists' reported absence of certain positive feelings in the countertransference when working with NPD, including a perceived urge to protect, to flirt with and become friends with the patient; having parental feelings for the patient, feeling an urge to self-disclose elements of their personal life with the patient and generally liking the patient very much (Tanzilli et al., 2017, p. 191).

The therapist's experiences and professional orientation

Generally, the found connections between the degree of pathological narcissism and countertransference emotions are independent of the participating therapists' theoretical orientation and applied treatment method. Thus, they are not just reported by, for example, psychodynamic therapists, and the participating therapists experience similar patterns of emotions in their countertransference, whether they believe that the phenomenon of countertransference actually exists or not and are trained in noticing and decoding it (Betan et al., 2005, p. 896). Furthermore, a few studies have found indications that the therapist's experience affects the perception of the described emotions in the countertransference. With experience, the therapist's countertransference in the work with patients with NPD becomes less dominated by negative feelings and characterized more by positive ones (Tanzilli et al., 2017, p. 189). This suggests that it will be helpful to refer patients with severe narcissistic pathology to more experienced – and highly specialized – therapists.

In relation to therapists' countertransference and likely stance in the encounter with patients with pathological narcissism, it is worth noting that a study based on a wide group of therapists found that a large majority of the participating professionals felt that it is important to provide treatment to people with NPD (Muir et al., 2021, p. 391). When asked whether they would be willing to work with this patient group themselves, however, the majority of them (78%) report negative or, at best, neutral feelings towards this question, while a little under half (42%) report having clearly negative feelings about the prospect of treating patients with NPD (p. 393). About a third of the respondents have a negative view of this patient group's ability to remain in treatment; cf. the relatively high risk of dropout that has been reported in several studies (see Chapter 4.1). Although the quoted study has some methodological weaknesses, it is worth noting that there are also indications of a certain link between professional expertise in treating NPD and greater confidence that it will be possible to have patients remain in a treatment that will benefit them; thus, therapists who are trained in and have experience with the treatment of NPD have a somewhat more positive view of the treatment prognosis of this group. This too supports the assumption that, whenever possible, the treatment of severe narcissistic pathology should be handled by experienced and specialist psychotherapists.

Psychotherapeutic attitude towards own countertransference

Overall, theoretical reflections, clinical experience and empirical studies all suggest that there is a considerable likelihood that therapists who work with patients characterized by pathological narcissism will experience a wide range of negative countertransference emotions. If the therapist acts out even a small part of this malignant countertransference, or if their behaviour in the interaction with the patient is otherwise – unconsciously, behind their back, so to speak – decisively influenced by negative countertransference aspects that are 'out of control', this may have significantly destructive consequences for the therapeutic process and the patient's ability to benefit of the treatment. More specifically, acting out negative countertransference dimensions may intensify destructive interpersonal processes in the therapeutic space and raise the risk of dropout considerably. There is even reason to fear that the patient will have a negative treatment outcome: that a series of negative relational experiences in the therapy will result in the patient's difficulties having been exacerbated at the conclusion of the treatment. Several researchers have pointed to the countertransference enactments as the most frequent cause when the treatment of pathological narcissism fails (Weinberg & Ronningstam, 2020, p. 134). Countertransference enactment is also inevitable, but, as mentioned above, the key is the therapist's ability to deal with it when it happens.

Without painting an overly grim picture of the possible negative consequences of therapists' lack of awareness about and capacity for dealing with the countertransference in a qualified and professional way, this does point to the key importance of the therapist not only adopting a psychotherapeutic stance in relation to the patient's way of being and acting in the therapeutic space but also to their own way of being and acting in the interaction with the patient. The therapist must always be able to take a step away from their own experiences, feelings and actions in the therapeutic space and reflect on (triangulate) how they may be understood in relation to – and contain significant information about – the patient's difficulties.

They may contain elements of repetition and enactment of relational patterns, powerful affects and yearnings as well as defences against these affects and yearnings, not just from the patient's relational life and history but also from the therapist's own life and history. What the therapist experiences in the countertransference contains important information about the patient's relational patterns, needs and narcissistic defence, just as affects and other mental states that are brought into play in the countertransference may provide an entrance to split-off or non-integrated parts of the patient's self that the patient is not fully aware of, let alone able to address verbally, but which the patient acts out and expresses in other ways through their nonverbal communication in the therapeutic space.

As a general rule, the therapist should always continually monitor their countertransference and use it as a basis for understanding the patient and how elements of the patient's difficulties are re-enacted in the therapeutic space. Ideally, countertransference, particularly negative countertransference, should not be acted out in the interaction with the patient. When it happens anyway, to some extent – which is inevitable, also for the good-enough therapist – the task is to notice and reflect on it, as much as possible, and to consider whether it may be helpful to include some parts of the concrete manifestations of the countertransference in the therapeutic work. This might be done, for example by explicitly addressing one's own concrete (unhelpful) reactions in the interaction with the patient and inviting the patient to speak about their perception of and reaction to them. For example, this may be the therapist who has a sense that he has been dominating recent sessions too much:

> After our last session I had a sense that maybe I was taking up too much room – that what I saw as an attempt to help you put difficult experiences into words might actually have been getting in the way of you having the time to sense and find a way to describe what was happening inside you. Does that make sense to you, and is it maybe something you recognized – both from our last session and perhaps also from other contexts in your life?

Or the therapist who is unsure whether, during their last sessions, he was too insistent in maintaining focus on painful experiences from the patient's life:

> After our last session, I was wondering if maybe, when I was asking about the difficult things you experienced from your former partner, I stayed on that for a little too long, making it uncomfortable and, in a way, invasive for you. Is that how you experienced it?

If the patient replies that she too had a similar experience of what happened during the last session, 'I'm sorry that you felt that I violated your boundaries in a way that was unpleasant for you. Is this an experience that you might recognize from other situations and relationships in your life?'

According to Kohut, the therapist's own unresolved narcissistic dynamics and disorders are perhaps the most significant source of the therapist's unhelpful reactions, particularly to the patient's idealizing transference in the treatment of pathological narcissism. He writes, 'the analyst's major reactions (including his countertransference) in the analysis of narcissistic disorders are rooted in the analyst's own narcissism and, especially, in the area of his own, unresolved narcissistic disturbances' (Kohut, 1971, p. 260). With this argument, Kohut is undoubtedly too radical in his normalization of severe narcissistic pathology. He is also stuck in an untenable one-person psychology, as the therapist's countertransference, remarkably, is traced back solely to the therapist themself. However, monitoring one's own countertransference also always involves continually noting how one's own narcissistic needs and defences may be activated in the therapeutic space, for example in the form of one's own yearnings for certain forms of contact or avoidance of contact, own grandiose perceptions, own narcissistic vulnerability and own perceived narcissistic injuries and defences, which may be activated in one's own attempt to evade and deal with one's own internal and relational processes.

The therapist's own narcissism

When the psychotherapist invests and uses themself in their work, they are very exposed if an intervention fails or is met with strong criticism. The competent psychotherapist has a particular sensitivity to interpersonal interactions, emotional exchanges and nonverbal communication. In many ways, this sort of sensitivity is a gift, but it is also associated with increased narcissistic vulnerability to attacks and injuries from others. This heightened sensitivity may mean that a greater susceptibility to these sorts of injuries and to being emotionally affected by them, particularly if it is not accompanied by a well-developed capacity for having nuanced thoughts about and understanding what can make others act and react the way they do – and about one's own reactions in interactions with patients. To maximize the benefits of therapy, the therapist has to be open to the patient and prepared to engage in deep emotional and psychological contact with them. This is only possible if the therapist is fully and authentically emotionally present and meets the patient with an open face and without significant activated defence strategies.

The therapist should always work from a position of a participating observer in the therapeutic space (see Chapter 4.1), which means being present with one's personal subjectivity and as a professional therapist who regularly takes a step away from and reflects on what is playing out in the relationship with the patient. However, the emotional contact with the patient that is the pivotal point of therapy will always be associated with a heightened level of narcissistic vulnerability, as the therapist's professional – and, to varying degrees, personal – identity and self-esteem may be brought into play and destabilized. This involves a heightened risk that the therapist might react in a way that is not therapeutically helpful in order to protect themself. Furthermore, the therapist should bear in mind that they are not just occupying the role of participating observer but are also being observed – put into the position of observed participant – by the patient, which can also be associated with narcissistic vulnerability and the risk of perceiving oneself as shamefully inadequate in the eyes of the patient's (and oneself).

Naturally, there are considerable individual differences among therapists, including variations in what therapists experience as narcissistic injuries and how strong an urge they might feel to have certain narcissistic needs met in their treatment work. In any case, remaining mindful of the risk that one's own narcissistic vulnerability and narcissistic needs may be activated and brought into play in the therapeutic space is a key part of the therapeutic task. As much as possible, the therapist has to prevent elements of their own narcissism from controlling their work and actions in the interaction with the patient. Again, this underscores the importance that the therapist persistently adopts an empathic but insistent psychotherapeutic stance to themself and their own actions in interactions with the patient.

Opening up and being emotionally present in the contact with the patient makes the therapist more vulnerable to being hurt, disappointed and humiliated by what the patient says, does or does not do (Maroda, 2022, p. 64). The therapist may be vulnerable to – and have difficulty dealing with – not feeling seen, appreciated and recognized as themself, as a person. These experiences may be associated with the therapist's own need to be the good, cherished object, feeling indispensable, omniscient, admired and appreciated by the patient. Investing so much of oneself in the therapeutic work and perceiving it as an important element of one's identity can make the therapist more sensitive to patients who express intense criticism and contempt for their treatment work and for them as a person (Chused, 2012, p. 899).

Other therapists may be more vulnerable to – or tend to be seduced into – uncritically accepting patients' idealization and fantasies about the therapeutic relationship that appeals to their own narcissism in various ways. They may also experience narcissistic injury later in the treatment process, as the patient's idealization wanes and is replaced by a more sober perception of the therapist (Kohut, 1971, p. 233). These types of issues are fairly likely to be actualized in the work with patients with pathological narcissism, including, particularly, patients with pronounced grandiose manifestations of narcissism, who often appear to ignore, look down upon and disparage the therapist, both as a person and as a professional (Luchner, 2013, p. 223). In this situation, the therapist's behaviour towards the patient may then – more or less unconsciously – be shaped or controlled by the therapist's urge to earn the patient's acceptance, recognition or even admiration (p. 223).

Therapists may benefit from reflecting on how they react when subjected to intense criticism from a patient, for example for not paying attention, being insensitive, not listening and 'not having a clue about anything' or for hiding behind a role as a professional therapist and not giving the patient what they explicitly want and believe they need – and feel entitled to. Does the therapist get hurt or defensive or react in ways that demonstrate that they might be more focused on maintaining their own self-image and defending their own destabilized self-esteem? Do they withdraw from contact with the patient, and get defensive – perhaps because they were scared by aggressive and abusive behaviour from the patient that they are not used to? Or do they manage to remain in contact with the patient and explicitly address and explore what it was specifically that brought on this intense criticism? And is the therapist ready, now or a little later, to share some of their own emotional reactions and parts of themself in relation to the patient's stated criticism and contempt – dimensions that may subsequently be used in the treatment work, in part to examine what reactions the patient evokes and encounters from others and what happens in interpersonal interactions generally when strong emotions are in play and people are narcissistically vulnerable?

The best possible way of dealing with an abusive patient who violates personal boundaries – or with an intensely idealizing patient – requires being good enough at preserving one's internal narcissistic balance (professional and personal self-esteem and so forth) in the encounter with these patients. The therapist should also avoid taking various defensive actions in an attempt to restore their destabilized narcissistic balance and, perhaps, their loss of face in relation to the patient. This involves, for example, not apologizing for an intervention that the therapist is convinced was well chosen, if the patient initially responds with intense rejection and aggressive criticism. Instead, the therapist should initially just remark that the patient was very angry about what the therapist said, express that this was not the therapist's intention and then invite the patient to engage in a joint exploration of what it was, specifically, that made the patient so angry and how they might understand this. When the therapist deals with narcissistic injuries and activated feelings of shame in the therapeutic space, they do so with the patient as an observer. The patient observes how the therapist deals with their narcissism and shameful experiences. Thus, the therapist models in vivo how to deal with the sorts of experiences that inevitably occur in interpersonal relationships (Bueckler, 2010, p. 122).

Contact with – and accepting – narcissistic vulnerability and needs

Coming into contact with one's own narcissistic vulnerability and narcissistic needs is a fundamental condition of working as a therapist. This is in no way a problem in itself, provided that it does not control the therapy process. Thus, therapists should not deny manifestations of their own narcissism but instead be open to them and reflect on them. Therapists are human beings with narcissistic (self-object) needs like everyone else, and these needs may be brought into play in the therapeutic space. If we deny this or treat it as taboo, we will only increase the risk of experiencing destructive shame and denying parts of our own subjectivity (Jaenicke, 2023, p. 323 ff.) – and we need to be able to draw on this subjectivity in our treatment work. All things being equal, a greater awareness of our own narcissistic needs will improve our ability to resist temptations to have these needs met by our patients and instead enable us to deal with these needs in other relationships. As therapists, we enhance our ability to function optimally by allowing ourselves to become aware of and explore it when our own narcissistic needs are activated in the therapeutic space – rather than prohibiting ourselves from coming into contact with and seeing these needs as part of our psychological reality (p. 327).

The risk of acting in unhelpful, unprofessional and unacceptable ways as a therapist are not removed by suppressing or denying one's countertransference and own narcissistic needs or striving for extraordinary distance in relation to the patient in an attempt to keep the countertransference down – on the contrary (Gabbard, 2024, p. 394). As therapists, we should instead strive to remain open to and examine our own narcissistic needs and vulnerability and explore how these parts of our selves may become a hindrance in the treatment work when these narcissistic processes are actualized in the therapeutic space. At the same time, we should be mindful of how acknowledging and examining one's own narcissism may be associated with shameful perceptions of being wrong or inadequate in one's work as a therapist. Thus, in practice, it is not always an easy task to acknowledge and reflect on how one's own narcissism pokes its head out in the therapeutic space. Particularly – but far from exclusively – younger and less experienced therapists may perceive their own narcissistic vulnerability as a weakness and a sign of professional deficiencies or of their failure and inadequacy as therapists. This may hamper their ability and readiness to examine what specifically happens in the therapeutic space when their narcissistic vulnerability or sensitivity becomes visible (Maroda, 2022, p. 68 ff.).

The therapist's own feelings of shame

One among many possible indications that the therapist's own shame and narcissism may be at play without the therapist being quite able or willing to acknowledge it is that the therapist keeps remembering and revisiting vaguely unpleasant or apparently emotionally significant experiences and patterns in the work with a patient without really reflecting on what this might be about. Another sign is if the therapist experiences recurring challenges in their work with a patient without addressing this in their supervision, even though they know, deep down, that they ought to. This is aligned with John Steiner's description of how we can turn a blind eye and deny parts of reality that we sensed but try to keep at a distance because they involve our own narcissism and are thus anxiety-provoking (see Chapter 3.6). If a therapist avoids bringing their own professional missteps and countertransference up in their supervision, this may be a sign that their own narcissism is in play. If a therapist tends to explain a patient's sudden dropout from treatment or prolonged lack of progress solely with reference to the patient's pathology or lack of treatment motivation – without considering possible problems in the treatment and their own role in them – this, too, may be an indication that the therapist is trying to protect their own narcissism (Chused, 2012, p. 908; Luchner, 2013, p. 228; Dittrich, 2024, p. 417 ff.). These dynamics stand in the way of the therapist's ability to reflect on and learn what they might have done differently in the work with a specific patient.

To become narcissistically injured and vulnerable in the therapeutic space is only really problematic when the therapist does not recognize or tolerate it. In that case, these narcissistic processes are denied, repressed, 'go underground' and may begin to control the therapist's actions behind their back, so to speak (Maroda, 2022, p. 66). Naturally, it is also not problematic in itself if the therapist perceives great joy and satisfaction in their work as a psychotherapist and if this in itself promotes their professional and personal self-esteem. In this sense, there is nothing problematic about having certain, more mature narcissistic needs met through one's work. However, it becomes a problem if the therapist needs to have more archaic narcissistic (self-object) needs met, for example being admired, idealized and very explicitly validated by their patients – and if the satisfaction of any of the therapist's needs happens at the expense of the patients (Maroda, 2022, p. 75).

More generally, pronounced narcissistic traits and self-perceptions in the therapist may increase the risk of sexual and other forms of transgressive behaviour and violations of the therapeutic framework. This includes the notion that standard ethical norms and rules do not fully apply to oneself, perhaps because the therapist believes that their extensive experience and expertise allow for special privileges. It may also happen because similar omnipotent perceptions of the therapist's own psychotherapeutic competencies 'convince' the therapist that it is acceptable to introduce highly 'unorthodox methods' into the treatment (Dittrich, 2024, p. 417 ff.; Gabbard, 2024, p. 387).

Furthermore, there are many needs that may prove problematic if they are too dominant in the therapist; for example, a therapist's need to be and be seen as the infinitely good and helpful Samaritan, the resilient therapist who is capable of containing and handling anything the patients might say or do, the very sensitive therapist who senses and sees everything in their patients, the insightful therapist who immediately grasps everything that is playing out in the therapeutic space, or the uniquely competent therapist capable of curing patients with virtually any form of psychological disorder. These types of obviously unrealistic perceptions, which are not necessarily fully conscious, may be associated with unrealistic ego ideals and may in that sense be embedded in more extensive narcissistic issues in the therapist. In any case, they will increase the risk that the therapist will perceive themself as shamefully inadequate when encountering the reality of the treatment work.

People who have made it their profession to help others will often, from an early age, have attained a position in their family and other social contexts where they have learned to read others' needs, decode how others feel and help persons who are struggling. This may contribute to the development of a level of emotional and relational empathy, sensitivity and responsiveness that is invaluable in many ways, not just in psychotherapeutic work. However, these same early experiences may also have taught the person to ignore or deny their own vulnerability and emotional needs, perhaps because there was no room for these parts of the self, let alone anyone else who might see and satisfy them. These internal psychological dynamics can lead to increased vulnerability to grandiose self-perceptions and unrealistic notions of one's own ability to solve any problem that the patient might present. This may make the therapist particularly susceptible to certain forms of idealization from the patient with the associated risk of failing to notice and instead playing along with this idealization rather than using it as a basis for understanding and helping the patient (Chused, 2012, p. 909). It may also be associated with a heightened risk of burnout.

Healthy vs problematic narcissism in the therapist

As in many other contexts, we need to distinguish between healthy and more problematic or actual pathological narcissism. Healthy narcissism in the therapist is defined, in part, by basically stable self-esteem that is realistically attuned to the self's actual characteristics and skills. This provides the foundation of strong and reality-based confidence in one's own professional competencies in combination with persistent critical reflection on one's own treatment work (Jørgensen, 2019). Without going overboard into grandiose self-sufficiency and disinterest in the patients' critic reactions to the self's way of being and acting in the psychotherapeutic space, healthy narcissism is associated with basic tolerance of and nurture for one's own self and inevitable missteps as a therapist. Moreover, these missteps are recognized and made the subject of professional reflection; cf. healthy doubt about and continual reflection on one's own professional work (see Nissen-Lie et al., 2017, p. 56).

This will help enable the therapist to deal with professional challenges – perceived criticism, contempt and devaluation as well as professional setbacks and failures – in the meeting with severely disorders patients. It will also help the therapist to strike a suitable balance in containing and reflecting on their own professional shortcomings, missteps and setbacks without falling into either excessive self-blame, self-contempt or grandiose defence strategies (Chused, 2012, p. 912). A therapist with healthy manifestations of narcissism is emotionally well prepared to deal with long periods of harsh criticism and a lack of recognition and validation from the patient without resorting to either feigned stoical impassiveness or profound doubt in their own abilities. They will also be equipped to preserve their ability continually to take a step away from and reflect on what it is that is playing out in the patient and in the therapeutic space that is causing the patient to be so critical and dismissive in the interpersonal contact – as well as how this might be related to the therapist's own actions in the therapeutic space, given that the therapist cannot legitimately protect their own narcissism by making themself impervious to criticism.

Healthy narcissism may also be an important driver in the work with more severely disordered patients. In this work, it is important that the therapist manages to preserve hope and faith in their own ability to help the patient – even during periods when the patient may be struggling or even deteriorating and is close to losing confidence in the treatment or treats any form of hope, in both themself and the therapist, with contempt, as a sign of naivety and weakness (Chused, 2012, p. 908). Furthermore, healthy narcissism also helps the therapist to accept that there may be times when the therapist does not fully understand what is playing out in the patient and in the therapeutic space or exactly where the therapeutic process is currently headed. The ability to contain and accept this uncertainty as a fundamental condition of therapeutic work with severely disordered patients is precisely what enables the therapist to remain confident that they are doing what it takes for the therapeutic process to be fruitful for the patient and to preserve their ability to reflect and engage in psychotherapeutic work. It enables the therapist to maintain the fundamental psychotherapeutic stance.

References

Abraham, K. (1999). Über eine besondere Form des neurotischen Widerstand Gegen die psychoanalytische Methodik [Of a particular form of neurotic resistance to the psychoanalytic method]. In K. Abraham (Ed.), *Psychoanalytische Studien*, vol. II (pp. 254–262). Psychosozial-Verlag. (Original work published 1919)

Alnæs, R., & Høglend, P. (1985). Overføring og motstand i behandling av patienter med narsisistiske personlighetsforstyrrelser [Transference and resistance in the treatment of patients with narcissistic personality disorders]. *Nordisk Psykiatrisk Tidsskrift*, 39, 119–127.

Altmeyer, M. (2003). *Im Spiegel des Anderen: Anwendungen einer relationalen Psychoanalyse* [In the mirror of the other: Applications of a relational psychoanalysis]. Psychosozial Verlag.

Balint, M. (1968). *The basic fault: Therapeutic aspects of regression*. Northwestern University Press.

Bateman, A. W. (1998). Thick- and Thin-skinned organizations and enactment I borderline and narcissistic disorders. *International Journal of Psychoanalysis*, 79, 13–25.

Bateman, A., & Fonagy, P. (2004). *Psychotherapy for borderline personality disorder: Mentalization-based treatment*. Oxford University Press.

Bateman, A., & Fonagy, P. (2016). *Mentalization-based treatment for personality disorders: A practical guide*. Oxford University Press.

Betan, E., Heim, A. K., Conklin, C. Z., & Westen, D. (2005). Countertransference phenomena and personality pathology in clinical practice: An empirical investigation. *American Journal of Psychiatry*, 162, 890–892.

Bion, W. R. (1967). *Second thoughts: Selected papers on psychoanalysis*. Karnac Books.

Bolm, T. (2021). Mentalisierungsbasierte Therapie für Patienten mit narzisstischer Persönlichkeitsstörung [Mentalization-based therapy for patients with narcissistic personality disorder]. In S. Doering, H.-P. Hartmann, & O. F. Kernberg (Eds.), *Narzisssmus: Grundlagen, Störungsbilder, Therapie* (2nd ed., pp. 658–668). Schattauer Verlag.

Boyer, M. F. M. (2022). Rupture or disruption: Identity diffusion and the therapeutic relationship. *Contemporary Psychoanalysis*, 58, 545–578.

Bradley, R., Heim, A. K., & Westen, D. (2005). Transference patterns in the psychotherapy of personality disorders: Empirical investigation. *British Journal of Psychiatry*, 186, 342–349.

Brauner, F., Müller, S., & Benecke, C. (2021). Scham, Neid und Wut – die zentralen Affekte des Narzissmus [Shame, envy and anger – the central affects of narcissism]. In S. Doering, H.-P. Hartmann, & O.F. Kernberg (Eds.), *Narzisssmus. Grundlagen, Störungsbilder, Therapie* (2nd ed., pp. 317–328). Schattauer Verlag.

Britton, R. (1998). *Belief and Imagination: Explorations in psychoanalysis*. Routledge.

Bromberg, P. M. (1998). *Standing in the spaces: Essays on clinical process, trauma and dissociation*. Analytic Press.

Broucek, F. J. (1982). Shame and its relationship to early narcissistic developments. *International Journal of Psychoanalysis*, 63, 369–378.

Bueckler, S. (2010). Overcoming our pride in the treatment of narcissistic patients. *International Forum of Psychoanalysis*, 19, 120–124.

Caligor, E., Levy, K. N., & Yeomans, F. E. (2015). Narcissistic personality disorders: Diagnostic and clinical challenges. *American Journal of Psychiatry*, 172, 415–422.

Caligor, E., & Stern, B. L. (2020). Diagnosis, classification, and assessment of narcissistic personality disorder within the framework of object relations theory. *Journal of Personality Disorders*, 34, 104–121.

Choi-Kain, L. (2020). Narcissistic personality disorder: A coming of age. *Journal of Personality Disorders*, 34, 210–213.

Choi-Kain, L. W., Simonsen, S., & Euler, S. (2022). A mentalizing approach for narcissistic personality disorder: Moving from 'me-mode' to 'we-mode'. *American Journal of Psychotherapy*, 75, 38–43.

Chused, J. F. (2012). The analyst's narcissism. *Journal of American Psychoanalytic Association*, 60, 899–915.

Colli, A., Tanzilli, A., Dimaggio, G., & Lingiardi, V. (2014). Patient personality and therapist response: An empirical investigation. *American Journal of Psychiatry*, 171, 102–108.

Crisp, H., & Gabbard, G. O. (2020). Principles of psychodynamic treatment for patients with narcissistic personality disorder. *Journal of Personality Disorders*, 34, 143–158.

DeYoung, P. (2022). *Understanding and treating chronic shame: Healing right brain relational trauma*. Routledge.

Diamond, D., Yeomans, F. E., Stern, B. L., & Kernberg, O. F. (2022). *Treating pathological narcissism with transference-focused psychotherapy*. Guilford.

Dimaggio, G. (2022). Treatment principles for pathological narcissism and narcissistic personality disorder. *Journal of Psychotherapy Integration*, 32, 408–425.

Dimaggio, G., & Attina, G. (2012). Metacognitive interpersonal therapy for narcissistic personality disorder and associated perfectionism. *Journal of Clinical Psychology*, 68, 922–934.

Dittrich, K. A. (2024). Die Zerstörung des analytischen Raumes in der Dynamik zwischen Marilyn Monroe und Ralph Greenson [The destruction of the analytical space in the dynamic between Marilyn Monroe and Ralph Greenson]. *Psyche. Zeitschrift für Psychoanalyse*, 78, 399–428.

Drozek, R. P., & Unruh, B. T. (2020). Mentalization-based treatment for pathological narcissism. *Journal of Personality Disorders*, 34, 177–203.

Drozek, R. P., Unruh, B. T., & Bateman, A. (2023). *Mentalization-based treatment of pathological narcissism*. Oxford University Press.

Ellison, W. E., Levy, K. N., Cain, N. M., Ansell, E. B., & Pincus, A. L. (2013). The impact of pathological narcissism on psychotherapy utilization, initial symptom severity, and early-treatment symptom change: A naturalistic investigation. *Journal of Personality Assessment*, 95, 291–300.

Ermann, M. (2020). *Narzissmus: Vom Mythos zur Psychoanalyses des Selbst* [Narcissism: From myth to psychoanalysis of the self]. Kohlhammer.

Fjermestad-Noll, J., Ronningstam, E., Bach, B., Storebø, O.J., Rosenbaum, B., & Simonsen, E. (2020b). Psychotherapeutic treatment of depressive symptoms in patients with narcissistic disturbances: A review. *Journal of Contemporary Psychotherapy*, 50, 21–28.

Freud, S. (1957c). *The dynamics of transference*. In J. Strachey (Ed. & Trans.), *The standard edition of the complete psychological works of Sigmund Freud* (Vol. XII, pp. 97–108). Hogarth. (Original work published 1912)

Freud, S. (1957d). The future prospects of psycho-analytic therapy. In J. Strachey (Ed. & Trans.), *The standard edition of the complete psychological works of Sigmund Freud* (Vol. XI, pp. 139–152). Hogarth. (Original work published in 1910)

Gabbard, G. O. (2024). Sexuelle Grenzverletzungen in der Psychoanalyse: Ein Rückblick auf 30 Jahre [Sexual boundary violations in psychoanalysis: A 30-year retrospective]. *Psyche. Zeitschrift für Psychoanalyse*, 78, 377–397.

Gabbard, G. O., & Crisp, H. (2018). *Narcissism and its discontents: Diagnostic dilemmas and treatment strategies with narcissistic patients*. American Psychiatric Publishing.

Gamache, D., Savard, C., Lemelin, S., & Villeneuve, E. (2017). Development and validation of the treatment attrition-retention scale for personality disorders. *Journal of Personality Disorders*, 31, 753–773.

Gazzillo, F., Lingiardi, V., Corno, F., Genova, F., Bornstein, R. F., Gordon, R. M., & McWilliams, N. (2015). Clinicians' emotional responses and psychodynamic diagnostic model adult personality disorders: A clinically relevant empirical investigation. *Psychotherapy*, 52, 238–246.

Green, A. (2004). *Die tote Mutter: Psychoanalytische Studien zu Lebensnarzissmus und Todesnarzissmus* [The dead mother: Psychoanalytic studies on life narcissism and death narcissism] (E. Wolff & E. Kittler, Trans). Psychosozial Verlag.

Grieser, J. (2015). *Triangulierung* [Triangulation]. Psychosozial Verlag.

Hilsenroth, S., Hamilton-Giachritsis, C., Garner, E., & Walker, J. (1998). The effects of DSM-IV cluster B personality disorder symptoms on the termination and continuation of psychotherapy. *Psychotherapy*, 35, 163–176.

Jaenicke, C. (2023). Eine inersubjektive Untersuchung der Bedürfniss der Psychotherapeuten. In M. Klöpper (Ed.). *Emotional – Refleksiv – Implicit. Wie wir in psychodynamischen Prozessen wirksam werden*. (pp. 323–338). Klett-Cotta Verlag.

Jørgensen, C. R. (2009). *Personlighedsforstyrrelser: Moderne relationel forståelse og behandling af borderlinelidelser* [Personality disorders: Modern relational understanding and treatment of borderline disorders] (2nd ed.). Hans Reitzels Forlag.

Jørgensen, C. R. (2019). *The psychotherapeutic stance* (D. Silver, Trans.). Springer. (Original work published 2018).

Jørgensen, C. R. (2024). *Understanding and working with shame: Psychotherapeutic, cultural and philosophical perspectives* (D. Silver, Trans.). Routledge. (Original work published 2023)

Karterud, S. (1995). *Fra narcissisme til selvpsykologi: En innføring i Heinz Kohuts forfatterskap* [From narcissism to self psychology: An introduction to Heinz Kohut's writings]. Ad Notam Gyldendal.

Kernberg, O. F. (1975). *Borderline conditions and pathological narcissism*. Jason Aronson.

Kernberg, O. F. (1984). *Severe personality disorders*. Yale University Press.

Kernberg, O. F. (2014). An overview of the treatment for severe narcissistic pathology. *International Journal of Psychoanalysis*, 95, 865–888.

Kernberg, O. F. (2018). *Treatment of severe personality disorders: Resolution of aggression and recovery from eroticism*. American Psychiatric Association Publishing.

Kernberg, O. F. (2019). Therapeutic implications of transference structures in various personality pathologies. *Journal of the American Psychoanalytic Association*, 67, 951–986.

Klein, M. (1975). Notes on some schizoid mechanisms. In *Envy and gratitude and other works 1946–1963* (pp. 1–24). (Original work published 1946)

Kohut, H. (1968). The psychoanalytic treatment of narcissistic personality disorders. *The Psychoanalytic Study of the Child*, 23, 86–113.

Kohut, H. (1971). *The analysis of the self*. The University of Chicago Press.

Kohut, H. (1977). *The restoration of the self*. The University of Chicago Press.

Kohut, H., & Wolf, E. (1978). The disorders of the self and their treatment: An outline. *International Journal of Psychoanalysis*, 59, 413–425.

Lecours, S., Briand-Malenfant, R., & Descheneaux, E. (2013). Affect regulation and mentalization in narcissistic personality disorder. In J. S. Ogrodniczuk (Ed.), *Understanding and Treating Pathological Narcissism*. American Psychological Association, 129–145.

Lee, T., & Levy, K.N. (2023). Treating narcissistic personality disorders: A case illustration of key contributions from TFP for psychoanalytic practitioners. *Psychoanalytic Psychotherapy*, 37, 179–192.

Lenzenweger, M. F, Clarkin J. F., Caligor, E., Cain, N. M., & Kernberg, O. F. (2018). Malignant narcissism in relation to clinical change in borderline personality disorder. An explorative study. *Psychopathology*, 51, 318–325.

Levy, K. N. (2012). Subtypes, dimensions, levels, and mental states in narcissism and narcissistic personality disorder. *Journal of Clinical Psychology: In session*, 68, 886–897.

Levy, K. N., Clarkin, J. F., & Crow, T. M. (2021). Narzisstische Persönlichkeitsstörung: Prävalenz und Verlauf [Narcissistic personality disorder: Prevalence and course]. In S. Doering, H.-P. Hartmann, & O. F. Kernberg (Eds.), *Narzisssmus: Grundlagen, Störungsbilder, Therapie* (2nd ed., pp. 189–200). Schattauer Verlag.

Lieberman, D. L. (2013). Kohut's self psychology approach to treating pathological narcissism. In J.S. Ogrodnickzuk (Ed.), *Understanding and treating pathological narcissism* (pp. 253–268). American Psychological Association.

Luchner, A. (2013). Maintaining boundaries in the treatment of pathological narcissism. In J. S. Ogrodniczuk (Ed.), *Understanding and treating pathological narcissism* (pp. 219–233). American Psychological Association.

Maroda, K. J. (2022). *The analyst's vulnerability: Impact on theory and practice*. Routledge.

McWilliams, N. (1994). *Psychoanalytic diagnosis*. Guilford.

Modell, A. H. (1975). A narcissistic defence against affects and the illusion of self-sufficiency. *International Journal of Psychoanalysis*, 56, 275–282.

Modell, A.H. (1976). The holding environment and the therapeutic action of psychoanalysis. *Journal of the American Psychoanalytic Association*, 24, 285–307.

Modell, A. H. (1980). Affects and their non-communication. *International Journal of Psychoanalysis*, 61, 259–267.

Modell, A. H. (1986). A narcissistic defence against affects and the illusion of self-sufficiency. In A. P. Morrison (Ed.), *Essential Papers on Narcissism*. New York University Press, 293–307.

Modell, A.H. (1991). Resistance to the exposure of the private self. *Contemporary Psychoanalysis*, 27, 731–736.

Morrison, A. P. (1986). Shame, ideal self, and narcissism. In A. P. Morrison (Ed.), *Essential papers on narcissism* (pp. 348–371). New York University Press.

Morrison, A. P., & Stolorow, R.D. (1997). Shame, narcissism, and intersubjectivity. In M. R. Lansky & A. P. Morrison (Eds.), *The widening scope of shame* (pp. 63–87). Psychology Press.

Nathanson, D.L. (1994). Shame, compassion, and the borderline personality. *Psychiatric Clinics of North America*, 17, 785–810.

Nissen-Lie, H. A., Rønnestad, M. H., Høglend, P. A., Havik, O. E., Solbakken, O. A., Stiles, T. S., & Monsen, J. T. (2017). Love yourself as a person, doubt yourself as a therapist. *Clinical Psychology and Psychotherapy*, 24, 48–60.

Pulver, S. E. (1986 [1970]). Narcissism: The term and the concept. In A. P. Morrison (Ed.), *Essential papers on narcissism* (pp. 91–111). New York University Press.

Ritter, K., Vater, A., Rüsch, N., Schröder-Abé, M., Schütz, A., Fydrich, T., Lammers, C. H., & Roepke, S. (2014). Shame in patients with narcissistic personality disorder. *Psychiatry Research*, 215, 429–437.

Ronningstam, E. (2022). Narcissistic personality disorder. In S. K. Huprich (Ed.), *Personality disorders and pathology: Integrating clinical assessment and practice in the DSM-5 and ICD-11 era* (pp. 375–389). American Psychological Association.

Ronningstam, E., & Weinberg, I. (2023). Narcissistic personality disorder: Patterns, processes, and indicators of change in long-term psychotherapy. *Journal of Personality Disorders*, 37, 337–357.

Rossberg, J. I., Karterud, S., Pedersen, G., & Friis, S. (2008). Specific personality traits evoke different countertransference reactions. An empirical study. *The Journal of Nervous and Mental Disease*, 196, 702–708.

Rosenfeld, H. (1971). A clinical approach to the psychoanalytic theory of life and death instincts: An investigation into the aggressive aspects of narcissism. *International Journal of Psychoanalysis*, 52, 169–181.

Sandler, J., Dare, C., & Holder, A. (1979). *The patient and the analyst*. Karnac.

Schalkwijk, F., Luyten, P., Ingenhoven, T., & Dekker, J. (2021). Narcissistic personality disorder: Are psychodynamic theories and the alternative DSM-5 model for personality disorders finally going to meet? *Frontiers in Psychology*, 12, 676733.

Steiner, J. (1993). *Psychic retreats: Pathological organizations in psychotic, neurotic and borderline patients*. Routledge.

Steiner, J. (2006). Seeing and being seen: Narcissistic pride and narcissistic humiliation. *International Journal of Psychoanalysis*, 87, 939–951.

Steiner, J. (2014). *Seelische Rückzugsorte verlassen. Therapeutische Schritte zur Aufgabe der Borderline-position* [Leaving psychic retreats: Therapeutic steps to abandon the borderline position]. Klett-Cotta.

Steiner, J. (2020). *Illusion, disillusion, and irony in psychoanalysis*. Routledge.

Symington, N. (1993). *Narcissism: A new theory*. Karnac.

Tanzelli, A., Muzi, L., Ronningstam, E., & Lingiardi, V. (2017). Countertransference when working with narcissistic personality disorder: An empirical investigation. *Psychotherapy*, 54, 184–194.

Vater, A., Roepke, S., Ritter, K., & Lammers, C.-H. (2013b). Narzisstische Persönlichkeitsstörung. Forschung, Diagnose und Psychotherapie [Narcissistic personality disorder: Research, diagnosis, and psychotherapy]. *Psychotherapeut*, 6, 599–615.

Volkan, V. (1979). The 'glass bubble' of the narcissistic patient. In J. Leboit & A. Capponi (Eds.), *Advances in psychotherapy for the borderline patient* (pp. 405–431). Jason Aronson.

Walter, M., & Bilke-Hentsch, O. (2020). *Narzissmus: Grundlagen, Formen, Interventionen* [Narcissism: Foundations, forms, interventions]. Kohlhammer.

Weinberg, I., & Ronningstam, E. (2020). Dos and don'ts in treatments of patients with narcissistic personality disorder. *Journal of Personality Disorders*, 34, 122–142.

Weiss, H. (2012). Utopien und Dystopien als Orte des seelischen Rückzugs [Utopias and dystopias as places of spiritual retreat]. *Psyche*, 66, 310–330.

Wolf, E. S. (1996). *Theorie und Praxis der psychoanalytischen Selbstpsychologie* [Theory and practice of psychoanalytic self psychology]. Suhrkamp Verlag.

Wurmser, L. (1987). Shame: The veiled companion of narcissism. In D. L. Nathanson (Ed.), *The many faces of shame* (pp. 64–92). Guilford.

Yakeley, J. (2018). Current understanding of narcissism and narcissistic personality disorder. *BJPsych Advances*, 24, 305–315.

Yeomans, F., Clarkin, J.F., & Kernberg, O. F. (2015). *Transference-focused psychotherapy for borderline personality disorder: A clinical guide*. American Psychiatric Publishing.

Young, J. E., & Flanagan, C. (2000). Schema-focused therapy for narcissistic patients. In E. F. Ronningstam (Ed.), *Disorders of Narcissism. Diagnostic, clinical, and empirical implications* (pp. 239–268). American Psychiatric Press.

Young, J. E., Klosko, J. S., & Weishaar, M. E. (2006). *Schema therapy: A practioner's guide*. Guilford.

5 Conclusion

This is a fake heading: delete at typesetting stage

In recent years, narcissism has been the subject of dramatically growing attention in the fields of psychology and psychiatry. It is a large and professionally highly interesting area with countless outstanding tasks and unanswered questions as well as a need for considerable professional clarification of the use of the term. During the 1970s and 1980s, the concept of narcissism came into widespread use. Applying an understanding of narcissism that must be characterized as vague at best, conservative culture critics in particular challenged what they saw as a new socialization practice that allegedly promoted the rise of narcissism among young people and the growth of a narcissistic culture. After this time, the concept all but disappeared from the public debate for a couple of decades, until its renaissance in recent years, when it has been used, in part, for the moral condemnation of persons and behaviours that are labelled as narcissistic, again without a precise definition of the concept.

As discussed in previous chapters, we need a more precise use of the term 'narcissism', moving away from the strong tendency to conflate what we might call healthy, adaptive or varying degrees of normal narcissism with severe personality pathology – clearly pathological narcissism – and we should seriously consider whether the concept of narcissism should be reserved for pathological conditions. At the very least, we need to get better at distinguishing between relatively trivial and clearly non-pathological – but in some cases perhaps somewhat repugnant or morally reprehensible narcissistic traits/behaviours – and clearly pathological narcissism. This should in no way be seen as an attempt to define or marginalize persons with pathological narcissism as radically different or 'non-human' (cf. 'othering'). Instead, it represents an effort to maintain – and take seriously – that individuals with pathological narcissism have certain psychological challenges that are qualitatively different and far more serious than more common narcissistic traits, which are not necessarily problematic and often associated with good mental health. We should also consider how behaviour driven by narcissistic traits and processes may be troubling to others – and subject them to various forms of intimidation and

DOI: 10.4324/9781003744962-5

injuries – even while the self perceives their own behaviour as unproblematic or even legitimate and appropriate.

It is remarkable that we generally seem inclined to perceive individuals with grandiose narcissism as more interesting and attractive, in part because they are typically extrovert, charismatic and express great confidence; these are all traits that may initially be seductive and difficult to resist (Lunbeck, 2014, p. 253 ff.). It is only upon closer contact, as we get to know them better, that we notice what may lie behind the grandiose facade. However, as long as they do not have an actual psychological disorder, meaning that they have poor psychosocial functioning and are in need of help – maybe psychiatric treatment – and harm people around them, perhaps we should not refer to them as 'narcissists'? Even though we will always face the challenge of where exactly to draw the line between what this book has described as healthy or normal narcissism and accentuated narcissistic traits versus pathological narcissism that requires treatment, it would arguably be helpful to develop a somewhat narrower and more clearly defined concept of narcissism, including a clearer demarcation from the problematic use of the concept of narcissism in social and personality psychology.

Directing your gaze at yourself and your own inner life and taking an interest in who you are and how you appear, act and are perceived by others may be described as narcissistic, in the sense that, to some degree, you are expending your mental energy on yourself rather than focusing on others and the world around you. What separates what we have so far referred to as healthy narcissism from the pathological variant is the ability to alternate between taking an interest in your own inner life and using this as a basis – and a precondition – of establishing deeper psychological and emotional contact with others and taking an interest in the external world, including what is bigger than us. Healthy and mature narcissism – and an interest in your own inner psychological and relational life – may serve as a basis of psychological growth and continued development of the ability to establish and be in contact with others and being open to the world. By contrast, pathological narcissism is an escape from contact and the external world, with exaggerated attention to your own self and how it is perceived by others, in an attempt to protect a vulnerable self that, in practice, blocks the self's ability to see and meet the world and other people (Parsons, 2022, p. 180). A self with healthy narcissism – balanced self-esteem and a nuanced self-image – is in contact with its own inner world and is able to move flexibly in and out of contact with both self and others – an ability that is disturbed in pathological narcissism.

Need for a revised diagnosis of NPD and qualitative studies

If we are to continue to apply categorical psychiatric diagnoses, we also need fundamental changes to the current diagnosis of NPD, which is much too narrowly defined and only includes grandiose manifestations of NPD but completely ignores the fairly common vulnerable manifestations of pathological narcissism. From a dynamic psychological perspective, pathological narcissism goes far beyond the NPD diagnosis in the *DSM* system and may co-exist, to varying degrees, in connection with a wide range of more severe psychological disorders, particularly including individuals with a personality organized at borderline level as defined by Kernberg (1984). It may thus be relevant to include the points of this book in the understanding and treatment of any form of personality pathology, not just NPD.

Ideally, we should first agree on a common definition of narcissism, including pathological narcissism and its basic elements, that includes both vulnerable and grandiose manifestations. This definition should also addresses how appearances can often be deceptive in people with grandiosity, whose self-assertive and perhaps superficially charismatic facade typically hides an unstable self-image and fragile self-esteem that are deeply dependent on persistent admiration and confirmation from others. In relation to this point, it is important to distinguish between what we might call the core of narcissism and the potential sequelae of pathological narcissism, for example dissocial behaviour. Only then – after we have established a form of professional consensus about what is the dynamic core of pathological narcissism – can we develop valid, concrete criteria for capturing pathological narcissism in diagnostic assessments. In these assessments, simply adding up diagnostic criteria can never stand alone and should be accompanied by a deeper and more nuanced understanding of the individual, for example in the form of a dynamic case formulation. Such a theoretically grounded multi-stage strategy may enable us to stop excluding key manifestations of pathological narcissism – based on legitimate but secondary regard for the precision of differential diagnostics – just as we will be able to limit unhelpful circular reasoning, such as, once we have defined NPD through a number of specific diagnostic criteria, we can conclude that the particular individuals – and only these individuals – who meet these criteria have a narcissistic personality disorder. This approach simply does not reflect the clinical reality, and as a result, individuals with pathological narcissism may be given diagnoses that fail or, at best, only partially capture the core of their difficulties, such as evasive and mixed PD or social phobia.

So far, the field of narcissism has had a remarkably strong emphasis on quantitative studies predominantly based on convenience samples of university students and other non-clinical populations. Based on typically fairly simple questionnaires for self-reporting narcissistic traits, these studies have attempted to document various elements of narcissism and their connection to various psychosocial challenges. Subsequently, these studies have been used, often with limited reflection, as a basis for understanding people with severely pathological narcissism. This involves generalizing data collected in one context and one population to apply to a different context and a group of people who, by all indications, face inherently different challenges, and may thus be quite problematic.

We need a heightened priority on research into pathological narcissism, including in particular the predominantly vulnerable manifestations of NPD and their psychotherapeutic treatment. We need a deeper understanding of the phenomenology of pathological narcissism – how are narcissistic disturbances expressed in the subjective experiences of the individual? And we need to explore the dynamic psychological connections between different elements of pathological narcissism, including, in particular, how vulnerable and grandiose manifestations of pathological narcissism are interrelated: how omnipotent self-perceptions and grandiose behaviour may be attempts to keep psychologically painful elements of narcissistic vulnerability in check and may also contribute to undermining relationships and thus exacerbating the narcissistic disorder and worsening the psychological pain in the people affected by pathological narcissism.

The significance of gender

With the feminist psychoanalyst Lynne Layton (1998, 2020), it can be argued that there is also a need to explore the significance of gender and possible gender differences in the development of and diverse manifestations of pathological narcissism. As mentioned earlier, prevalence studies based on the *DSM* system have found that NPD is more common in men than in women. However, there is reason to assume that this is in part related to the chosen diagnostic criteria and to the definition of NPD in the *DSM*, which does not include more vulnerable manifestations of pathological narcissism. Gender inequality, gender-based distribution of household work, gender-based socialization, differences in the cultural representations of men and women that individual children and young people may feel are misaligned with how they view themselves and their subjectively perceived gender identity – their 'true self' – which, thus, is not seen, represented and recognized may influence the development of pathological narcissism and, not least, how the narcissistic core pathology manifests itself in the individual's self-perception and behaviour. Layton (1998, p. 33 ff.) speaks of classic binary and hegemonic perceptions of masculinity and femininity that may contribute to gendered manifestations of pathological narcissism – and to disturbances in the capacity for mature dependence and the balanced separation of self and others that Layton (2020, p. 237) considers key elements of narcissistic disorders.

Even though this is an area of modern culture that has undergone considerable change, particularly in recent decades, prevailing perceptions of masculinity still mainly centre on notions of a degree of agency, autonomy, strength and self-reliance, while emotional needs and parts of the self that are associated with vulnerability and dependence on others may be split off – which are all features that are associated with more grandiose manifestations of narcissism. By contrast, our perception of what is 'feminine' still revolves around notions such a high priority on relationships and concern for the needs of others – in part at the expense of the self's own needs and autonomy – an inclination for passive submission and confirmation of the self for these traits, while a desire for individuation and insistence on a separate self are commonly met with various forms of disapproval. This may mean that the need and striving for autonomy may be split off or hidden (cf. more vulnerable and masochistic manifestations of pathological narcissism).

Certain biologically based gender differences will always exist, but whole and healthy human beings need to contain and integrate elements from both these classic perceptions of feminine and masculine qualities. A continued socialization practice and cultural discourses that stand in the way of this may contribute to the development of narcissistic difficulties and various manifestations of pathological narcissism. In extension of this point, it is worth considering whether the development of narcissistic personality pathology might in some cases be associated with deficient internal integration of gender-related identity elements (Layton, 2020, p. 244). At one extreme, this would have the primary manifestation of exaggerated conformity, passivity, dependence and self-disparagement, corresponding to a pathological distortion of classic perceptions of feminine qualities and of the fundamental human need for contact and embeddedness in social communities. These manifestations are characteristic of predominantly vulnerable narcissism and would be likely to occur more frequently among women. At the other extreme, we would see overt grandiosity, self-overvaluation, pseudo-autonomy, tendency towards dissociality, an urge to take action and demonstrate agency, independence of others and rejection of the demands and expectations of the external environment, corresponding to pathologically distorted manifestations of classic notions of masculinity and the basic human need for self-definition. These are characteristics of predominantly grandiose narcissism and would be more likely to occur among men.

Narcissism clarifies basic elements of the human psyche

As a broad concept, narcissism – and our encounter with and attempts to understand pathological narcissism – may be seen as presenting challenges that confront us with certain fundamental elements of the human psyche: basic conflicts and challenges related to the human condition and life in the late modern Western culture that make it even more interesting to explore the basic elements of narcissism. As discussed in the previous chapters, narcissism relates in part to challenges with striking the right balance between dependence and independence, interpersonal separation and connectedness, the urge to merge with idealized others and to attain separation from/control over the same idealized others, the need for self-definition/autonomy and attachment to others/embeddedness in safe and obliging social communities.

In addition to these challenges, which are universally familiar to all of us, to varying degrees, even if their specific manifestations vary widely, we can also associate narcissism with a shameful gap between our own ideal and real selves, our need to be seen, positively mirrored and recognized by others and our urge to evade or control others' evaluating gaze on the self. Narcissism can also be related to our persistent attempts to strike the right balance between, on the one hand, hedonism and the urge for immediate gratification and, on the other hand, necessary dismissal or delay of the gratification of our own needs and challenges with striking an appropriate level of – and the right balance between – love of self and love of others, which also involves the readiness to waive the satisfaction of our own immediate needs and the exclusive pursuit of our own narrow individual interest in favour of others and of concerns that go beyond ourselves.

If we associate narcissism with deficiencies in our ability to look beyond ourselves and our own immediate needs, we may also understand our current approach to the increasingly visible changes in earth's climate as expressions of narcissism in the sense that we – meaning the current generations of adults and those in power – so far have not been able to look beyond ourselves and our own convenience and hedonistic needs and do what we know is necessary to secure our common home and a reasonable existence for the people and other living beings who are going to follow us. Viewed through a fairly dark lens and gloomy predictions, we can easily point to a disturbing list of current global crises and threats the world peace and the survival of the human race.

This includes, for example, the many tangible manifestations of ongoing climate change, migration crises, the consequences of increasingly obvious overpopulation and escalating polarization and violent conflicts, both internally in modern societies and among societies/cultures driven, in part, by mutual narcissistic injuries and the resulting narcissistic rage, the undermining of the capacity for mutual empathy, and technological innovations that we seem incapable of controlling. In addition, there are grandiosely narcissistic leaders whose main concern is themselves, their own needs and appearance, and how they can promote their own grandiose self-image and fragile self-esteem by scoring victories in simplistic political power struggles and looking out for the narrow interests of their own social group. Meanwhile, they have little interest in what it will take for us to work together to solve the serious crises we are facing, right now and in the near future. Although many of these crises have been ongoing for a long time, we have yet to step up and develop a common strategy as a global community. Leaders who wish to make a real contribution to dealing with disagreements about the best way to solve common problems need to be able to push their own narcissistic needs aside – including their insistence on always being right, knowing the truth and having others confirm this – and instead meet their negotiation partners with humility, respect, openness and willingness to listen to and understand their perspectives on reality, even if it might differ significantly from their own. Like competent psychotherapists, leaders need to not take themselves too seriously and they have to be ready to meet others' missteps with the graceful willingness to forgive and avoid being driven by resentment and anger when they experience narcissistic injury because others might fail to see, confirm and admire their person and work the way the feel they deserve.

The growing number of unresolved crises presumably bear witness to and illustrate the limitations of our own intelligence, rationality and capacity for long-term thinking. In addition, the increasingly visible deficiencies in the ability demonstrated by humanity so far to deal with these ever more severe crises and threats to the survival of our species may be viewed through the lens of our inherent narcissism, in a broad sense, and show us the consequences we might face unless we improve our ability to understand and deal with toxic and pathological narcissism. Among other manifestations, this toxic narcissism is expressed in a lack of recognition of our own basic vulnerability, aggressive and grandiose defences against (recognizing) this vulnerability, greed, lack of mutual empathy, tendency to take offence and to react with narcissistic rage to perceived narcissistic injuries rather than engage in curious exploration of what is happening inside us and between us when crises and social conflicts escalate.

References

Kernberg, O. F. (1984). *Severe personality disorders*. Yale University Press.

Layton, L. (1998). *Who's that girl? Who's that boy? Clinical practice meets postmodern gender theory*. Jason Aronson.

Layton, L. (2020). *Toward a social psychoanalysis: Culture, character, and normative unconscious processes*. Routledge.

Lunbeck, E. (2014). *The Americanization of narcissism*. Harvard University Press.

Parsons, M. (2022). *Lebendigkeit in der Psychoanalyse* [Vivacity in psychoanalysis]. Psychosozial-Verlag.

Index

Note: locators in **bold** indicate tables.

For Product Safety Concerns and Information please contact our EU representative GPSR@taylorandfrancis.com Taylor & Francis Verlag GmbH, Kaufingerstraße 24, 80331 München, Germany